DEVELOPMENTAL BIOLOGY

Developmental Biology

M.A. SUBRAMANIAN

Former Principal
Sree Amman Arts and Science College
Erode, Tamil Nadu

MJP PUBLISHERS

Chennai New Delhi Tirunelveli

Cataloguing-in-Publication Data
Subramanian, M.A (1949 –).
Developmental Biology / by M.A. Subramanian.-
Chennai : MJP Publishers, 2023
xiv, 232 p.; 24 cm.
Includes Glossary, References and Index.
ISBN 978-81-8094-151-1 (hb.)
1. Biology Developmental 2. Biology, Reproduction I. Title
571.8 SUB MJP 130

ISBN 978-81-8094-151-1

Printed and bound in India

MJP PUBLISHERS
New No. 5, Muthu Kalathy Street
Triplicane
Chennai 600 005

Publisher : J.C. Pillai
Managing Editor : C. Sajeesh Kumar
Project Editor : P. Parvath Radha
Acquisitions Editor : C. Janarthanan
Editorial Team : B. Ramalakshmi, V.R. Padma, C. Devi, N. Yamuna Devi, S. Jeevasruthi, B. Annalakshmi, Lissy John
CIP Data : Prof. K. Hariharan, Librarian
RKM Vivekananda College, Chennai.

Preface

Developmental biology is one of the major disciplines of biological sciences and fundamentally it requires the understanding of the basic concepts. Accordingly, this endeavour has been made to present the basic ideas and facts of animal development, especially the chordate animals. Though this field is very vast and its diversified functional knowledge is rapidly increasing, emphasis has been given to the descriptive embryology of selected animals with small number of examples as well as to certain principles and historical background to some extent. The work is mainly a collection from lectures over the years and contains a broad range of topics on gamete formation, fertilization, early as well as later embryonic development of animals including organogenesis, embryonic adaptations, metamorphosis, regeneration and so on. Attempts have also been made to illustrate the basics of invertebrate development as well as to give practical guidelines including a few selected embryological methods. The subject matter has been written concisely and compactly in clear and understandable language illustrated by appropriate simplified figures. This book would provide good references as a core text for the developmental aspects of animals, thus fulfilling the needs of biology students.

I profoundly express my thanks to my family members and friends for their help to make this effort a great success. The friendly encouragement to carry out the project and the timely publication of this by MJP Publishers, Chennai, are greatly acknowledged. Valuable criticisms and helpful suggestions are welcomed for the future improvement of the book.

M.A. SUBRAMANIAN

CONTENTS

1

INTRODUCTION

Developmental biology is the study of the processes of the development of adult organisms and so it deals with the ontogenetic development which may be either embryogenetic or blastogenetic development. Embryogenesis is sexual reproduction by which a new individual is developed from the fertilized egg or zygote which is formed by the fusion of male and female gametes. On the other hand, blastogenesis is asexual reproduction by which a new individual is formed from the somatic cells of the parent body. In short, ontogenetic development refers to the growth, differentiation and development of a cell into a highly integrated multicellular organism. During the developmental process, the young individuals undergo progressive changes by which they mature into adults with the capability of reproduction and the adult animals face degenerative changes through which they ultimately die due to ageing. In other words, the life history of higher animals includes two distinct phases namely **embryonic** or **prenatal development** which occurs within the egg or the womb of the mother until hatching or birth and **postembryonic** or **postnatal development** which is the period from hatching or birth to natural death of individuals. Thus developmental biology deals with growth and development of animals with an emphasis on cell growth, differentiation and morphogenesis whereas embryology is a field involving the study of organisms between the cell stage (zygote) and the end of the embryonic stage.

Developmental biology is one of the fastest growing areas in Life Sciences and it has exploded in so many directions in the past decades. Modern developmental biology requires an understanding of classical embryology. Embryology is a term derived from the Greek words namely *embryon* meaning embryo and *logia* meaning discourse. Developmental biologists have discovered the basic biological processes of embryogenesis, polarity of the cells, neurogenesis, organogenesis, ageing and so on. This branch occupies a central position in modern biology as it combines and makes use of disciplines like cell and molecular biology, genetics, morphology, physics, chemistry, microbiology, mathematics, and psychology. It has the following divisions:

Descriptive embryology It involves an elaborate description of developmental sequences of embryos.

Comparative embryology It deals with the comparative study of ontogenic development of vertebrate organisms. The comparison of development of embryos of two or more species is greatly useful in taxonomic and phylogenetic studies.

Experimental embryology This is an important division of descriptive embryology in which the developmental hypotheses are tested using genetic and embryo manipulations.

Chemical embryology It is the discipline of embryology which deals with the study of various developmental phenomena in molecular terms by incorporating biochemical and physiological techniques.

Analytical embryology It is the branch which deals with the study of the basic principles and processes of development by means of sophisticated modern equipment like electron microscope and techniques such as chromatography, electrophoresis, ultracentrifuge, isoelectric focusing, autoradiography and so on. These studies can be made only on the basis of knowledge from descriptive embryology, comparative embryology and experimental embryology.

Molecular embryology This is a new field of embryology which deals with the study of differential expression of the inherited genes in different populations of cells.

Ecological embryology This branch deals with the possible effects of environmental alterations due to global warming, pesticides and other pollutants leading to disruption of development in organisms as well as the resultant formulations of environmental regulations.

Evolutionary embryology or evolutionary developmental biology ('evo devo') This branch offers some indirect evidences for evolution as it deals with comparative study of developmental processes of different animals and plants in order to know the ancestral relationship between organisms and the evolution of developmental processes.

Teratology It is an interdisciplinary field encompassing embryology, pathology and basic medical science, and focuses on abnormal development and congenital malformations in higher mammals especially in humans.

ROLE OF DEVELOPMENTAL BIOLOGY IN THE FIELD OF MEDICINE

Developmental biology plays a prominant role in the field of medicine. In general, certain pathological conditions and malformations can be explained as failures in growth, development and differentiation. The phenomenon of onset of ageing and age-related diseases in man could be peeped out on the genetic basis. More recently, the origin, functions and uses of stem cells have been the major developmental issues as these cells have inherent property of renewing themselves continuously, giving rise to cells necessary for the formation of an organ. The methods of purification of more specialized stem cells of haemopoietic system form the basis for treatment of leukaemia and other types of cancer as well as for organ transplantation. Stem cells of neurons are useful in the treatment of many degenerative diseases of the nervous system. The incorporation of developmental biology into biotechnology has paved the way for regeneration of spinal neurons and bones for the first time in man. Moreover, many congenital and other genetic diseases could only be treated by gene therapy and many investigations are on the way to introduce genes into mice and human beings in order to correct the genetic diseases.

In the last ten years, knowledge with regard to the developmental mechanisms has grown elaborately by employing techniques of genetics and molecular biology. At present, it is known that billions of cells of a large animal like a mammal have the same genotype which is similar to that of the single-celled zygote from which the animal develops. Developmental biologists were the first to clone animals showing that the adult nuclei contain all genetic information and to provide an understanding of the differential control of gene expression. They have discovered micro-RNAs and morphogens as well as the fundamental principles of differential gene regulations. The recent cloning of **Dolly**, a lamb (Wilmut, *et al.*, 1997), the Cumulina mouse (Wakayama, *et al.*, 1998) and a non-human primate (Chan *et al.*, 2000) confirm the fact that the specialized cell carries the genes for all other kinds of cells of animals. Thus, altering of development by embryonic stem cells, cloning and even the enhancement of our genetic constitution is now theoretically possible. However, an entire field of bioethics has now emerged, as the cloning of Dolly has resulted in controversial views throughout the world. In recent times, work is on progress to explore pathways of communications for the eventual organization of cells within a tissue or organ. As these studies continue and expand, developmental biology would definitely be a core discipline of Life Sciences.

2

HISTORICAL REVIEW AND THEORIES OF DEVELOPMENTAL BIOLOGY

Observation of embryos of different stages and their development have been the subject of discussion and can be traced back to the ancient Greek Philosophers.

Empedocles (500 BC) He conceived that an embryo arose partly from female and partly from male gametes through sequential developmental events.

Hippocrates (460–377 BC) He noticed the developmental processes in chick.

Aristotle (384–322 BC) He was the first person who recorded different stages in the development of embryos and recognized that the organisms reproduce in multiple ways. He described the development and reproduction of many animals and laid the foundation for the basic principles of **Epigenesis**. Thus he established embryology as an independent biological science.

Willian Harvey (1578–1657) He expanded and corrected Aristotle's work and proved that many aspects of Aristotle's theory were wrong. Modern embryology might have begun with his work on the development of chick (1651). He postulated that all animals came from eggs, thus favouring **Preformation hypothesis**.

Malpighi (1672) He opined that an ovum was found to contain a miniature of its adult animal and the miniature creature unfolded and increased in size by development.

von Leeuwenhoek (1632–1723) He first discovered the sperm of man and other mammals at the invention of microscope (1677) and believed that the miniature organism was not present inside the egg but in the head of the sperm.

Charles Bunnet (1720–1793) Like Malpighi, he also believed that the ovum contained an unobservable miniature organism which was stimulated for further development by the seminal fluid.

Spallanzani (1729–1799) He successfully carried out the first artificial insemination using frog's eggs, thus putting an end to Preformation theory.

Friedrich Wolff (1738–1794) He put forward the **Epigenetic theory** (1759) and was the first man to demonstrate morphogenesis in animals. By his concept, he argued that the organs of the body did not exist at the beginning of gestation but formed from some originally undifferentiated material through a series of steps.

Pandar (1814) He discovered the three primary germ layers in chick embryo.

Dumas (1824) He was the first to describe the cleavage of eggs as building units in the embryos.

Karl Ernst von Bear (1792–1876) He was considered as the founder of comparative embryology and put forward **Baer's law** (1828). He first identified the mammalian egg (1827) but was not able to explain its significance in development. He made significant studies in descriptive embryology and noted many similarities between the embryos of vertebrates, particularly of amniotes.

Ernst Haeckel (1834–1919) He named the 'Baer's law' as **biogenetic theory** or **recapitulation theory** or **law of phylogeny** (1864) and evidenced the concept "Ontogeny recapitulates phylogeny".

Van–Beneden (1883) He showed that equal number of chromosomes were contributed by the male and female gametes during fertilization.

August Weismann (1834–1914) He put forward the **germplasm theory** (1904) and suggested that the self-reproducing determinants located on the chromosomes were the guiding agents in morphogenesis. He believed that cell differentiation was the result of cells acquiring different chromosomes during replication.

Oscar Hertwig (1849–1922) and Richard Hertwig (1850–1937) They were the first to demonstrate the major events of fertilization in sea urchin's egg. They discovered the existence of polar bodies and made significant advances in the study of meiosis.

Wilhelm Roux (1850–1924) He put forward the **mosaic theory** (1888) according to which each and every part of the egg was predetermined to develop into a particular organ.

Hans Driesch (1867–1941) He disproved the mosaic theory of Roux by his **regulative theory** (1891) according to which different parts of the eggs are not predetermined but they have potentiality to develop into any type of organs.

Hans Spemann (1869–1941) He discovered the process of induction through experimental procedures in living embryos for the first time (1918) and won Nobel Prize in 1935 for his discovery of the organizer effect using the dorsal lip of the blastopore of the developing embryo **(Organizer theory).**

Embryological thoughts have prevailed since the Greek civilization periods. In general terms, developmental biology explains the ontogenic development of organisms. At present, **Developmental Genetics**, a distinct biological science, helps us to know the expression of genes during development and the mechanisms of cell division. Even as early as the 1930s, it was known that different genes are involved in different aspects of embryonic development. With developments in the field of molecular biology after the 1950s, it was clear that genes are responsible for each morphological change that takes place in an embryo. During 1970–1980, gene manipulation techniques were invented and this aided in the investigation of genetic control of development in organisms. **Stem cell research** started growing from the works of **Mc Culloch** and **Till** (1960) and now stem cells can be grown and transformed into specialized cells. The embryonic cell lines generated through **molecular cloning** seem to be promising tools for future therapies. They could be a potential source for regenerative medicine and tissue replacement. Adult stem cell research is mainly involved in the treatment of leukaemia and related bone/blood cancers through bone marrow transplants. In addition, pluripotent stem cells equivalent to embryonic stem cells have been developed using genetic reprogramming with the resultant success to create the first cloned sheep, **Dolly**. However, a widespread controversy exists with regard to human embryonic stem cell research and the existing debate regarding stem cell research has resulted in the formulation of regulatory frameworks so that it represents a social ethical challenge.

IMPORTANT THEORIES OF DEVELOPMENT

Preformation Theory

Swammerdam (1637–80), a Dutch scientist, proposed that the gametes contain preformed embryos (miniatures of the adults). He along with biologists like **Malpighi** (1673), **Haller** (1708–77), **Bonnet** (1720–93) and **Spallanzani** (1729–99) believed that an ovum contained a miniature of its adult animal and the development consisted of unfolding and increase in size of that miniature creature. In human beings, this miniature creature was called **homunculus.** On the other hand, people like **Leeuwenhoek** (1682–1723), **Hartsoeker** (1656–1725), *et al.* believed that the miniature organism was not present in the egg but in the head of the sperm called **animalcule**. Thus the followers of the Preformation theory were split into two groups namely **ovists** who believed that the embryo was inside the ovum and **spermists** or **animalculists** who opined that the preformed embryo was inside the sperm.

Epigenetic Theory

This theory was proposed by **Friedrich Wolff** (1759) and accepted after the discovery of protoplasm. According to this theory, the egg contains granular substances which arrange themselves to form germinal layers, giving rise to the body of an embryo during development. He experimentally proved that there was no preformed embryo in chick, and that the chick embryo developed through the progressive transformation of germinal layers into various organs. This theory was strongly opposed by **Haller** and **Bonnet** but was supported by the embryologists of the early 19th century like von Baer, and is today accepted.

Pangenesis Theory

This theory was put forward by Darwin (1817) who opined that each somatic cell of an organism would produce a minute copy of its own called **gemmule** or **pangene** and all the **gemmules** were deposited in the testis or ovary via the blood and then concentrated in the germ cells. He believed that each germ cell was a minute replica of the parent's body and was capable of developing into the same type of body.

Germ Layer Concept

This theory was given by **Pander** (1817) and **von Baer** (1827) based on the observation of the three germ layers in early chick embryo. This theory envisages that these three germ layers are formed during the development of all embryos.

Baer's Law

The first embryological data was given by **Karl Ernst Von Baer** (1828) in the form of a theory called **Baer's law**. According to this theory, more general characters that are common to all the members of a group of animals, develop earlier than the more specialized characters which differentiate the various members of the group. In this way, in vertebrates, the common general characters such as brain, notochord, muscles, etc. develop first during development followed by the characteristics of various classes such as limbs, hairs, feathers, etc. and the features of the families, genera and species develop last. In this way, early embryo basically possesses common characteristics of all members of a large group of the animal kingdom.

Biogenetic Law or Recapitulation Theory

Fritsz Muller and **Oscar Haeckel** (1864) renamed the Baer's law as **biogenetic law** or **recapitulation theory**. According to this theory, the ontogeny of each and every individual repeats or recapitulates to some extent its phylogeny. In other words, the characteristics of ancient origin develop earlier during embryonic development whereas the characteristics of newer origin (species) develop later. Baer's law and the biogenetic law made embryologists to investigate the development of animals of all major groups of the animal kingdom systematically. Thus these two concepts paved way for the growth of descriptive embryology and comparative embryology.

Mosaic Theory

By his experiments in frog's eggs, **Wilhelm Roux** (1888) propounded the mosaic theory and concluded that the ontogenic development consists of differentiation of cells from a more or less undifferentiated and homogeneous egg. At the event of cleavage, the blastomeres gradually become smaller and smaller with the demarcation of more areas for specific tissues and organs in the blastula. As a result, the blastula now resembles a mosaic pattern with regard to the potencies of its blastomeres. In other words, each and every part of the egg is predetermined to develop into a particular organ. The eggs which undergo this type of development are known as **mosaic eggs**.

Regulative Theory

Hans Driesch (1891) made experiments on sea urchin's eggs and put forth the **Regulative theory** according to which the blastomeres of the egg at an early stage possess equal potentiality (**equipotent**). As a result, a cleaving egg is a harmonious and equipotential system with its every part capable of developing into a whole organism. In other words, different parts of the eggs are not predetermined but they have potentiality to develop into any type of organs. The eggs which undergo this type of development are known as **regulative eggs**. Similar results were also obtained by **Endres** (1895) and **Spemann** (1901, 1903) in newt's eggs and by **Schmidt** (1933) in frog's eggs. Thus, this theory disproves the mosaic theory.

Germplasm Theory

In 1904, **August Weissmann** proposed the **Germplasm theory**. This concept postulates that the body of an organism is formed by two types of cells namely **somatic cells** and **germ cells**. The changes which are brought in the germ cells are inherited to the offspring whereas those in the somatic cells would not be inherited. Moreover, the nuclei of the germ cells contain **determinants** for each part of the body of an organism so that a complete set of determinants would be handed over from one generation to another. But the determinants are distributed unequally in the blastomeres during cleavage and so each blastomere contains only one type of determinants. However, this theory has no supporting evidence at present.

Gradient Concept

This theory was put forward by **Boveri** (1910) who believed that the vegetal region of the egg exerts a control over the animal region and this influence decreases from the vegetal pole towards the animal pole. But he was not able to explain the reasons for these variations. In 1940, **Child** found that the cytoplasm of animal pole of the eggs divide with high frequency and the frequency gradually decreases towards the animal pole. He demonstrated the existence of differences in the rate of general metabolism in the ooplasm of animal and vegetal pole of oocytes and cleaving eggs. This implies that the ooplasm in the animal pole has high metabolic rate which gradually decreases towards the vegetal pole. Thus he showed that a single physiological gradient namely **metabolic axial gradient** exists along the animal–vegetal axis. **Horstadius** (1955) and **Runnstrom** (1967) put forth the modified version of the gradient concept. According to them, morphogenesis and differentiation in the early development of eggs are under the control of a double gradient system namely **animal gradient** and **vegetal gradient.** When the animal gradient is suppressed, the vegetal gradient becomes dominant and the embryo is vegetalized (**vegetalization**). When the vegetal gradient is suppressed, then the animal gradient becomes dominant and the embryo is animalized (**animalization**). Therefore, normal development could result only when there is an equilibrium between these two gradients. In 1969, **Horstadius** and **Josefsson** have shown that the animal substance of the egg contains tryptophane and the vegetal substance, a nucleotide.

Organizer Concept

Spemann (1918) received the Nobel Prize for his **Organizer concept** which was put forth by observing the induction of the entire process of development by the dorsal lip of an early embryo. In 1924, **Spemann** and **Hilde Mangold** established the organizing action of the dorsal lip, thus showing the **concept of induction** as the basic mechanism in embryonic development. When an embryonic tissue evokes the development of a structure from another tissue, it is called **inductor** or **organizer** and this effect is called **induction.**

REVIEW QUESTIONS

1. Give an account of the historical background of developmental biology.
2. Write notes on the following:
   - i. Preformation theory
   - ii. Epigenetic theory
   - iii. Pangenesis theory
   - iv. Germ layer theory
   - v. Baer's Law
   - vi. Recapitulation theory
   - vii. Mosaic theory
   - viii. Regulative theory
   - ix. Germplasm theory
   - x. Gradient concept
   - xi. Organizer concept
3. Give short notes on the major contributions of the following embryologists:
   - i. Aristotle
   - ii. Swammerdam
   - iii. Leeuwenhoe
   - iv. Wolf
   - v. von Baer
   - vi. Darwin
   - vii. Haeckal
   - viii. Wilhelm Roux
   - ix. Hans Driesch
   - x. August Weissman
   - xi. Boveri
   - xii. Child
   - xiii. Horstadius
   - xiv. Runnstorm
   - xv. Spemann

3

GAMETOGENESIS

In animals, the first phase of embryogenesis is gametogenesis which starts at sexual maturity. During the process of gametogenesis, two specialized sex cells called **gametes** are produced namely **egg** or **ovum** in females and **sperm** or **spermatozoon** in males. When both types of gametes are produced by separate individuals of the same species, then they are called **unisexual** or **dioecious organisms**. Those animals in which a single individual is capable of producing both gametes are called **hermaphrodites** or **monoecious** organisms.

In animals, the functional male gametes are the sperms or spermatozoa and the sex organ which gives rise to sperms is the **male gonad** or **testis**. The functional female gametes are the ova or eggs and the sex organ which gives rise to ova is the **female gonad** or **ovary**. Both the testis and ovary in vertebrates have two main functions namely production of gametes and secretion of sex hormones appropriate to male or female. **Gametogenesis** can be defined as the formation of gametes and in general, it is uniform throughout the animal kingdom. Both male and female gametes have haploid or 'n' number of chromosomes.

ORIGIN OF GERM CELLS

The germplasm is possibly set aside early in embryonic development and later it gives rise to the germ cells which reach the gonad. The germ cells may probably be extragonadial in origin. That is, the germ cells may arise outside the gonads. Techniques by using both natural and artificial markers have helped to determine the origin of germ cells. For example, in birds and reptiles, the germ cells are said to have an endodermal origin (**extragonadial**).

It is believed that these cells move into the developing gonad via the blood. Experimentally when the germ cells are destroyed, the gonads develop in chick without germ cells. In mammals also such studies have shown an extragonadial origin of germ cells. These studies thus clearly evidence that the germ cells arise outside the gonads and subsequently migrate to the gonads. However, there is also possibility of the germ cells arising in gonads themselves. This is because, new germ cells continue to form the tissues of the gonad in birds during each breeding season. Therefore, new germ cells arise from the tissues of the gonads as well. The question is thus very much open for further study.

SPERMATOGENESIS (FORMATION OF SPERM)

The sperms are formed in testis which is made up of **seminiferous tubules** separated by interstitial tissue. These tubules contain different cell types of which the most important types of cells are the primordial germ cells. They are found within the cellular layer along the margin of the seminiferous tubules. The other cells within the tubules either help to support or nourish the germ cells. The **primordial germ cells** have diploid or '2n' number of chromosomes and they undergo repeated mitotic divisions, thus increasing the volume of the testis. The cells which are formed by repeated divisions are called the **spermatogonia.** This stage of spermatogenesis is called **multiplication phase.** Now the spermatogonia absorb more food and increase in size. At this stage, the cells are called as **primary spermatocytes** and the stage is called **growth phase**. Then the primary spermatocytes undergo meiotic division and this stage is called **maturation phase.**

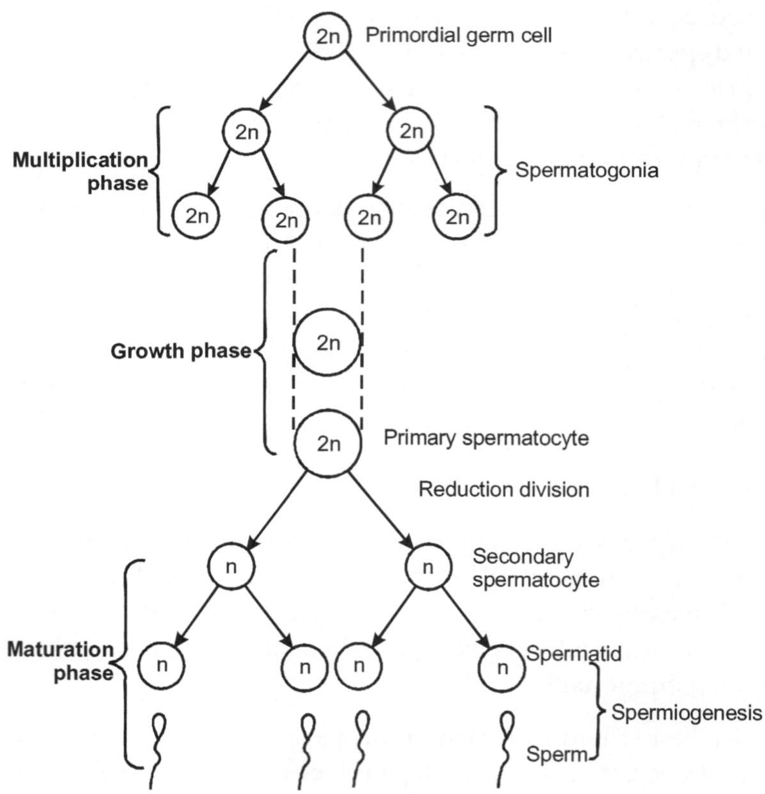

Figure 3.1 Diagram showing the events of spermatogenesis

The first meiotic division is the reduction division in which the two daughter cells get only haploid or 'n' number of chromosomes. Each daughter cell is called **secondary spermatocyte** which now undergoes the second meiotic division (mere mitotic division). Thus, the resulting two daughter cells retain the same 'n' number of chromosomes and are called **spermatids**. In this way, each primary spermatocyte gives rise to four spermatids each with haploid number of chromosomes. Then each spermatid undergoes various changes and ultimately gives rise to a sperm. This process of transformation of spermatids into sperms is called **spermiogenesis** or **spermateleosis**. All the events that occur during spermatogenesis are shown in Figure 3.1.

Morphology of a Sperm

It is necessary to know the morphology of a sperm for an easy understanding of spermiogenesis. Even though the sperms show great variations, each sperm appears to have a basic structure in relation to its function. Figure 3.2 shows the organization of the sperm cell.

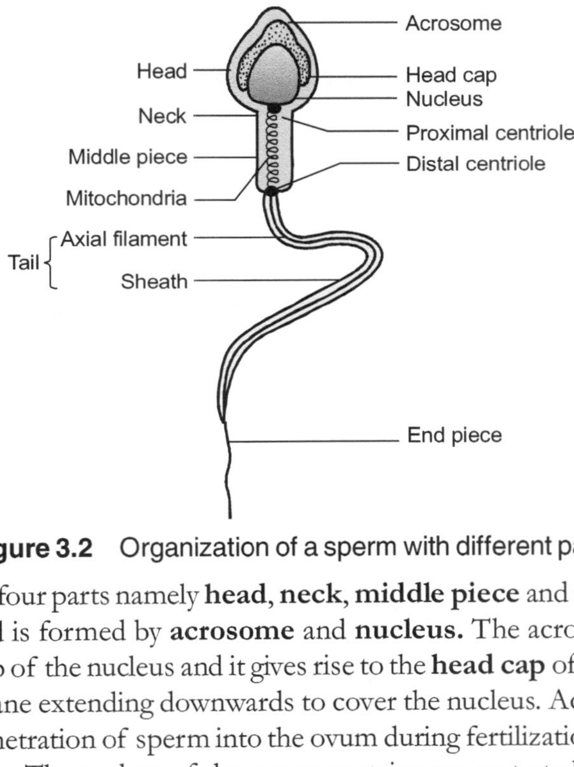

Figure 3.2 Organization of a sperm with different parts

A typical sperm has four parts namely **head, neck, middle piece** and **tail**. Electron microscopy has shown that the head is formed by **acrosome** and **nucleus.** The acrosome is in the form of a compact mass on the top of the nucleus and it gives rise to the **head cap** of the sperm. The head cap is a two-layered membrane extending downwards to cover the nucleus. Acrosome seems to play an important role in the penetration of sperm into the ovum during fertilization and in the activation of the egg to develop further. The nucleus of the sperm contains concentrated DNA and protein and all other materials in the spermatid are lost during its formation.

The neck of the sperm is that part which contains the **proximal** and **distal centrioles**. The two centrioles lie at right angles to one another. The proximal centriole has an important part to play in the first division of the fertilized egg. The distal centriole forms the axial filament of the sperm tail. The axial filament is attached to the distal centriole.

The middle piece of the sperm is occupied by mitochondria which may be in the form of compact clumps or in the form of a sheath surrounding the distal centriole and the proximal part of the axial filament. The mitochondria contain oxidative enzymes and so play a key role in sperm metabolism by providing the necessary energy.

The axial filament forms the main central structure in the tail. It is surrounded by a small amount of cytoplasm and the cell membrane. The axial filament exhibits many modifications in different animals. For example, the mammalian sperm contains extra filament surrounding the axial filament. In fishes, the tail is provided with an undulating membrane. The tail forms the basis for the movement of the sperm because the sperm has to travel distances to meet the ovum. The locomotion of the sperm is due to the lashing movement of the tail. There are of course some invertebrates that produce sperms without flagella.

Spermiogenesis or Spermateleosis

Each spermatid consists of cytoplasm, a nucleus with the gametic chromosomal number, a pair of centrioles, Golgi bodies, chondriosomes and other cellular inclusions. The process of spermiogenesis mainly involves a series of changes in nucleus, mitochondria, Golgi bodies and centrioles as shown in Figure 3.3.

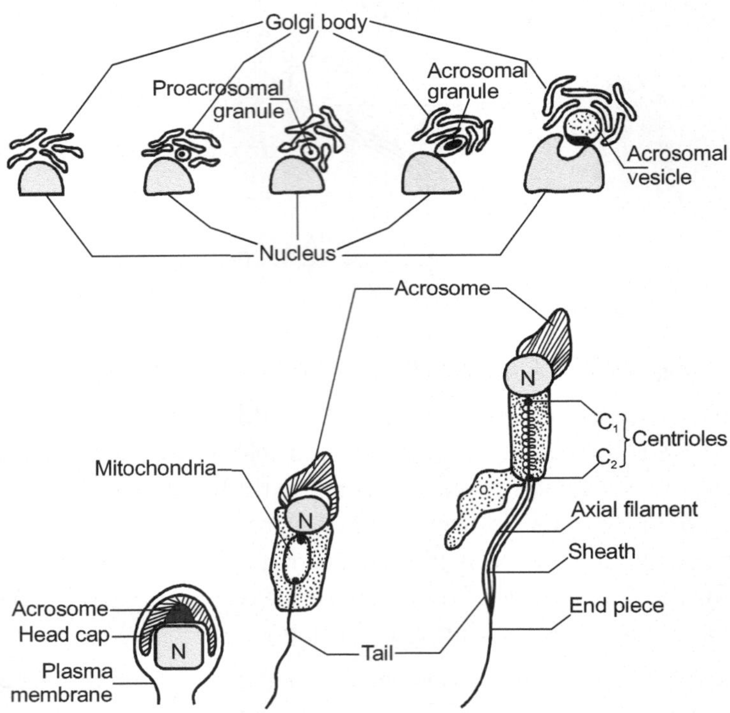

Figure 3.3 Changes in organelles during spermiogenesis

Changes in the nucleus The nucleus loses water from the nuclear sap and the chromosomes become short and compact. This has a functional significance in that it reduces the weight to be carried by the flagellum. This facilitates increased motility of the sperms. The RNA becomes scarce in the nucleus especially in the nucleolus and only the DNA concentrates in the nucleus. The shape of the nucleus is also changed and it becomes elongated and narrow. Such a shape is useful for the movement of spermatozoa in a liquid medium. The shape of the head of the sperms is variable and these shapes are perhaps related to movement.

Changes in the Golgi bodies The acrosome of the sperm is derived from the Golgi bodies which are arranged as a series of membranes around small vacuoles. One or more vacuoles begin to enlarge and a dense body is formed inside the vacuole. This dense body is called **proacrosomal granule**. When there are more than one granule, they fuse together and eventually one large vacuole containing a large dense granule is formed. This vacuole with its granule moves close to the tip of the nucleus and contacts it. The granule further increases in size and now it is termed as **acrosomal granule** which forms the core of the **acrosome**. The vacuole loses water and its wall spreads out covering the front half of the nucleus and the acrosome. This is the **head cap** of the nucleus and the rest of the Golgi bodies are now lost (Figure 3.3).

Changes in the centrioles Both the centrioles come out of the microcentrum in the cytoplasm of the spermatid. One of the centrioles reaches the periphery and throws off the **axial filament** which forms the axial structure of the sperm tail. Then the two centrioles move towards the nuclear membrane. In some cases, both the centrioles remain near the nuclear membrane. In others, one of the centrioles migrates apart from the other centriole which remains attached to the nuclear membrane. The migration of this centriole is along the axial filament up to a distance. Thus the region between these two centrioles forms the **middle piece**. In some other cases, one of the centrioles become plate-like with a pore in the middle through which the axial filament passes. Here, the axial filament arises from the other centriole which is attached to the nuclear membrane and is granular (Figure 3.3).

Changes in the mitochondria In mammalian spermatids, the mitochondria become grouped in a region near the posterior pole of the nucleus. In this region, they form a compact sheath near the proximal portion of the axial filament as a spiral forming the **middle piece**. In the spermatids of insects, the chromosomes usually unite into a single large mass called **Nebenkern**. This structure divides soon and elongates as two long strands which either remain lengthwise or coil about at the region of the middle piece (Figure 3.3).

Formation of tail The axial filament grows and becomes the main part of the flagellum. It is surrounded by a thin layer of cytoplasm and plasma membrane. Much of the cytoplasm of the spermatid is finally discarded (Figure 3.3).

In this way, a functional sperm is formed and is well-adapted for propulsion in a liquid medium. It carries only the essential materials namely the paternal DNA essential for fertilization, the centrioles essential for initiating cell division, the mitochondria essential for the supply of energy for movement and the flagellum essential for locomotion.

Factors Controlling Spermatogenesis

In vertebrates, the testis is under endocrine control particularly under the control of pituitary gland. The anterior lobe of the pituitary gland produces hormones called **gonadotropins** that maintain the functions of the gonads. Thus spermatogenesis is under hormonal control. It is also known that the pituitary gland is subjected to 'external influences'. For example, in birds and in rodents like squirrels and rats, the pituitary secretion is influenced by the length of the day. This is referred to as **photoperiod influence**. Even in some invertebrates, the formation and liberation of gametes is influenced by or is dependent on light. The way light affects the pituitary body seems to be as follows: In the beginning, the influence of light is on the retina of the eye of the animals. Then optic nerves take the information to the brain leading to the release of the secretion from the pituitary body into the blood. Now the hormones influence the gonadial activity.

OOGENESIS (FORMATION OF EGG OR OVUM)

The eggs or ova are formed in the ovary. The first cells which give rise to the mass of the ovary are called **primordial germ cells** as in the case of testis. In some features, the early formation of the ova and sperms can be compared. But the later history of the unfertilized egg is quite different. The entire process of oogenesis is shown in Figure 3.4.

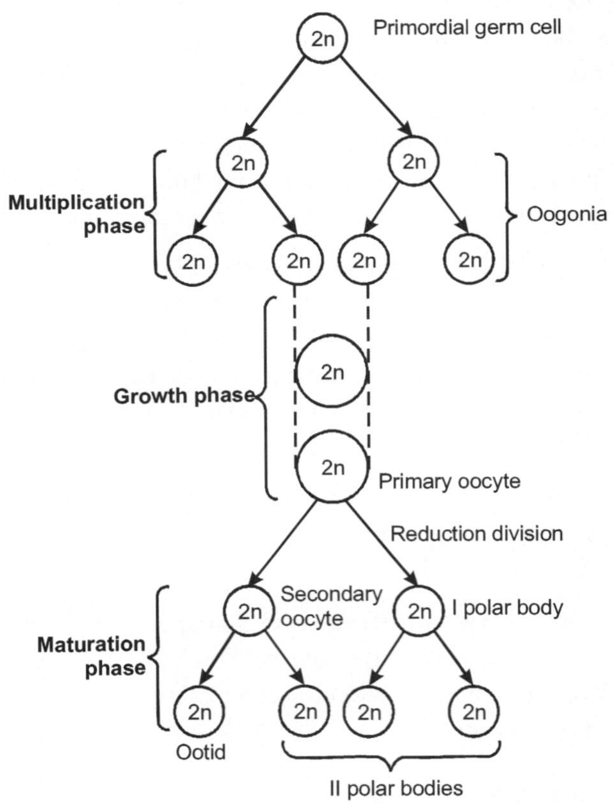

Figure 3.4 Diagram showing the events of oogenesis

Each primordial germ cell undergoes repeated mitotic divisions and gives rise to the cells called **oogonia.** This period is called as the **multiplication phase** of oogenesis. Some of the oogonia enlarge in size periodically and become what are called **primary oocytes**.

This stage is called the **growth phase**. Each primary oocyte now undergoes first meiotic division resulting in the formation of large and small cells. The larger cell is the **secondary oocyte** and the smaller one is the I **polar body**. Both these cells get only 'n' or haploid number of chromosomes. The secondary oocyte now undergoes the second meiotic division which is almost mitotic so that each daughter cell gets the same 'n' number of chromosomes. Among these cells, one daughter cell is larger and becomes the **ootid** and the other one is smaller called **polar body** (II). At the same time, the I polar body also divides and gives rise to two daughter polar bodies (II). All these polar bodies will be lost and the ootid grows into the functional ovum. Thus only one egg is formed from each primary oocyte and this stage is called as the **maturation phase**.

When the haploid ovum unites with the haploid sperm, a diploid fertilized egg results. Thus we see that the early formation of the ovum is similar to the main events that occur during spermatogenesis and the later history of the ovum is different. In vertebrates, the ovum is shed during the breeding season and this shedding of ovum is known as **ovulation**. The process of ovulation in animals is a seasonal and rhythmic one. The ovum is released into the body cavity and then transported from there into the oviduct and then to the outside as in non-mammals or to the uterus in mammals.

During oogenesis, enormous qualitative and quantitative changes occur in the cytoplasm and nucleus of the oocyte. The primary oocyte acquires large size through progressive growth which can be studied under two phases namely **previtellogenesis** and **vitellogenesis**.

Previtellogenesis

In general, there is a tremendous increase in the volume of the nucleus and the cytoplasm of the oocyte during the previtellogenic phase of the oocyte.

Changes in the nucleus A large quantity of nuclear sap is produced by the nucleus which increases in size. The nucleus undergoes the first meiotic division and synthesizes messenger RNA which controls protein synthesis in the cytoplasm. Now the nucleolus synthesizes ribosomal RNA and proteins and it becomes enlarged in size. The chromosomal DNA undergoes its own duplication.

Changes in the cytoplasm The cytoplasm becomes finely granular due to the accumulation of ribonucleoproteins and DNA material. The mitochondria increase in number so that the quantity of mitochondrial DNA is higher than the nuclear DNA. The Golgi bodies aggregate as spherical masses around the centrioles and are involved in the production of cortical granules. The endoplasmic reticulum are in the form of annulated lamellae which act as storage organs for RNA in the cytoplasm.

Formation of Yolk in the Oocyte (Vitellogenesis)

It was long-believed that the production of yolk in the oocytes is the result of the activities of a special body called **yolk nucleus** or **yolk nucleus of Balbiani.** This special body was first noticed in the oocytes of spiders. It was later shown to be present in the oocytes of amphibians and mammals. This yolk nucleus is found next to the nucleus in the early stage of oocyte development (Figure 3.5). But later on, it breaks up into fragments which get distributed in the cytoplasm of the egg. But this simple view of the formation of yolk in the oocyte has been questioned.

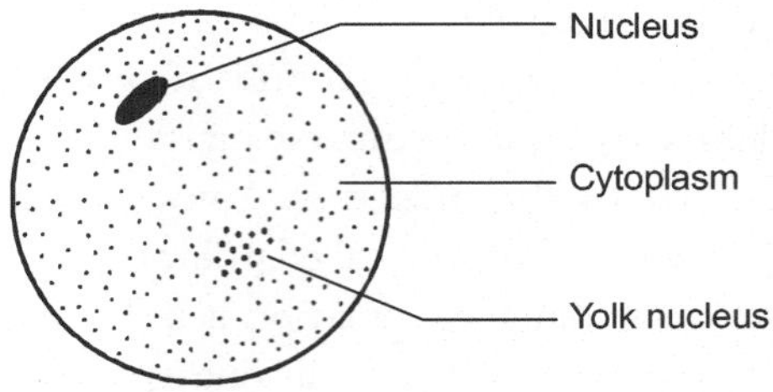

Figure 3.5 Yolk nucleus in the developing amphibian oocyte

Apart from yolk nucleus, other cellular organoids have also been considered to be responsible for yolk formation. The best results are from the studies of amphibian oocytes. There is good evidence in amphibians based on electron microscopy that yolk platelets are formed from the **modified mitochondria**. In this process, the inner mitochondrial membrane becomes arranged in a concentric manner and the interior of the mitochondrion is taken up by yolk platelets.

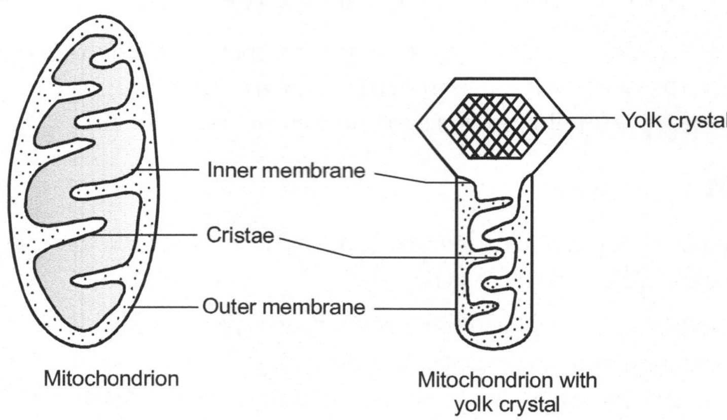

Figure 3.6 Typical mitochondrion and a mitochondrion containing a yolk crystal

Figure 3.6 shows a yolk crystal within the mitochondrion and the rest of the organelle with the usual structures. As more and more yolk platelets are formed, they fill the cytoplasm of the oocyte from the outside inward. In the later stages of growth of the oocyte, the yolk platelets are formed around the nucleus and the cytoplasm is filled with yolk platelets of different sizes. At the vegetal pole of the oocyte, they are large and closely packed.However, the yolk is probably shown not to be synthesized in the egg itself. In vertebrates, the yolk is found to be formed elsewhere in the liver and then transported in a soluble form via the blood. It is then absorbed by the oocyte from the follicle cells and finally deposited in the form of platelets. The following enzymatic reaction makes possible the formation of insoluble yolk from the soluble form. This reaction is reversible, and protein kinase is the mitochondrial enzyme. This explains the mechanism of deposition of yolk in the mitochondria.

$$\underset{\text{(Soluble form)}}{\text{Partially phosphorylated protein}} + \text{ATP} \underset{Mg^{++}}{\overset{\text{Protein kinase}}{\rightleftharpoons}} \underset{\text{(Insoluble form)}}{\text{Fully phosphorylated protein}} + \text{ADP}$$

It is observed that the yolk proteins and phospholipids are synthesized in the liver and then transported to the oocyte. This has been revealed by experiments in amphibians using radioactive substances. When such a material is injected into the body of the animal, the radioactivity is initially highest in the liver and the lowest in the oocytes during the first 8 hours after injection. About 12 hours after injection, the radioactivity of the liver is decreased and that of the ovary has been increased. This suggests that the initial synthetic process takes place in the liver and there is a subsequent transfer of these compounds to the oocytes.

Characteristics of Yolk

Vitellogenesis is the process by which the egg cytoplasm gets packed with the reserve food material namely **yolk** or **deutoplasm** or **vitellin**. In general, yolk is formed of **water** (48.7%), **proteins** (16.6%), **phospholipids** in the form of phosphatides and cholesterol, **neutral fats** (32.6%), and **carbohydrates** (1.0%). Depending on the chemical nature, two types of yolk namely **protein yolk** and **fatty yolk** occur in animal eggs. In some eggs (echinoderms, amphioxus, tunicates), protein yolk occurs in the form of fine granules which are evenly distributed throughout the egg cytoplasm. This type of yolk is described as **granular yolk.** On the other hand, the yolk is in the form of large granules in most of the vertebrate eggs and is denoted as **yolk platelets.** The yolk platelets contain a highly phosphorylated protein called **phosvitin** and a bound lipid called **lipovitellin.** In addition, lipids and glycogen are also found in the yolk platelets of amphibian eggs. In the eggs of almost all animals, the yolk material contains enzymes namely **phosphoprotein phosphatase** and **cathepsin** which are used for the breakdown of phosphate and yolk proteins to be utilized by the embryo after fertilization.

External Membranes of the Egg

All eggs are covered by the cell membrane called **plasmalemma.** In addition, the eggs of all animals except a few are surrounded by special egg membranes. Depending on their origin, the egg membranes are of two major types namely **primary membranes** and **secondary membranes**. The primary egg membranes develop in the ovary from the ovum itself. The secondary membranes are formed from the follicles, oviducts and other accessory parts of the genital organs while the egg is passing from the ovary to the exterior.

1. ***Primary egg membranes*** The primary membranes include the following types.

Vitelline membrane It is formed of mucopolysaccharides and some fibrous proteins. It is a thin and transparent membrane closely applied to the underlying plasma membrane. It is found in the eggs of insects, molluscs, amphibians and birds.

Zona radiata It has a stratified appearance and is found in sharks, some bony fishes, amphibians and reptiles. In fishes, this membrane has perforations called **micropiles** through which the sperms enter into the egg during fertilization.

Zona pellucida This membrane is nothing but a modified zona radiata. It is secreted by both the follicular cells and the ovum and is found in mammals.

Jelly envelop In the eggs of many marine invertebrates, the primary egg membrane is thick and jellylike.

2. ***Secondary egg membranes*** The secondary egg membranes include the following types:

Chorion In insects, a second thicker membrane is secreted by the follicular cells around the vitelline membrane and is called chorion.

Corona radiata In mammals, the escaping egg from the ovary has larger follicular cells around the zona pellucida and this layer is called corona radiata.

Egg Membranes in Birds

In birds, the egg has many complicated egg membranes as shown in Figure 3.7.

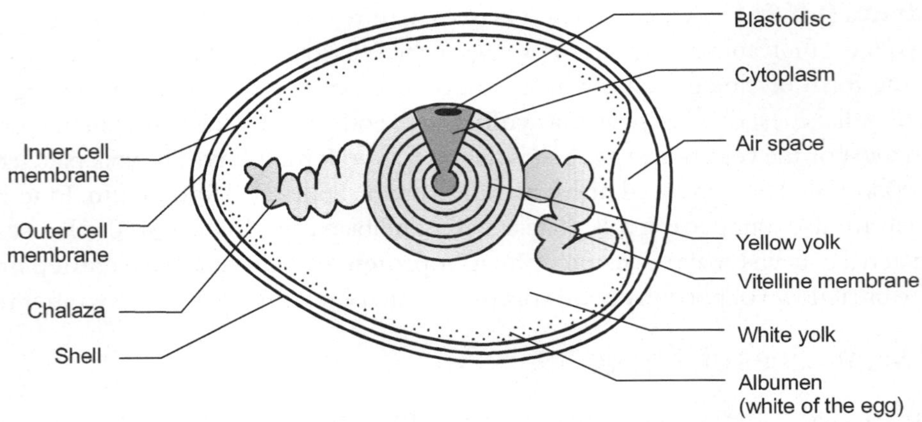

Figure 3.7 T.S. of hen's egg to show secondary egg membranes

The innermost membrane is the vitelline membrane, next to which is the white of the egg surrounded by the inner and outer cell membranes.

Membranes of Graafian Follicle

In mammals, the developing egg with its associated membranes is called **graafian follicle** which is covered by both follicular and egg membranes (Figure 3.8). The follicular membranes comprise two connective tissue layers namely **theca externa** (external fibrous layer) and **theca interna** (cellular layer containing blood capillaries). Inner to the follicular membranes are the three egg membranes which comprise the outer **basement membrane** on which rest many layers of epithelial cells forming the **membrana granulosa** and the innermost **zona pellucida** or **zona radiata**.

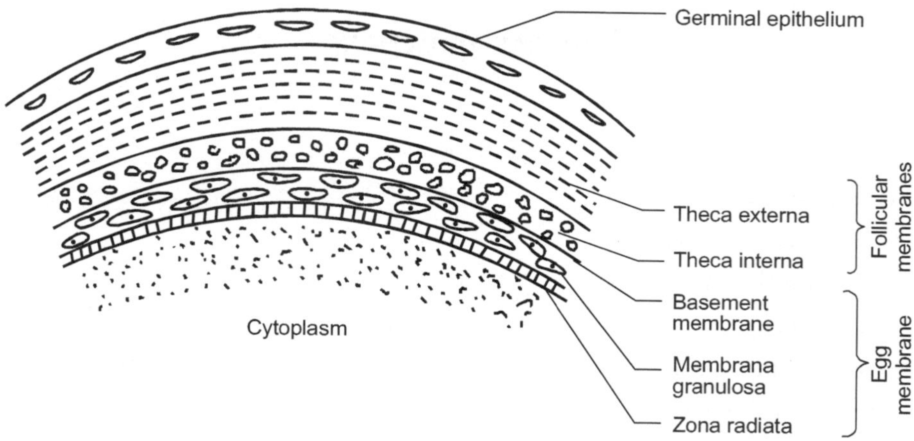

Figure 3.8 Diagrammatic structure of a portion of a graafian follicle showing its membranes

HORMONAL CONTROL OF GAMETOGENESIS

In vertebrates, the pituitary gland links the neurosecretory centres of the brain to the endocrine tissues of the gonads through its gonadotropic hormones. It is proved that **gonadotropin-releasing hormone** (Gn-RH) is responsible for the release of FSH and LH in mammals. In all groups of vertebrates, hypothalamic factors regulate the pituitary activity and the seasonal changes in the environment is found to regulate reproduction. In experimental vertebrates, removal of pituitary gland results in the regression of reproductive function, i.e., gametogenesis is blocked at the spermatogonial or oogonial stage. Though the gametogenic cells continue to divide, maturation does not occur. In female animals, vitellogenesis stops or is not initiated in the eggs and the yolk-filled ova degenerate with the removal of yolk.

The anterior pituitary secretes three different hormones in mammals namely FSH (**follicle stimulating hormone**), LH (**luteinizing hormone**) and **prolactin** in female and **testosterone** in male, which regulate gametogenesis. **Sertoli cells** of testis and the **granulosa cells** of ovary are under the control of FSH. In mammals, LH stimulates synthesis and secretion of androgens which, in turn, stimulate spermatogenesis. It is experimentally proved that FSH stimulates spermatogonial divisions and LH completes spermatogenesis. Hormones comparable to mammalian FSH and LH have also been found in most tetrapods. For example, a hormone namely **maturational hormone** secreted from the pituitary in fishes induces oocyte maturation and ovulation in females and spermiation in males. Another hormone namely **vitellogenic hormone** induces vitellogenesis and accumulation of yolk in the ovary. **Androgens** from testes, **estrogens** from ovarian follicle and **progestrone** from corpus luteum are also involved in vertebrate gametogenesis. Androgens are steroids, low doses of which suppress spermatogenesis in rats by inhibiting the pituitary gonadotropins whereas higher doses stimulate and maintain spermatogenesis even though the pituitary FSH and LH are absent. In man, high concentrations of androgens from testes are required for the maintenance of spermatogenesis. The mammalian estrogens help to prepare the uterine mucosa in females to receive the embryo and **progestrone** regulates the pituitary body with feedback effect. In the case of frog, estrogen inhibits maturation of oocytes and ovulation, and progestrone stimulates these processes.

REVIEW QUESTIONS

1. Give a brief account of the process of gametogenesis.
2. Write an essay on spermatogenesis.
3. Write an essay on oogenesis.
4. Describe the morphology of a typical spermatozoan.
5. Enumerate the changes that occur in cellular inclusions during spermiogenesis.
6. What are the previtellogenic changes during the growth of the primary oocyte?
7. What is vitellogenesis? Discuss the process of yolk synthesis in the growing oocyte.
8. Brief the hormonal control of gametogenesis.
9. Write notes on the following :
   i. Germ cells ii. Spermatids iii. Head cap
   iv. Oocytes v. Yolk
10. Give an account of types, structure and functions of egg membranes.

4

ORGANIZATION OF EGG—POLARITY, SYMMETRY AND GRADIENTS

The egg is the female gamete containing all the materials necessary for the entire process of development of the embryo. It has three major functions namely supply of haploid set of maternal chromosomes to the offspring, supply of almost all the cytoplasm of the egg and supply of food resources for the embryo until it begins to feed on food. Morphologically, the size and shape of the eggs are variable. The egg cytoplasm consists of **yolk, pigments, cortical granules**, etc. in addition to the **cell organelles**. These are unequally distributed in the egg cytoplasm resulting in the development of polarity in the eggs. The yolk is usually present in the vegetal pole of the egg. The pigments of the egg may be brown, black, red, yellow, green or grey. The distribution of these pigment granules aids us in knowing the fate of each of the organ-forming areas of the egg. The cytoplasm of the egg is divided into an outer surface layer and an inner layer. The inner region is more fluid, containing nutritive substances and cell organelles. This layer is called **endoplasm** and the surface layer with the plasma membrane is called **ectoplasm** or **egg cortex**. The ectoplasm is more viscous, gelatinous and static and its thickness varies from 2–3 μ. In annelids, sea urchins, fishes, frogs and some mammals like man and rabbit, the cortex of the egg contains **cortical granules.** These granules are absent in insects, gastropods, urodeles, birds and in some mammals and are spherical in shape with a thin membrane, filled with acid mucopolysaccharides. At the time of fertilization, these granules swell and burst so that their products accumulate into the perivitelline space as a fluid and play a vital role in the activation of the egg.

POLARITY

Even a superficial examination shows that the egg cytoplasm is not a homogeneous mass of protoplasm and has a definite internal organization. It contains a variety of substances like yolk, pigments, RNA and other cellular organelles which exhibit an unequal distribution in fully developed advanced oocytes. These materials are distributed in such a way that two opposite poles can be identified in the egg namely the **animal pole** and **vegetal pole**. The line connecting these two poles through the centre of the egg is called **polar axis** or **egg centre** or **median axis**. The unequal distribution of these egg constituents establishing the two opposite poles of the egg is called **polarity**. The upper half of the egg usually forms the **animal pole** towards which the nucleus is always located. The polocytes or polar bodies are eliminated only through this pole and this distinguishes the animal pole in oligolecithal eggs in which the concentration of the yolk in the vegetal pole is not very distinct. Usually, the distribution of the yolk in this pole is negligible, if it is present. In contrast, the lower half of the egg forms the vegetal pole containing abundance of yolk especially in telolecithal eggs. This is because the yolk is heavier than the other inclusions in the ooplasm. The yolk accumulated at this pole serves as the nutrient for the developing embryo.

SYMMETRY

In addition to polarity, many animal eggs also possess an obvious **bilateral symmetry** which is not visible in most cases until after fertilization. In many amphibian eggs, a zone of lighter pigmentation called grey crescent develops on one side of the egg in the first few hours of fertilization (Figure 4.1). This structure marks the dorsal side of the egg and later, of the embryo, thus showing the bilateral symmetry of the egg. **Ancel** and **Vintemberger** (1948) have demonstrated that the formation of grey crecent is due to shifting of the egg cortex to the deeper layers of the cytoplasm. Investigations have shown that the cortical changes determine the plane and position of the symmetry in the egg. The local differences in the composition of the egg cytoplasm duto to the uneven distribution of physicochemical properties within the egg cytoplasm determine polarity and symmetry. As a rule, these distributions could be qualitatively and quantitatively different. The regional cytoplasmic variations in the egg may be interpreted as qualitative differences in the chemical composition of the parts of the egg. The developmental part of the egg may be determined by the nature of the substances contained within that part of the egg. These materials are often referred to as **morphogenetic substances.**

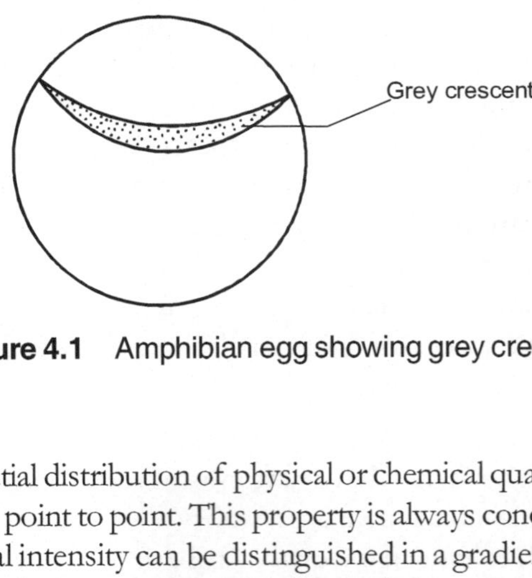

Figure 4.1 Amphibian egg showing grey crescent

GRADIENT CONCEPT

This concept explains the spatial distribution of physical or chemical quantity in the egg and the gradual changes of this quantity from point to point. This property is always concerned with the so-called scalar quantities and planes of equal intensity can be distinguished in a gradient field. Thus several different types of gradient fields can be distinguished in animal eggs. If the scalar quantity (gradient) is maximum at one end of the egg and minimum at the opposite end, then it is described as **linear gradient system**. If the direction of the gradient coincides with one of the axes, then it is called as **axial gradient system**. On the other hand, a gradient may extend over a flat or curved surface (**surface gradient system**) or may extend in all directions (**spatial gradient system**). In many eggs, the gradient systems have been found to be correlated with polarity and symmetry. It is well known that there is an increase in yolk concentration along the main axis of many eggs and this can be ascribed as **yolk gradient**. **Child** and his co-workers (1940) have suggested the importance of local differences and the intensity of metabolism in animal eggs for the occurrence of a gradient system. As a rule, the intensity of metabolism is greatest at the animal pole of the eggs and it decreases gradually in the direction of the vegetal pole along the main axis of the egg.

Spek (1930) measured the pH of the egg protoplasm and found that most of the eggs had more or less uniform pH. But he noticed a bipolar differentiation in the egg protoplasm shortly after the beginning of development, ie., the animal pole cytoplasm was alkaline in nature and the vegetal pole cytoplasm was acidic in nature. He believed that the colloidal particles with positive and negative electric charges were originally mixed throughout the egg cytoplasm. Later the positive particles moved to one pole and the negative particles to the opposite pole so that the mixture would thereby be separated and particles of the same size would be concentrated at each of the poles. He assumed that this migration of particles was by an electrical field due to differential penetration of certain ions from the environment to the egg. However, later investigators showed that this bipolar differentiation is rather due to the shifting of the egg yolk. In other words, yolk material consisting of fat and protein granules now assumes its final position with regard to the egg axis. That is why the acid yolk proteins accumulate at the vegetal pole and their disappearance in the animal pole causes the pH to shift in the direction of alkalinity.

The gradient system is found to play an important role in animal development. **Driesch** (1908) has shown that sea urchin's blastomeres, when separated at the four-cell stage, can develop into complete larvae. This has stimulated several other investigators to study the developmental potencies of blastomeres. When developing sea urchin's egg was separated into animal (A_1 and A_2) and vegetal (V_1 and V_2) halves, the isolated animal half developed into a holoblastula with long cilia over the entire larva but it had no further development. In the same way, the isolated vegetal half failed to survive but it developed a gut with rudimentary skeletal parts and ill developed ectoderm without ciliary covering (Figure 4.2). From these experiments, it was concluded that the animal field contains a set of factors responsible for the development of animal structures namely ectoderm and long cilia and the vegetal field contains a set of factors for the development of gut and skeletal part. On the intact egg, the animal and vegetal poles are balanced so that a normal embryo develops. When the embryo was treated with lithium chloride, the animal cells actually developed the vegetal structures and on treatment with sodium thiocyanide, the vegetal cells developed animal structures (Figure 4.2). It was also found that a few micromeres are also formed due to high activity of the vegetal field in the vegetal pole. If an isolated animal half was supplied with the micromeres of the vegetal pole, the animal cells developed vegetal structures so that a normal but smaller larva was formed. On the other hand, if the animal cells were supplied with V_2 cells alone, then the resulting larva had ill-developed gut and apical tuft of animal half. Similarly, the animal half combined with V_1 cells developed very little gut but the apical tuft was much extensive (Figure 4.3).

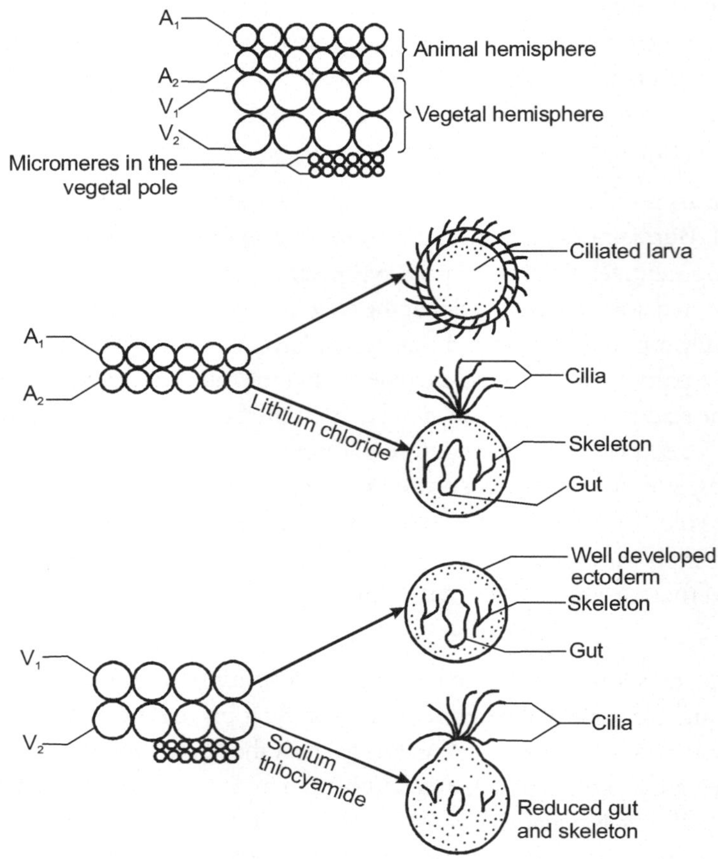

Figure 4.2 Isolation and development of animal and vegetal hemispheres in sea urchin's egg

The above experiments show that there is a gradient of vegetalizing activity which is the highest at the vegetal pole and it progressively decreases towards the animal pole. Similarly, the animal field has an opposite gradient which is high at the animal pole and progressively reduces towards the vegetal pole. It is possible to combine two sea urchin's embryos to form a double-sided larva which are attached together with their animal and vegetal gradients coinciding. When a sea urchin's blastula is cut into two halves passing through both animal and vegetal poles, then each half will develop into a complete larva. Based on this, **Runnstrom** (1928) proposed that there are two oppositely directed gradients in the eggs namely **animal–vegetal gradient** and **vegetal–animal gradient**. Therefore, the fate of each cell will be determined by the interaction of the two gradients. Thus, lithium suppresses the animal–vegetal gradient and sodium thiocyanide suppresses the vegetal–animal gradient.

According to **Lyndahl** (1936), the above two gradients are closely related with two different metabolic differences, ie., the animal gradient is concerned with carbohydrate metabolism which is inhibited by lithium whereas the vegetal gradient is concerned with protein metabolism which is influenced by sodium thiocyanide. The earliest symmetry of the ovum is marked by the polar axis or the primary axis. According to the **Gradient theory** put forward by **Boveri** (1910), the vegetal region of the sea urchin's egg exerts a dominant influence. **Child** (1940) viewed that there is a marked difference in the rate of metabolism in between the animal and vegetal poles and the metabolic vigour is the greatest at the animal pole and diminishes gradually towards the vegetal pole where the rate of metabolism is lesser. This hypothesis of Child is generally called as **metabolic axial gradient theory**. Furthermore, it is shown that certain areas containing organ-forming substances of the future embryo are prelocalized in the polar axis even before fertilization has occurred. Thus the materials in the area of the animal pole will mainly give rise to the anterior parts and that in the area of the vegetal pole to the posterior regions of the embryo. Thus, the animal pole always develops into the head region and the vegetal pole into the posterior region of the animal.

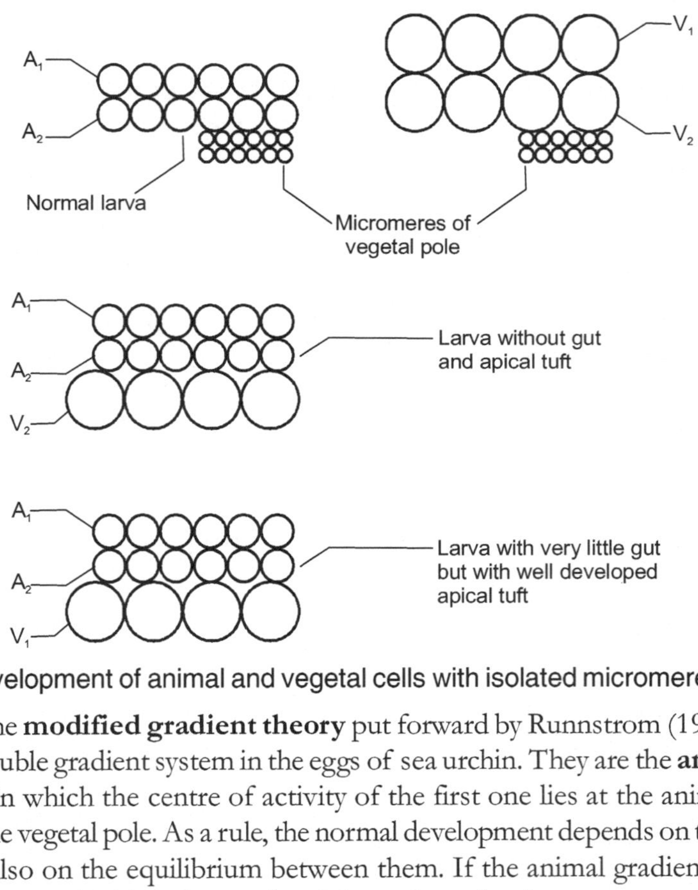

Figure 4.3 Development of animal and vegetal cells with isolated micromeres of vegetal pole

According to the **modified gradient theory** put forward by Runnstrom (1967) and Horstadius (1969), there is a double gradient system in the eggs of sea urchin. They are the **animal gradient** and **vegetal gradient** in which the centre of activity of the first one lies at the animal pole and of the second one lies at the vegetal pole. As a rule, the normal development depends on the presence of both the gradients and also on the equilibrium between them. If the animal gradient is suppressed, the vegetal gradient becomes highly influenced and the embryo develops excess parts related to vegetal gradient (**vegetalized embryo**). On the other hand, if the vegetal gradient is suppressed, then the animal gradient becomes highly influenced and the embryo develops excess parts related to animal gradient (**animalized embryo**). The equilibrium between the two gradients may be altered by a number of means. For example, the animal gradient can be made weak by altering its centre of activity either through removing the blastomeres at the animal pole or with the action of lithium salts. Similarly, the vegetal gradient may be weakened either by removing the blastomeres at the vegetal pole or by the action of sodium thiocyanide. Horstadius and Josefson (1969; 1972) have shown that the animal gradient in the eggs is due to tryphtophane which prompts the synthesis of RNA and protein and the vegetal gradient is due to nucleotide which inhibits the synthesis of RNA and proteins.

If the polarity of the egg is determined by the axial gradients, then the disturbances of the inside gradients might cause changes in the polarity. Centrifugation of the egg would bring profound modifications in its structure. As a rule, the protein yolk is heavier and the fatty yolk is lighter than the clear cytoplasm, so they would accumulate at opposite poles. However, the polarity of such eggs, in majority of cases, has remained unchanged. The egg materials displaced by centrifugation, often within a short time, return to the normal positions with regard to their original egg axis. This clearly evidences that the factors governing polarity have not been altered by centrifugation but they must be inherent in the components of the egg. Presumably, polarity depends on factors localized in the egg cortex and the axial gradients arise only as a result of these factors with some exceptions. For example, the yolk gradient in amphibian eggs seems to be the decisive factor for directing the later development of the embryo. In general, just as the cortical factors are of importance for polarity, so also are they for symmetry. While working on amphibian eggs, **Pasteels** (1962) has proved that the localization of the primordia of the future embryo and the direction of its plane of symmetry depend on the interaction of two factors namely **yolk gradient** localized in the internal cytoplasm and a gradient field in the cortex called **cortical field**.

In summary, it can be stated that the directional organization of the egg is governed by the interaction of axial and cortical gradient fields. These fields determine the polarity and symmetry of the egg and thereby simultaneously determine the main direction of the future embryo. Thus there is a definite relationship between the polarity and symmetry of the egg and the organization of the future embryo.

REVIEW QUESTIONS

1. Define the terms polarity and symmetry. How do they become established during the development of egg ?
2. Write an essay on gradient concept.
3. Write notes on the following:
   i. Egg cytoplasm
   ii. Animal and vegetal poles
   iii. Morphogenetic substances
   iv. Gradient systems
   v. Modified gradient theory
   vi. Animalization and vegetalization
   vii. Cortical field.

5

OVULATION AND EGG TRANSPORT

Periodical shedding of the ovum from the ovary is known as **ovulation.** The shed ovum is then transported from the ovary to the site of fertilization. The process of ovulation is under the control of both the season (breeding season) and the internal hormones (pituitary hormones).

OVULATION IN AMPHIBIANS

In frog, the ovary contains large number of eggs and is attached to the body wall. The ova are about 2 mm in diameter and they are inside the follicles. When the eggs become ripe, they break out of the follicles and get into the ciliated body cavity. The rhythmic beating of the cilia in the body cavity will move the ova forward to the oviducal openings. As the ova come down the oviduct, they are coated with jelly and come to rest in the ovisacs. As a result, a mass of eggs collects in the ovisacs, and this egg mass is released at the time when the male liberates the sperm. After ovulation, the germ cells in the ovary begin to grow to form the next batch of eggs. Here the fertilization is external.

OVULATION IN MAMMALS

In mammals, the egg grows within the follicle which is composed of cuboidal epithelial cells. As the follicle grows, a cavity develops within the follicle. This cavity is the **antrum** of the follicular space and is filled with a fluid called **follicular fluid**. When the developing ovum gets attached to the wall of the follicle, it is surrounded by two layers of follicular cells namely an inner layer of cells called **corona radiata** and an outer layer of cells called **cumulous oophorus**. The follicular cells lining the antrum form the **stratum granulosum**. The whole follicle is surrounded by two fibrous coverings namely **theca interna** and **theca externa**. Surrounding the ovum, there is a thin membrane with radial canals called **zona radiata** or **zona pellucida**. When the follicle is fully formed, it projects on the surface of the ovary and is now called as **Graafian follicle**. At this stage, a small area of follicular wall is deprived of blood supply. This point is called **stigma** where the follicle breaks and releases the ovum surrounded by some follicular cells into the body cavity. When the ovum is discharged from the ovary **(ovulation)**, the oviduct shows increased motility and it almost moves over the surface of the ovary. In this way, the ovum gets into the oviduct and the cilia in the oviduct transport the egg down the tube. The peristaltic movement of the oviduct also helps in transporting the ovum. The process of ovulation in mammals is depicted in Figure 5.1.

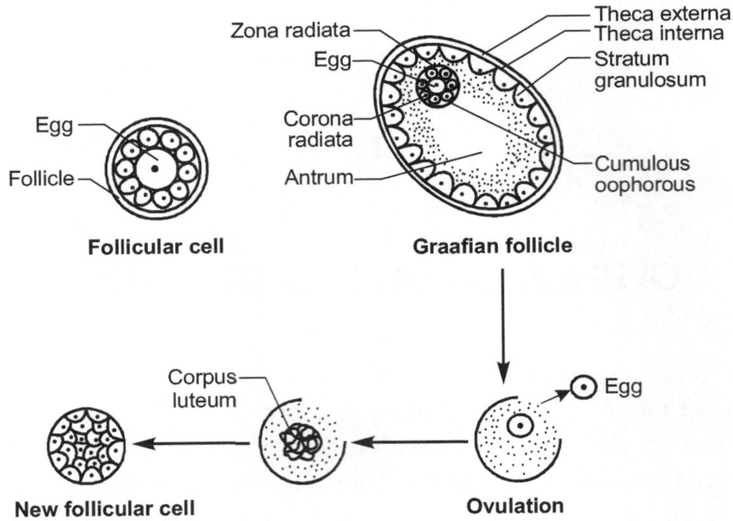

Figure 5.1 Diagram showing the structure and transport of graafian follicle in mammals

In mammals, fertilization is internal, usually occurring in the oviduct. After ovulation, the follicle is filled up with connective tissue in the form of a solid body called **corpus luteum**. In the absence of fertilization, the corpus luteum regresses and degenerates and a new ovarian follicle begins to develop in some other parts of the ovary. If the ovum is fertilized, the corpus luteum remains functional as an endocrine gland concerned with the implantation of the ovum and early development. In the absence of pregnancy, the reproductive cycle is repeated.

Hormonal Regulation of Ovulation in Mammals

In the ovarian cycle of mammals, there are two major processes namely (1) growth of follicle to ovulation and (2) formation of corpus luteum. These two events are under the control of three gonadotropins (hormones) produced by the pituitary body—**Follicle stimulating hormone** (FSH) induces the growth of the follicle, **luteinizing hormone** (LH), in combination with FSH induces the ovulation and the formation of corpus luteum, and **luteotrophic hormone** (LTH) is responsible for milk secretion and maintains the corpus luteum. While the ovarian activity is controlled by the pituitary gland, in turn, the pituitary is influenced by two ovarian hormones namely **estrogen** and **progesterone.** Figure 5.2 explains the hormonal control of the ovarian cycle in mammals. The FSH stimulates the growth of the follicle and together with the LH stimulates the production of estrogen in the ovary. Estrogen has a feedback effect on the pituitary gland and induces it to secrete more of LH and LTH and less of FSH. Under these conditions, ovulation occurs and corpus luteum is formed. The corpus luteum produces **progesterone** and is maintained by LTH. When this body degenerates, the ovarian hormones are reduced. As a result, the pituitary produces more FSH to start the cycle again. When the corpus luteum degenerates, it is replaced by connective tissue and is known as **corpus albicans**.

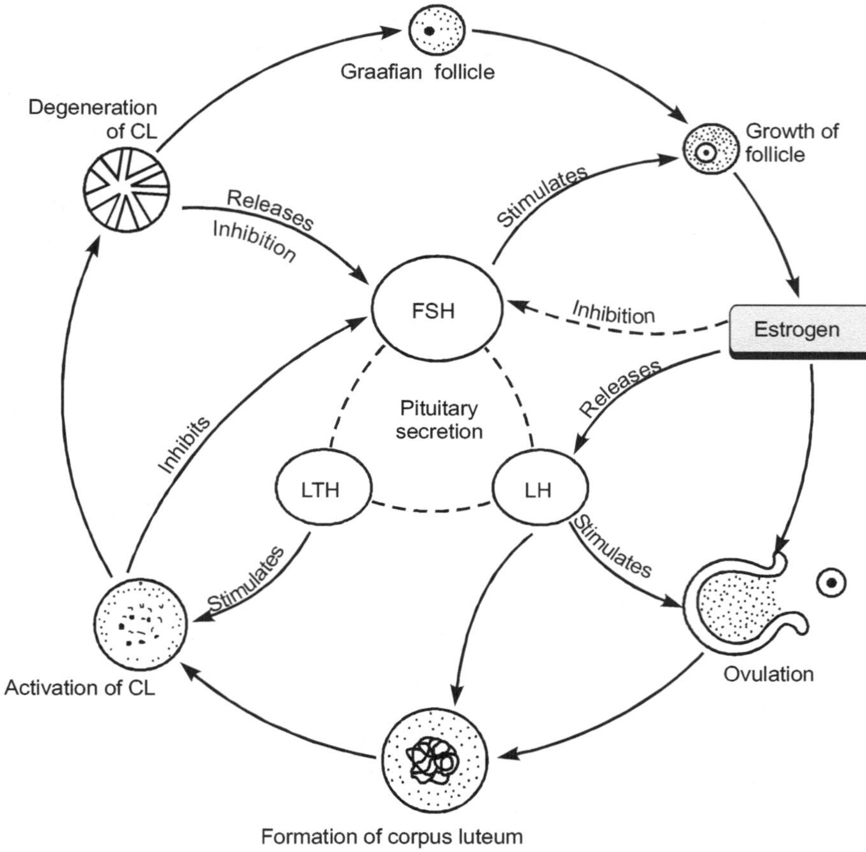

Figure 5.2 Hormonal control and ovarian cycle in a mammal

ESTROUS/MENSTRUAL CYCLE

In mammals, at the event of pregnancy, the placental hormones maintain the corpus luteum, intact, inhibiting FSH and preventing ovulation throughout the gestation period. If there is no pregnancy, the corpus luteum degenerates so that the secretion of progesterone is reduced along with the production of more FSH by the pituitary. Now the ovarian cycle is started once again. These are the two phenomena associated with ovulation in mammals.

The **estrous cycle** begins with estrous which is a period of sexual urge coinciding with ovulation and is seen in all mammals except higher primates. During this period, the uterine wall becomes spongy, thick and soft because of the proliferation of the epithelial layers, and the vaginal lining becomes cornified. If fertilization takes place, the uterus is ready to receive the zygote which becomes implanted in it. In the absence of fertilization, the uterine lining is shed. This shedding of uterine lining takes place within a short period and is known as **metestrum** which is followed by a period of rest and repair called **diestrum**. Just before the next estrus, there is a short period known as **proestrum** during which the wall of the uterus undergoes changes and prepares for the estrous. The length of the estrous cycle varies in different mammals.

The human estrous cycle is called as **menstrual cycle** because it occurs almost monthly. In general, it takes place in about 28 days. The menstrual cycle can be studied under the following phases:

Menstruation

From first to fifth day, menstruation occurs lasting for five days during which the proliferated thickened **endometrium** (inner wall of the uterus) gets sloughed off. The entire sloughed endometrium is thrown out along with blood from the uterus.

Repair During the fifth and sixth day (one day), the uterine lining and the broken blood capillaries get repaired.

Proliferation After seven days of commencement of menstruation, the uterine wall becomes proliferated and the proliferation lasts up to the fifteenth day. Now the endometrium becomes much thickened.

Ovulation From the fourteenth to sixteenth day, ovulation takes place at the end of the proliferation period.

Secretion From the sixteenth to twenty-eighth day, the uterine glands secrete a fluid rich in glycogen.

The various phases of the menstrual cycle are represented in Table 5.1.

Table 5.1 Various phases and duration of menstrual cycle in humans

Phases	Duration (days)
Menstruation	1–5
Repair	5–6
Proliferation	7–15
Ovulation	14–16
Secretion	16–28

From the above account, it is clear that the process of ovulation, the preparation of the uterus for implantation, gestation and birth or parturition in mammals are under the control of various hormones.

GESTATION

This is the retaining period of a young one within the uterus of the mother and it includes two phases namely **luteal phase** and **placental phase**. After fertilization, the zygote gets attached with the inner surface of the uterine wall which is already receptive due to histological alterations. The implanted zygote becomes surrounded by the uterine tissues, suppressing the menstrual cycles throughout the pregnancy. After implantation, the chorion of the embryo develops a large number of villi which branch extensively into the spongy uterine wall. Thus the placenta is formed for the exchange of materials between the foetus and mother. All these events constitute the **luteal phase** of gestation. The fully developed placenta also acts as an endocrine gland and secretes hormones (**estrogen and progesterone**), thus providing major hormonal control of pregnancy starting from the 12th week of gestation. This is the **placental phase** which exists up to the 9th month of pregnancy. The gestation periods of certain mammals are given in Table 5.2.

Table 5.2 Gestation periods of some mammals

Animal	Gestation period (days)
Rat and mouse	21
Rabbit	32
Dog	60
Cat	63
Lion	110
Pig	120
Goat and sheep	150
Tiger	155
Monkey	180
Bear	183
Man	280
Cow	284
Horse	330
Camel	390
Elephant	640

SEXUAL PHOTOPERIODICITY (ENVIRONMENTAL EFFECT ON OVULATION)

In addition to hormonal control, ovulation is also affected by the environmental condition via the nervous system. It is known that changes in the climatic conditions would lead to variations in the time of ovulation in domestic animals. For example, when mice are exposed to light at night and kept in the dark during daytime, they will change their habits of ovulation. When they are continuously exposed to light, ovulation is found to be inhibited. Thus variations in the amount of light regulate the activity of the gonads. In this way, one can regulate ovulation by controlling the ratio of light to dark period in each day. This periodicity in light controlling the sexual cycle is called as **sexual photoperiodicity**.

However, the effect of light on the sexual cycle is not a direct one on the ovary but the action is through the pituitary gland. This can be evidenced by simply removing the pituitary where any increase in light has no effect on ovulation. In this process, the eyes play an important role as they are the organs which receive light stimuli leading to sexual activation. Therefore one could expect the optic nerve to be important in the process of ovulation. Again, this can be shown by transecting the optic nerve and abolishing the effect of light. From the available evidence, the steps in inducing ovulation can be explained as is illustrated in Figure 5.3.

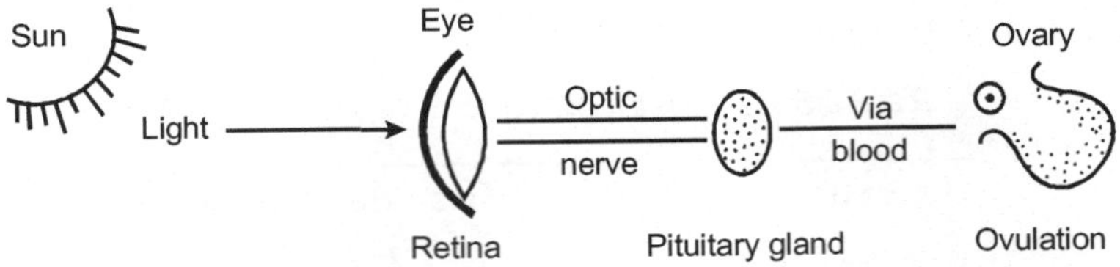

Figure 5.3 Diagrammatic structure to show the steps in inducing ovulation

The initial stimulus is the ratio of light to darkness. The retina of the eye fixes up the light stimuli which pass to the brain centre through the optic nerve. In the brain, the impulses stimulate the pituitary gland to release the hormones into the blood. The hormones travel via the bloodstream to act on the ovary resulting in follicle growth and ovulation. The pituitary body, is in turn, under nervous control. The nerve fibres from the hypothalamus of brain end in the posterior lobe of the pituitary body. The connection between the posterior lobe and the anterior lobe is through a portal system called **the hypophyseal portal system**. The stimuli from the hypothalamus pass through these nerve fibres which ultimately reach the blood capillaries. At this point, substances could enter the bloodstream and reach the anterior lobe which is now stimulated to release its hormones such as FSH, LH and LTH. This photoperiodicity is characteristic of most of the birds and of a few mammals.

A similar mechanism also seems to control the activity of the male gonad or testis. However, this type of photoperiodicity in males is not characteristic of all animals. For example, man has internal control independent of light and other controls.

REVIEW QUESTIONS

1. Give an account of ovulation and egg transport in animals?
2. Write an essay on hormonal control of ovulation in mammals.
3. Explain the processes of estrous and menstrual cycles in mammals.
4. Write notes on the following:
   i. Antrum
   ii. Graafian follicle
   ii. Corpus luteum
   iv. Gestation
   v. Sexual photoperiodicity and ovulation.

6

FERTILIZATION

It is believed that the essential features of fertilization are the entrance of the sperm into the egg and the mere coming together of the nuclei of the male and female gametes. But fertilization is much more than the surface reactions between two gametes to start embryonic development. In other words, it induces the next step of further development of the egg namely **cleavage**. i.e., the further development of the ovum depends on the entry of the sperm into it. For a successful fertilization, two prerequisites are needed as far as the spermatozoa are concerned. One requirement is that sperm must be in an active or motile stage and the another one is that the sperm must not be too young or too old, i.e., the sperm must not be overripened or underripened. The sperm and the ovum may be considered as defective cells but are complementary to each other at the time of fertilization. The ovum provides the basic general cytoplasm as well as plenty of nourishment. The sperm, on the other hand, provides the functional centrosome, a very essential organoid for cleavage of the egg. Both the spermatozoan and ovum provide chromatin structure, Golgi substance and mitochondria during fertilization.

EVENTS OF FERTILIZATION

The union of two different types of sex cells namely male and female gametes is called **fertilization** which is prevalent not only in animals but in plants too. The act of fertilization can be divided into three phases namely (1) attraction (2) penetration and (3) conjugation.

Attraction

When sperms come into the vicinity of the egg, they usually assemble around it. This constitutes the attraction which is accomplished by different methods in animals. Several factors such as chemotaxis, thigmotaxis and enzyme action are believed to be involved in this process.

Chaemotaxis It is the movement of sperms towards the egg attracted by the liberation of some chemical substances. **R.S. Lillie** (1918) has found that the sea urchin's egg and sperms produce **fertilizin** and **antifertilizin** respectively and these chemicals interact and neutralize, attracting or keeping the sperms towards the egg, when the sperms come to the vicinity of the egg.

Thigmotaxis The sperms are capable of spiral movement brought about by the tail. This movement makes the sperms to be attached to the egg. Experiments have proved that the sperms will move directly towards a small solid body, even a sand grain when they come in contact with it.

Enzyme action **Lillie, F.R.** (1919) has shown that the sea urchin's egg emits an enzyme towards the sperms to bring about agglutination.

Recent view According to the recent view by **Bishop** (1998), the sperms are pushed up by the contractions of the uterine wall in higher vertebrates. The movement of the sperms from the site of deposition to the site of fertilization usually involves only little active swimming of the sperms themselves. The movement of the sperms is also believed to be brought about by the countercurrents in the backwardly flowing liquid contents of the reproductive tract.

Penetration

It was formerly believed that the penetration of the sperms into the ovum was an active process. But later experiments have proved that the sperm entry into the egg is a passive process. At the time when the sperm penetrates through the egg envelop, it apparently comes to rest against the plasma membrane of the egg. In some invertebrates, the acrosomes are smooth and are not pointed for poring the egg membrane. Here, the acrosome produces a chemical substance which will dissolve the egg membrane so that the cytoplasm is thrown to form a **fertilization cone** or even a **long filament**. When the sperm head comes in contact with this structure at the surface of the egg, the cone or filament retracts drawing the sperm into the egg. In some other invertebrate eggs, a funnel-like structure is formed through which sperm entry is possible. The mature unfertilized egg contains a chemical substance called **fertilizin** which makes the sperm enter the egg. When the sperm enters the egg, fertilizin counteracts with the substance called **antifertilizin** present in the sperm. By the physical contact of each other, a **chemical lock** is established between the fertilizin molecules of unfertilized egg and the antifertilizin molecules of spermatozoan. This chemical lock prevents the entry of other sperms though they may be near the surface of the egg.

Fate of supernumerary sperms In some cases, multiple sperm invasion or **polyspermy** occurs by which more than one sperm make their entry into the ovum. The additional number of sperms are called **supernumerary sperms** and this is common in the megalecithal eggs of reptiles and birds. In such cases, only one sperm nucleus unites and the others are usually degenerated and discarded.

Mechanism of sperm entry Once the sperm has become attached to the egg, it must be able to penetrate the egg envelope. It has been shown that the spermatozoa of various species of invertebrates and vertebrates possess the property of dissolving the egg membrane. These lysins are proposed to be secreted by the acrosome of the sperms. On making contact with the surface of the egg membrane, the acrosome breaks, giving rise to a rigid and straight filament. This structure pierces the egg envelop and reaches the surface of the egg shell proper (**Colwin** and **Colwin**, 1957). At the same time, the lysin liberated by the egg membrane erodes the membrane barrier in the sperm head and the sperm is engulfed through the surface projection of the egg (fertilization cone). The situation in mammals deserves special mention here. When leaving the ovary, the mammalian egg is surrounded by a layer of follicle cells which are kept maintained by a viscous substance, probably **hyaluronic acid**. It has been proved that the sperm contains an enzyme namely **hyaluronidase** which reacts with hyaluronic acid, thereby causing the disintegration of the coronal cells. As a result, the sperm gains free entry into the egg surface.

Changes in the sperm structure within the ovum In general, the entire sperm enters into the ovum and in rare cases, the tail is left outside the egg. After getting inside the ovum, the sperm head detaches itself from the flagellum and its nucleus loses compactness and becomes large and vesicular. At this stage, the sperm head constitutes **male pronucleus** and the sperm now rotates 180^0 so that the centrosome and the middle piece go first followed by the male pronucleus.

Reactions in the ovum (cortical changes and formation of fertilization membrane) The entry of the sperm into the egg induces certain reactions in the egg to begin the process of development (activation of the egg). The unfertilized egg is surrounded by the vitelline membrane. Following the penetration of the sperm into the egg, a change occurs in the cortex of the egg and it spreads from the point of the entry of the sperm. As a result of this cortical change, the vitelline membrane becomes lifted off due to the accumulation of expelled substances by the egg in the space between the egg surface and membrane. This is the **perivitelline space** which soon increases in size rapidly. This space is filled with a fluid called **perivitelline fluid** which sets fertilization membrane starting from the point of the sperm contact (Figure 6.1).

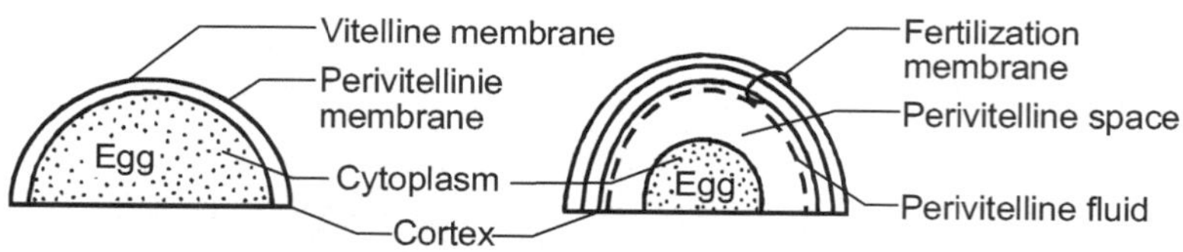

Figure 6.1 Formation of fertilization membrane

The fertilization membrane has been considered to be an obstacle to the entry of extra-sperm cells. It is also believed that the perivitelline fluid might have **Antifertilizin** which prevent the entry of another sperm. Apparently, after the fertilization membrane is formed, the egg decreases in diameter owing to the secretion of the perivitelline fluid. In vertebrates, the egg undergoes the second maturation division and gives rise to two polar bodies after the entry of the sperm. The nucleus of the ovum which is now large and vesicular is called as **female pronucleus** found situated near the animal pole. The centromeres of the egg generally disappear after the entry of the sperm.

Conjugation

The union of the two pronuclei (male and female) is known as **conjugation.** During this process, they come together by a route which may be analysed in the following components:

The sperm penetration path When the migration of the male pronucleus towards the female pronucleus takes place, the granules of the cytoplasm found on the way are cleared off and a line is formed. This is called the **penetration path** which is usually the radius of the egg at which the sperm entered.

The sperm copulation path Soon after a local gelation, the ooplasm once again liquifies so that the sperm migrates freely in this path towards the point at which the pronuclei will meet. This path is often at a considerable angle to the penetration path.

The egg copulation path This is the passage along which the female pronucleus moves towards the meeting point.

The cleavage path This is the pathway along which the two pronuclei move to their final position on the egg axis. This will be often slightly nearer the pole.

At this time, the two pronuclei unite to form a common zygote. The centromeres of the zygote are generally derived from the centromeres of the sperm or they are probably newly formed. Thus fertilization is completed and the mitochondrial elements of the sperm become fragmented and distributed throughout the cytoplasm of the zygote. The entire mechanism of the events of fertilization are shown in Figure 6.2.

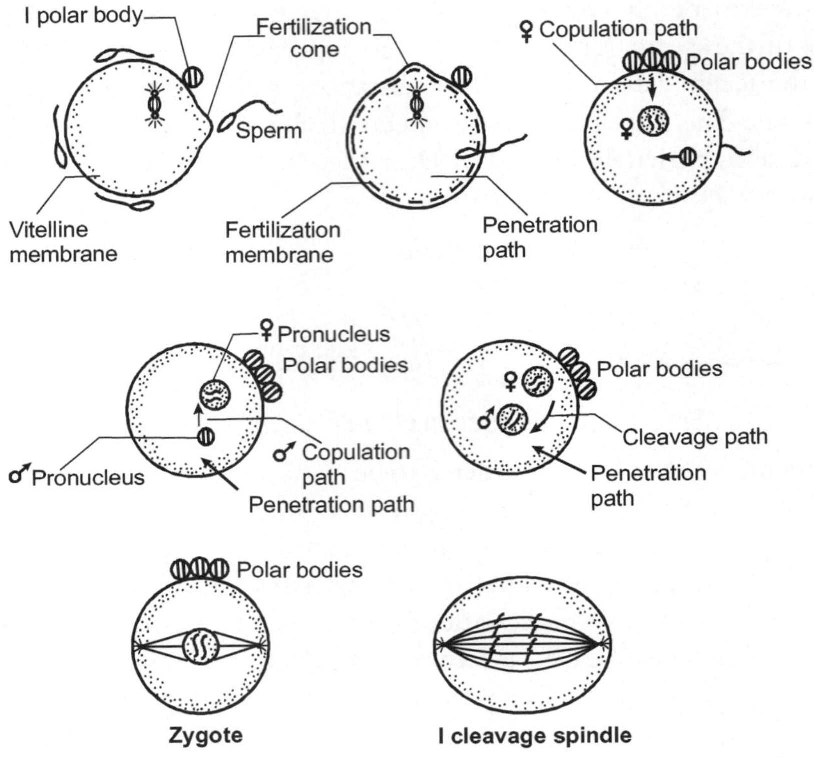

Figure 6.2 Diagrams showing the major events of fertilization

EFFECT OF FERTILIZATION

The actual process of fertilization induces the ovum for further development through cortical reactions **(activation of the egg)** with the resultant formation of fertilization membrane. Experiments have proved that at least two conditions must be fulfilled during conjugation. The first one is the maturation of the egg and secondly, the sperm must have traversed the egg cortex. Sperms that have been artificially injected into the egg remain completely inactive. The same is also true of sperms which have penetrated into the egg without cortical plasm. Evidently, the sperms are activated during their passage through the cortex and it is this activation which enables the two pronuclei to complete the process of fusion. In somatic mitosis, the division centre or centrosome is handed down from cell to cell. But in the development of the female gamete, the division centre degenerates or becomes physiologically incapable of continuing the division of the egg. The mature egg thus contains all the essentials for the development other than a potent division centre. The sperm on the other hand lacks the cytoplasmic conditions necessary for development but possesses an active division centre which it introduces into the egg at fertilization. Fertilization, therefore, restores the diploid number of chromosomes to the egg. However, this view has been questioned and it has been shown that cytoasters can also be produced in the cytoplasm.

Metabolic Changes During Fertilization

The following are the major metabolic changes that occur in the event of fertilization:

i. During the cortical reactions, there is a breakdown of cortical granules with an increase in the viscosity of the cortex and in the permeability to water and K^+ ions.

ii. There is a rapid change in membrane potential. The potential difference prior to fertilization between the inside and outside of the cell is 30–60 mV, which decreases immediately after fertilization.

iii. The intracellular concentration of cations especially Na, K and Ca undergo changes in which the change in Ca ion concentration has great significance in the activation of the egg.

iv. Many synthetic pathways in the fertilized egg are initiated as NADP and NADPH contents increase during fertilization.

v. In the fertilized eggs, the rate of respiration fluctuates and an increased oxygen uptake is related with the oxidation of glycogen and other foodstuff in the egg and with the synthesis of enormous ATP molecules.

vi. Even though the mature unfertilized egg has a complete protein synthetic machinery, some inhibitor or repressor proteins inactivate the protein synthesis in them. These inhibitor proteins are removed by some proteolytic enzymes during fertilization so that active protein synthesis is started in fertilized eggs.

vii. The most important metabolic change is the initiation of mitosis for cleavage of the fertilized eggs.

SIGNIFICANCE OF FERTILIZATION

The act of fertilization has many consequences which have been found to be of vital significance. However, these consequneces may not necessarily depend or fertilization.

i. Reproduction

The main significance of fertilization is to bring about reproduction by activation (except parthenogenetic eggs) and by restoring the diploid number of chromosomes in the zygote. This is because of the introduction of the male haploid chromosomes by the sperm into the ovum resulting in **amphimixis** of maternal and paternal chromosomes.

ii. Rejuvenation

Experiments on some protozoans show that cell division will gradually become less frequent and will finally cease in the absence of fertilization.

iii. Variations in Young Ones

In reality, variations are brought about in the genes of offspring by mutations and recombinations through meiotic division during fertilization.

iv. Sex Determination

In higher vertebrates, the event of fertilization enables the determination of the sex by the contribution of X or Y chromosome by the sperm.

REVIEW QUESTIONS

1. Describe the major events that occur during the processes of fertilization.
2. How could polyspermy be prevented at the time of fertilization?
3. Explain the mechanism of sperm entry into the egg and its changes in structure within the ovum.
4. Give an account of cortical reactions and formation of fertilization membrane.
5. Write an essay on metabolic changes and significance of fertilization.
6. Write notes on:
   i. Fertilization cone
   ii. Fertilizin–antifertilizin complex
   ii. Pronuclei
   iv. Fertilization membrane
   v. Amphimixis

7

EGG CORTEX AND DEVELOPMENT—CORTICAL REACTIONS AND THEORIES OF FERTILIZATION

We already know that fertilization is not just the mere coming together of the female and male pronuclei, but involves much more complex reactions between the two gametes to start embryonic development. Once the sperm has become attached to the egg, it must be able to penetrate the egg envelop. It is shown that the sperms of various species of invertebrates and vertebrates contain lytic agents possessing the property of breaking down the egg membrane. These lytic substances are secreted by the acrosome. On making contact with the surface of the egg membrane, the acrosome gives rises to a rigid and straight filament which pierces the egg envelop and reaches the surface of the egg cell proper. At the same time, the egg membrane also liberates lytic agents which erode the membrane barrier in the sperm head. Thus the egg is stimulated with the acrosome filament. In the fusion of the egg and sperm, substances secreted by each of these cells play a major role. The ovum produces a highly complex substance called **fertilizin** with a molecular weight of 3,00,000. Chemically, fertilizin is a glycoprotein in which the carbohydrate part is formed by one or more monosaccharides and the protein part by many different types of amino acids. On the other hand, the sperm produces **anti-fertilizin** which is much smaller than fertilizin and has a molecular weight of about 10,000. It is an acidic protein and has got the capacity to react with the fertilizin of the egg of the same species. This reaction is known as **fertilizin–antifertilizin reaction,** which is intended mainly to limit the spermatozoa number at the vicinity of the ovum, thus preventing the entry of two or more spermatozoa into the egg. The entry of sperm causes certain reactions in the egg to begin development. The first reaction is the **cortical reaction** in the egg and the **formation of the fertilization membrane**.

CHANGES IN THE EGG CORTEX

When the spermatozoan enters into the ovum, there is an alteration of the membrane potential inside the egg. This change spreads to the whole of the egg, starting from the point of sperm entry. By this cortical change, the vitelline membrane of the egg is lifted off from the plasma membrane and is expanded and transformed into a fertilization membrane which acts as an obstacle for **polyspermy**. Now substances expelled by the egg accumulate in the space between the egg surface and the membrane, called the **perivitelline space**. Soon the perivitelline space increases and the membrane-bound **cortical**

granules produced by the Golgi bodies of oocytes swell up, burst and liberate a fluid of mucopolysaccharides. This fluid absorbs more and more water and completely fills up the perivitelline space as **perivitelline fluid** (Figure 7.1).

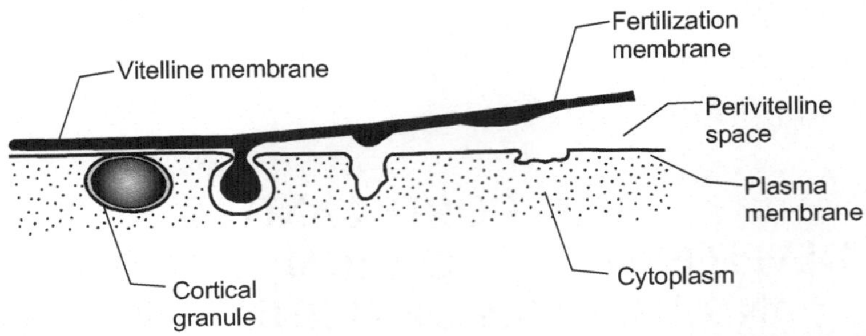

Figure 7.1 Changes in the egg cortex and formation of fertilization membrane

As a result, the egg decreases in diameter. It is shown that the perivitelline fluid contains antifertilizin which also prevents polyspermy. Some of the cortical granules remain intact on the surface of the egg and they are applied to the fertilization membrane, thus making the membrane much thicker and stronger. In frog, the perivitelline fluid fills the space between the egg plasma membrane and vitelline membrane and in bony fishes, the space between the egg plasma membrane and the chorion. The cortical granules are absent in many mammals except a few like hamsters, rabbits and humans. In these mammals, the perivitelline fluid is found in the space between the egg membrane and zona pellucida. Mammals like rat, guinea pigs, etc., urodele amphibians and insects do not possess cortical granules and the cortical reaction is found to be absent at the time of fertilization. Obviously the extrusion of perivitelline substance is due to sudden changes in the cortex of the egg and this phenomenon of cortical reactions is even visible in the eggs of sea urchin. In these eggs, there is a radical colour change immediately after sperm contact. The entire surface of the egg becomes changed from yellow to white. This is found to occur at the point of sperm contact and to spread all over the surface within 20 seconds. Experiments have proved that the sperms are activated during their passage through the cortex and it is this activation which enables the two pronuclei to complete the process of fusion and amphimixis. When the sperm is artificially injected into the egg, there are no further changes, thereby proving the importance of the egg cortex.

Theories of Fertilization

The normal development of the egg requires two changes namely **cortical changes** and the **formation of amphiaster** which are so interwoven that they cannot be seen separately. But it is possible to study the above phenomena in the case of artificial parthenogenesis. Based on these two processes, various theories have been put forward to explain the role of cortex and its changes in the activation of the egg. Among them, the following important theories have been explained.

Loeb's Theory (1913)

He worked on sea urchin's eggs. When the eggs were first treated for a few minutes in a weak solution of butyric acid in sea water, they immediately developed the fertilization membrane, though the eggs were unfertilized. After 15 to 20 minutes, they were brought for a period of 30 to 60 minutes into the sea water made hypertonic by the addition of NaCl. Finally they were returned to the normal sea water. Now many of the eggs cleaved and developed into normal larvae.

From the above experiments, Loeb believed that two factors are involved in the activation of the egg. The first one is **superficial cytolysis** (cortical changes) of the egg cortex which leads to sudden increase in the oxidative processes of the egg. The second is the one which corrects cytolysis and egg's activation, thus restoring the egg to normal chemical condition. Thus he placed much emphasis on superficial cytolysis of the egg cortex with resultant elevation of fertilization membrane.

Bataillon's Theory (1910–1913)

He discovered that frog's eggs extruded perivitelline fluid and developed the fertilization membrane when they were punctured with a fine needle. However, cleavage occurred only when the eggs were previously moistened with blood and then punctured. In this way, he found that cleavage could be provoked in a great number of eggs and a certain percentage of normal development would take place.

Like Loeb, Bataillon also emphasized two steps in the activation process of the egg. The first treatment, whether it is the puncture of the frog's egg by a fine needle or butyric acid treatment of the sea urchin's egg, causes the elevation of the fertilization membrane and also the formation of the **monaster.** The second treatment, whether it is blood in the case of frog's egg or hypertonic sea water in sea urchin's egg, introduces a catalyser which converts the monaster into an **amphiaster** thus rendering the egg capable of cleavage. Bataillon gave much importance to the exudation substances into the perivitelline space and the elevation of the fertilization membrane. He believed that the unfertilized egg was inhibited due to the accumulation of metabolic products and that the activation or fertilization led to the release of these substances to the exterior of the egg.

Theory of Lillie, F. R. (1919)

He postulated that a substance called fertilizin present in the cortex of the egg exerts two kinds of action in the activation process namely an activating, attracting and agglutinating action on the sperm and an activating effect on the egg itself. He believed that the inactive fertilizin produced by the egg is released into the surrounding water and it activates, attracts and agglutinates the sperm and the egg sruface. As the sperm touches the egg, it combines with the fertilizin and this **fertilizin–sperm complex** is the activating principle. This spreads throughout the egg, activating it towards development. The complex is thought to work especially on the cortex of the egg producing cortical changes including the formation of the fertilization membrane.

Theory of Lillie, R.S.(1918)

Like Loeb, Lillie, R.S. also contended that the cortical changes bring out the main aspects of activation. According to him, an activating substance (A), comparable to the growth hormone, auxin, is found in the egg. The production of this substance is due to the interaction of the substances S and B found in the egg. (S is formed from a synthetic process and B is a product of the hydrolytic process in the egg). Thus he believed in a single factor as an initiator of development. If A is produced in adequate concentration, then complete activation of the egg would occur. On the other hand, partial activation would result when A is present in a quantity below the optimum concentration.

Theory of Heilbrunn (1920)

He believed that an increase in the viscosity with the resultant coagulation or gelation of the egg cytoplasm is directly involved in the initiation of development. He proved that this process is similar to the clotting of the blood and recorded that calcium is the main agent in bringing about this effect. According to this view, calcium is bound to protein molecules in the egg cortex. At the time of activation either artificially or by sperm contact, part of this calcium is liberated which in turn produces coagulation of cytoplasm, initiating development.

Theory of Runnstrom (1952)

He contended that an inhibitor of proteolytic enzymes might be present in the vitelline membrane and in the cortex of the egg. He assumed that the inhibitor, probably fertilizin, would be identical with a heparin-like substance. The enzyme kinase which acts on proenzymes may be released when the sperm unites with the inhibitor. This would result in the production of an enzyme or enzymes which initiate development.

Theory of Monroy (1965)

His hypothesis is a recent one and he has given some convincing explanation in molecular terms regarding the activation of the egg. According to him, the energy-yielding systems are blocked during maturation of the egg so that all the reactions which require a large amount of energy are also inhibited **(Repressor theory)**. This theory has been supported by many modern embryologists. There are also many evidences that the repressor substances found in the egg during the maturation phase inhibit both the metabolic activities in the cytoplasm and the genetic activities in the nucleus. The act of fertilization removes the repressors releasing the cytoplasmic metabolic activities and the activity of the nuclear genetic system at a time.

PRINCIPLES OF BIPOLARITY

The egg cytoplasm generally contains all the materials except the cytocentres (centromeres). On the other hand, the sperm produces an amphiaster during fertilization with the help of well-developed cytocentres and they lack cytoplasmic materials. But this view has been proved to be wrong. In the case of **Ciona**, the egg also develops cytoasters. To explain this phenomenon, various views have been put forward by different workers.

Dalcq (1930) has proposed that "the principles" are carried in the sperm nucleus which produces the amphiaster for cleavage. Experimentally, he has proved that the egg develops a monaster when the two pronuclei are separated, preventing union with each other. On the other hand, the sperm nucleus undergoes normal mitotic division by the production of amphiaster. The same phenomenon has been noticed in sea urchin's egg by Wilson (1901) and in frog's egg by Bataillon (1911). However, this view has been much questioned and there are many possibilities for the formation of amphiaster in the egg cytoplasm by different stimuli. To get over this problem, Bataillon came forward to explain the following phenomenon. He proposed that the formation of amphiaster is due to the removal of 'anachronism' between the development of nucleus and the asters in the egg. The entry of the sperm mediates the difference between the nucleus and the asters. He also believed that when the cytoplasm gelates, the sperm asters are formed and this spreads as an "*on-de-degelification*" in all directions. At the same time, the centre of the cytocentre isolates and then only the amphiaster is formed. Thus the anachronism between the nucleus and the asters is abolished by the "*on-de-degelification*".

In summary, it may be concluded that the whole cytoplasm has the capacity for aster formation but normally this capacity is strongest in the region of the cytocentre. The division of the cytocentre and thereby the formation of an amphiaster is somehow dependent on the presence of a nucleus especially of its nucleoplasm. After the extrusion of the polar bodies, the egg nucleus and the cytocentre are, as a group, unable to form a bipolar spindle. But they may regain this capacity when an "*on-de-degelification*" has passed through the cytoplasm. Therefore it is worth mentioning that the egg must have matured and the sperm must have traversed the egg cortex to ensure fertilization.

REVIEW QUESTIONS

1. What is the role of egg cortex in the activation of the egg?
2. Give an account of various theories regarding the act of fertilization.
3. Write notes on the following:
    i. Cortical granules
    ii. Amphiaster
    iii. Superficial cytolysis
    iv. Repressor theory
    v. Principles of bipolarity
    vi. "on-de-degelification".

8

PARTHENOGENESIS—VIRGIN BIRTH

In sexually reproducing animals, a new individual is produced from the egg that is fertilized by the spermatozoan. However, many plants and animals are capable of developing from the eggs without fertilization. This type of development of an egg into an embryo without fertilization is known as **parthenogenesis**. In other words, it is the development of a female gamete into an organism without genetic contribution from the sperm (the male gamete). The individuals that are produced by parthenogenesis are called **parthenotes.** Parthenogenesis is most prevalent and sporadical in large number of plant species but never seen as widely in any major animal groups. This phenomenon is frequently found to occur in certain orders of **insects** namely **Hymenoptera** (bees and wasps), **Homoptera** and **Coleoptera** (beetles), **rotifers** and **lower crustaceans**. While certain individuals reproduce exclusively by parthenogenesis, it seems to occur as a regular feature and alternates with the sexual generation in some groups. In animals like **annelids, molluscs, echinoderms** and **amphibians** including a few **mammals**, parthenogenesis can be artificially induced. Therefore, the process of parthenogenesis can be studied under two major heads namely **natural parthenogenesis** and **artificial parthenogenesis.**

NATURAL PARTHENOGENESIS OR OBLIGATORY PARTHENOGENESIS

Here, an individual is formed in normal course without any artificial induction. This occurs naturally in the life cycle of animals in which the adults possess only a haploid number of chromosomes. In some species, natural parthenogenesis is the only means of reproduction whereas it also plays a role in reproduction as well as sex determination in others. If the individuals reproduce exclusively by parthenogenesis with no sexual generation, then it is **complete parthenogenesis**. This type is seen in minor animal groups in which the individuals that are developed from the unfertilized eggs are exclusively females. As a result, in complete parthenogenesis, there is no possibility for sexuality and recombination of genes as noticed in rotifers and in some helminth worms and insects. In some cases, the parthenogenetic generation alternates with a sexual generation as seen in some insects like aphids, wasps and bees. This type is know as **incomplete** or **partial** or **cyclic parthenogenesis** in which the life cycle includes two generations, one alternating with the another one. However, in some cases, the unfertilized eggs develop parthenogenetically into males so that they are haploid in nature whereas the fertilized eggs develop into females which are diploid in nature. Thus natural parthenogenesis is in general distinguished into two types namely 1) **haploid parthenogenesis** and 2) **diploid parthenogenesis**.

Haploid or Arrhenotokous Parthenogenesis (Arrhenotoky)

Here the egg develops typically with one reduction division along with two polar bodies. This haploid egg develops into an embryo without fusion with the sperm so that the embryo and adult are haploid. These haploid individuals devlop into males. On the other hand, the females develop from the fertilized eggs in the normal manner and so they are diploid as given below:

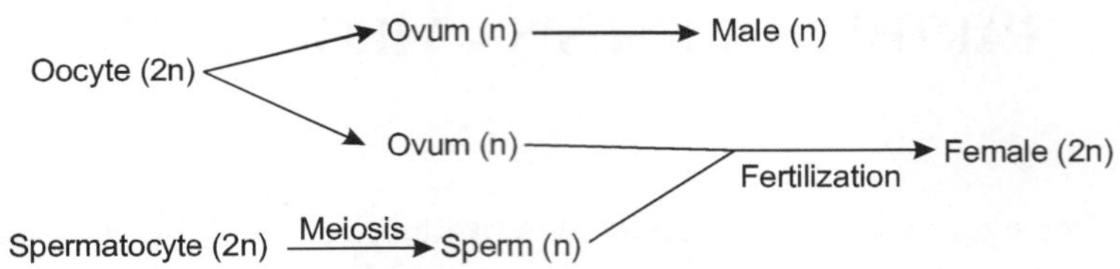

Thus haploid parthenogenesis also forms a method of sex determination in addition to reproduction. In this type of reproduction, the frequency of the developing male individuals depends on the production of number of unfertilized haploid eggs and sex ratio varies from species to species. This type of parthenogenesis is more common in insect groups like hymenopterans, homopterans, coleopterans and thysanurans as well as in arachnids and rotifers.

Diploid or Thelytokous Parthenogenesis (Thelytoky)

Here, the developing ovum retains the diploid number of chromosomes by the loss of reduction division or restores secondarily the diploid nature by fusing with one of the polar bodies. As a result, the individuals which arise from the unfertilized eggs are diploid. In Daphnia, weevils and long-horned grasshoppers, the normal reduction division is completely suppressed during oogenesis so that the egg has diploid number of chromosomes and develops into diploid individuals.

This type of parthenogenesis is called **ameiotic** or **apomeiotic parthenogenesis**. But in some parthenogenetic insects, the eggs are formed by the normal process of oogenesis with haploid number of chromosomes ('n' number of chromosomes). However, the eggs retain diploid number through a process called **diplosis** either through **restitution** or through **autofertilization**. In the process of restitution, cytokinesis fails to occur during the I maturation division of an oocyte which now produces two daughter cells, each with diploid number of chromosomes by II maturation division. Of these two cells, one becomes the egg and the another one develops into polar body (Figure 8.1a).

This diploid egg produces the diploid individual as in parthenogenetic lepidopterans. During **autofertilization**, any one of the polar bodies fuse with the ovum so that the original diploid number of chromosomes is restored (Figure 8.1.b). This type of mechanism is found in lepidopteran insects and in some hymenopteran wasps.

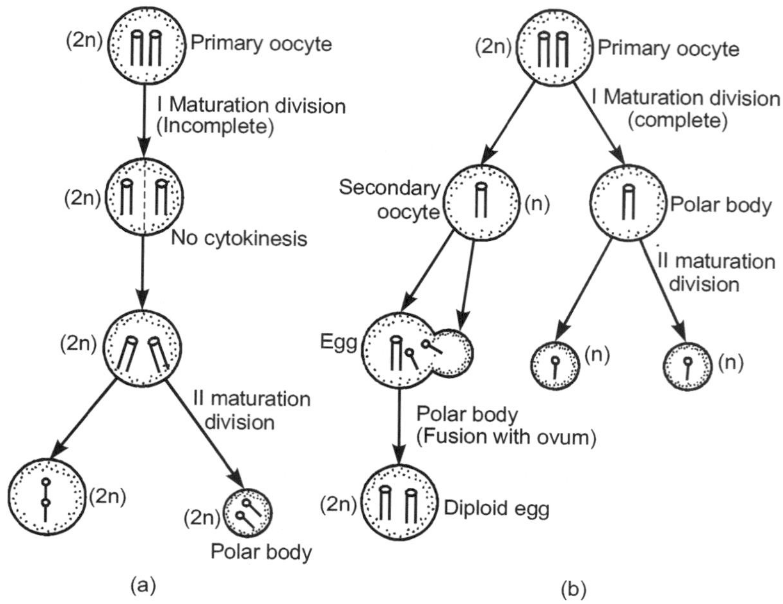

Figure 8.1 Meiotic thelytoky (a) Restitution process (b) Autofertilization

Special Types of Natural Parthenogenesis

In aphids, the males are not produced during summer season but females are produced parthenogenetically only for two generations. In these insects, no males are produced sexually but winter females develop sexually (Figure 8.2).

During winter and summer, the eggs with '2n' chromosomes develop only into females through diploid parthenogenesis. But this diploid female generation produces two types of eggs during spring. One type of eggs is larger in size with diploid number of chromosomes and the other type is smaller with 2n–X chromosomes in which one X chromosome is less. The larger eggs develop parthenogenetically into females which produce eggs containing 'n' number of chromosomes (haploid eggs). On the other hand, the smaller eggs develop into males which produce two types of sperms. One type of sperms contain 'n' number of chromosomes and the other type without 'n' number is abnormal and does not survive. The sperms with 'n' number of chromosomes fertilize the haploid eggs resulting in the formation of diploid zygotes which develop into females.

In some flies, larval **parthenogenesis** or **paedogenesis** is witnessed. The word "paedogenesis" literally denotes **reproduction by the young ones**. Here, the sex organs mature even at the larval stage and produce eggs which develop into daughter larvae for several generations. Later, these larvae undergo metamorphosis, developing into few mature adults. They produce new larvae which repeat the cycle once again. In some sexually reproducing animals like grasshoppers, cockroaches, silkworms, butterflies and fruit flies, an unfertilized egg may undergo normal development and this phenomenon can be considered as **accidental parthenogenesis**.

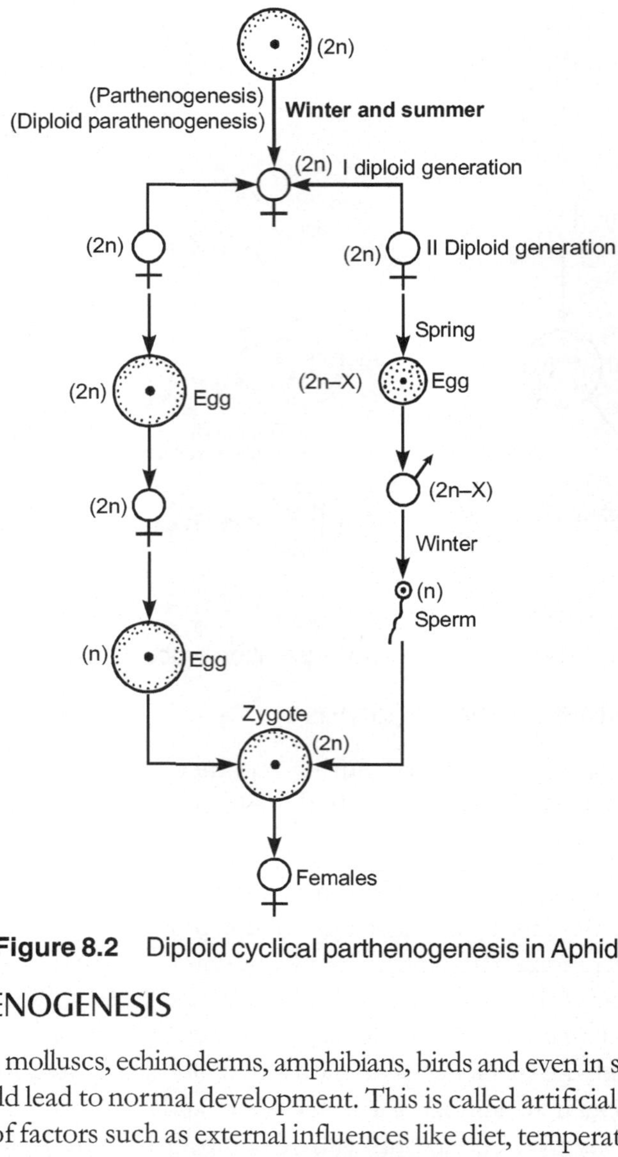

Figure 8.2 Diploid cyclical parthenogenesis in Aphids

ARTIFICIAL PARTHENOGENESIS

In animals like annelids, molluscs, echinoderms, amphibians, birds and even in some mammals, artificial activation of eggs would lead to normal development. This is called artificial parthenogenesis which depends on a number of factors such as external influences like diet, temperature, crowding, etc., and the nature of activators. However, the artificially induced parthenotes would rarely attain maturity with few exceptions. The development of unfertilized eggs can be induced by a number of stimuli. The chemical substances which induce the development of the egg include hypertonic or hypotonic sea water, chlorides of potassium, calcium, sodium, magnesium, etc., weak organic acids like butyric acid, lactic acid, fat solvents like toluene, ether, alcohol, etc. and also ammonia. Recently, calcium ions are found to be more effective in activating the development of eggs in molluscs, sea urchins, tunicates, amphibians and mammals. Warm water (32°C) or cold water (0–10°C), electric shock as well as ultraviolet light are also found to activate the eggs. Pricking of the eggs with a fine glass needle dipped in blood is found to be more effective in inducing normal whole development in frog. Rabbit's eggs are shown to be activated when they are kept in ordinary tissue culture medium. The unfertilized eggs of some species can be induced by making the entry of sperms of another species as in the case of fertilization of echinoderm eggs with annelidan sperms or of sea urchin's eggs with the sperms of starfish.

SIGNIFICANCE OF PARTHENOGENESIS

1. It is a simple, easy and well established method of reproduction and it also helps in sex determination.
2. It is found that the individuals which develop parthenogenetically multiply faster than those which arise through sexual reproduction.
3. In organisms, parthenogenesis results in polyploidy which prevents gamete formation leading to sterility. But these individuals reproduce successfully through parthenogenesis. Therefore, parthenogenesis is a device to escape from sterility.
4. It helps to transmit the mutated characters from one generation to another in which the mutated characters remain as such.
5. Parthenogenesis prevents variations in organisms so that they are more alike and resemble their parents, thus eliminating variety in populations.
6. It helps to restrict the harmful mutated combinations of genes through natural selection.
7. However, the parthenotes are not so successful in survival and do not produce new and advantageous combinations of genes in organisms, but are with restricted adaptability leading to either extinction or to reversal of sexual reproduction.

REVIEW QUESTIONS

1. What is parthenogenesis? Classify and characterize it with suitable examples.
2. Write an essay on natural parthenogenesis.
3. What do you mean by artificial parthenogenesis?
4. Explain cyclical parthenogenesis in detail.
5. Give brief notes on the following:
   i. Arrhenotoky
   ii. Thelytoky
   iii. Restitution
   iv. Autofertilization
   v. Significance of parthenogenesis

9

CLEAVAGE

The fertilized egg or the zygote undergoes a series of repeated mitotic cell divisions resulting in a large number of cells. This process of division of the unicellular fertilized egg by mitosis into a group of increased number of cells with decreased size is called **cleavage** or **segmentation**. The cells thus formed are called **blastomeres**. In this way, cleavage results in the formation of a ball of cells called **morula** which is in turn transformed into a single layered **blastula**. Formation of blastula is the final stage of cleavage. During cleavage, the embryo does not grow in size as the resulting cells undergo progressive decrease in size. In other words, the blastomeres in each division will possess only half of their original size. In general, the shape of the embryo does not change during cleavage, which depends on the cytoplasm rather than the nucleus. Though the nucleocytoplasmic ratio is very low in the beginning of cleavage, normal level as in the somatic cells has been maintained at the end. No new materials are forward in dividing cells during cleavage but the reserve food substances like yolk, glycogen, etc. are converted into active cytoplasm. The cytoplasm, in turn, synthesizes the nuclear substances such as DNA, RNA and nucleoproteins. RNA and nucleoproteins. In dividing egg cells, the organization of the ooplasm is maintained the same as in the fertilized egg but the ooplasmic substances are redistributed in such a way as to promote further development. The rate of cleavage varies in different species and is influenced by temperature, oxygen and carbon dioxide. The rate of respiration increases considerably during cleavage. The divided cells or the blastomeres become attached with each other at the time of cleavage by a number of means such as the egg membrane, hyaline layer of fertilized egg, sticky coating and so on.

MECHANISM OF CLEAVAGE

The cleaving eggs, especially those of invertebrates, have been frequently used to study the general mechanism of cell division. The series of events by which a blastomere is divided into two cells are normally initiated by nuclear division which is usually followed immediately by cytoplasmic division. During this process, the egg substances divide qualitatively and quantitatively into equal parts. The movement of the pronuclei and the arrangement of the amphiaster are very useful for this purpose. In some eggs, these mainly depend upon the general organization of the egg cytoplasm. According to **Swann** and **Mitchison** (1958), there are a number of theories proposed by different workers to explain the formation of the **cleavage furrow**. A few theories include **astral growth theory, spindle elongation theory, cortical gel contraction theory, expanding membrane theory, growth theory** and the **theory of amoeboid movement**. Most of these theories have been based on the study of cleavage of sea urchin's egg. However, none of these theories have explained the mechanism of cytokinesis in cleaving eggs. The recent investigation by **Lovtrup** (1974) suggests that the egg cortex along with the cytoplasmic organelles such as microfilaments, microtubules, Golgi complex and endoplasmic reticulum of the ooplasm play their significant roles in the formation of cleavage furrows in the cleaving eggs.

CLEAVAGE PLANES

A regular cleavage pattern occurs in the eggs due to the formation of the cleavage furrows which bisect the egg at different angles. The plane of the cleavage is determined by the position of the spindle fibres immediately after fertilization. In general, the plane of division lies always at right angles to the long axis of the spindle which as a rule is formed at the centre of the yolk-free cytoplasm near the animal pole. The following types of cleavage planes are met with in various kinds of eggs.

Meridional Plane of Cleavage

Here the cleavage furrow passes through the centre of the main axis of the egg. In other words, it bisects the animal–vegetal pole through the egg centre. In most eggs, the furrow develops first in the animal pole but there are instances where it may also develop from vegetal pole. The first cleavage furrow in the egg of chick and the first and second cleavage furrows in the eggs of Amphioxus and frog occur through the meridional plane.

Vertical Plane of Cleavage

Here the furrow passes in the same direction as in the meridional plane. ie., from animal to vegetal pole but it appears on the one side of the axis not passing through the median axis of the egg. For example, the third cleavage plane in chick's egg is vertical which is parallel to the first meridional one.

Equatorial Plane of Cleavage

Here the furrow bisects the egg at right angles to the median axis and half way between the animal pole and the vegetal pole. This condition, in a typical way, cannot be seen anywhere among the chordates but the nearest approach to this condition is met in the first cleavage plane of the eggs in higher mammals.

Latitudinal Plane of Cleavage

It is otherwise called as **transverse plane** or **horizontal plane** which is somewhat similar to the equatorial plane. But in this plane, the cleavage furrow passes through the egg cytoplasm on either side of the equatorial plane. This is seen in the third cleavage of the eggs in Amphioxus and frog.

CLEAVAGE TYPES

The period of cleavage is one in which the egg divides into a number of cells until the movement of cells bring about the other process namely gastrulation. Cleavage is a very well-coordinated process which depends on two major factors namely cytoplamic factors (which induce the formation of spindle) and the quantitative distribution of yolk in the ooplasm. Cleavage produces more cells that are smaller, in the less yolky animal region than in the more yolky vegetal end. When the stored yolk is very large, the most heavily laden regions may not divide at all during cleavage. In fact, in the eggs of reptiles and birds, a small superficial area in the animal pole where alone there is appreciable amount of cytoplasm and cleavage is confined only to this area. Therefore, the cleavage types can be classified as follows:

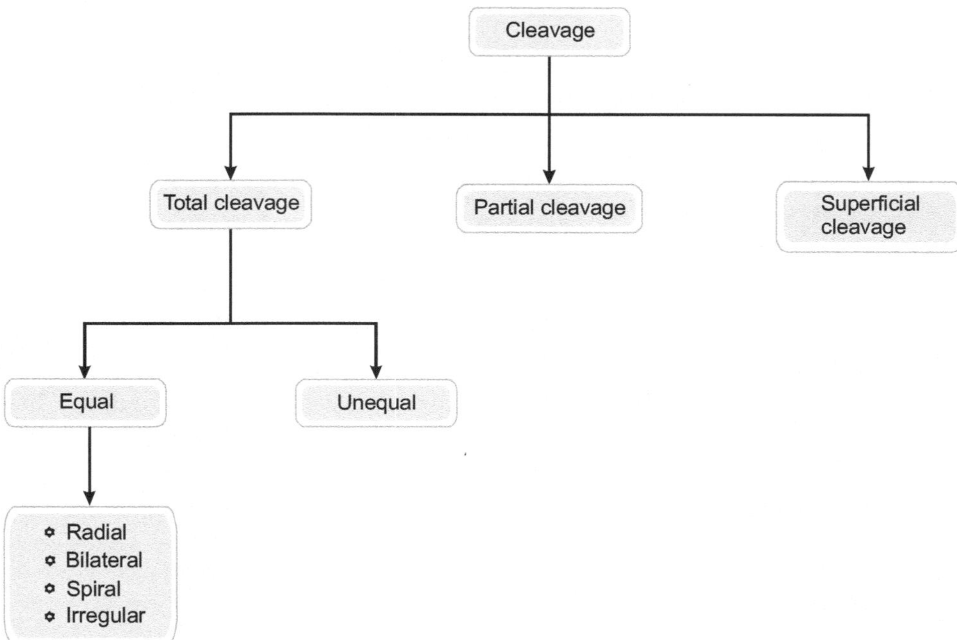

Total Cleavage

This type occurs in the smaller non-yolky eggs of most marine invertebrates. In the eggs of many species of echinoderms, molluscs, coelenterates, worms, etc. only very little yolk can be seen. The first cleavage in such eggs usually cut them into cells of equal size. In most cases, the equality between the cells is not very exact and it usually does not occur throughout many cleavage divisions. The division of these eggs result in characteristic patterns of large and small cells. Many eggs possess an organizational pattern which plays a more important role in controlling cleavage irrespective of the presence of yolk. The main patterns of total cleavage include the following types.

Radially symmetrical cleavage When successive cleavage planes cut straight through the egg at right angles to one another and the resulting blastomeres become symmetrically arranged around the polar axis, then it is called **radial cleavage**. This is best seen in echinoderms in which the first cleavage is horizontal and the second and third are vertical. But a more complicated pattern appears at the fourth division in which the cleavage plane is vertical in the animal half and horizontal in the vegetal half resulting in the formation of lowering of micromeres. In this pattern, each of the blastomeres of the upper tier lies over the corresponding cells of the lower tier (Figure 9.1).

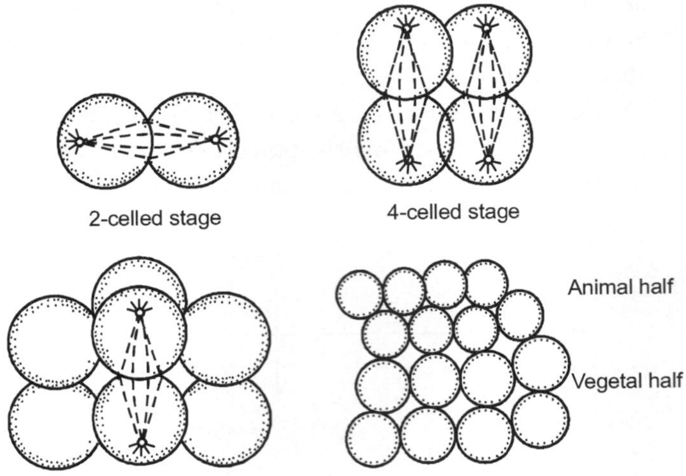

Figure 9.1 Radially symmetrical cleavage in echinoderm egg

Bilaterally symmetrical cleavage Here the spindles and planes remain bilaterally arranged with reference to a plane of symmetry which coincides with the median plane of the embryo. In a number of eggs, the first two cleavages are vertical, passing through the animal and vegetal axes and cut off four cells. These cells are not equal and are arranged with a bilateral symmetry (Figure 9.2). This is true, for instance, in some coelenterates, ascidians, amphioxus and in some vertebrates where the accumulation of yolk is not so large.

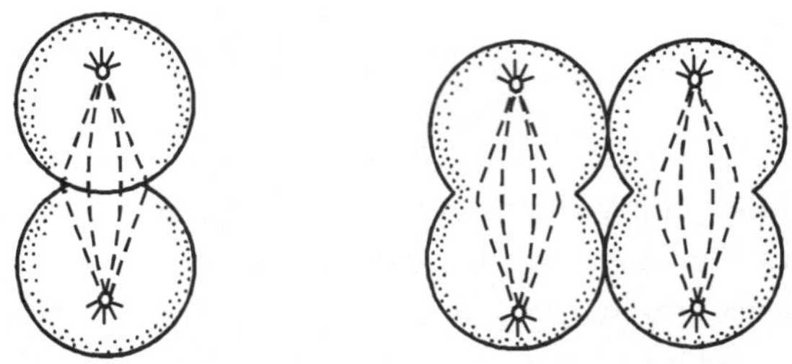

Figure 9.2 Bilaterally symmetrical cleavage in Ascidian egg

Spirally symmetrical cleavage When the axes of the early cleavage spindles are oblique to the polar axis, it is called **spiral cleavage**. In the eggs of a number of invertebrates (nemertines, annelids and molluscs), the first two cleavages are not quite vertical but slightly inclined so that when looked at from the animal pole, the first four cells are arranged in a single spiral twist. The third cleavage plane is more or less horizontal and cuts off a ring of micromeres at the animal end. These cells again do not lie immediately above the lower ring of four cells but are twisted (Figure 9.3). As this pattern is due to the formation of oblique spindles, it is otherwise called as **oblique cleavage**. If the turn of the spiral lies in the clockwise direction, it is **dextral cleavage** and if in counterclockwise direction, it is called **sinistral cleavage**.

Various cells formed after the first five or six cleavages regularly develop into definite parts of the embryo. Thus, this cleavage pattern is very intimately involved in the developmental process.

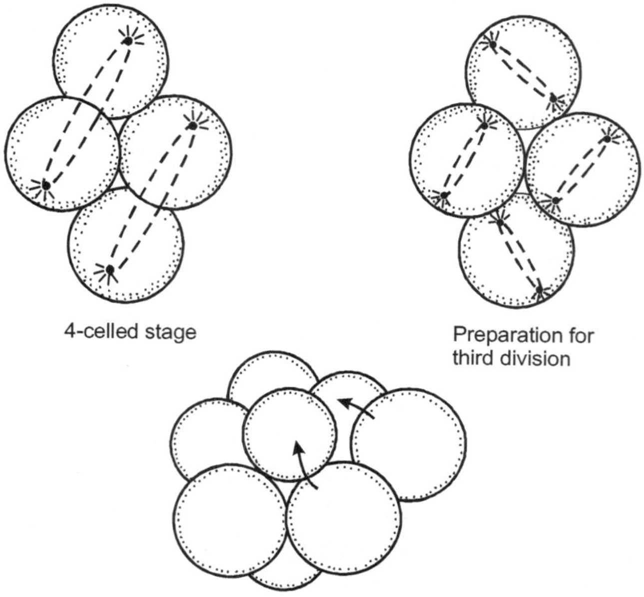

Figure 9.3 Spiral cleavage in molluscan egg

Irregularly symmetrical cleavage In some coelenterate eggs, the cleavage pattern is quite irregular and the blastomeres tend to fall apart. They are held only loosely together by the jelly in which they are loosely embedded. The pattern of cleavage found in insects can also be considered as irregular cleavage in which the division only involves the separation of daughter nuclei within the sub-divided mass of the yolky egg (Figure 9.4).

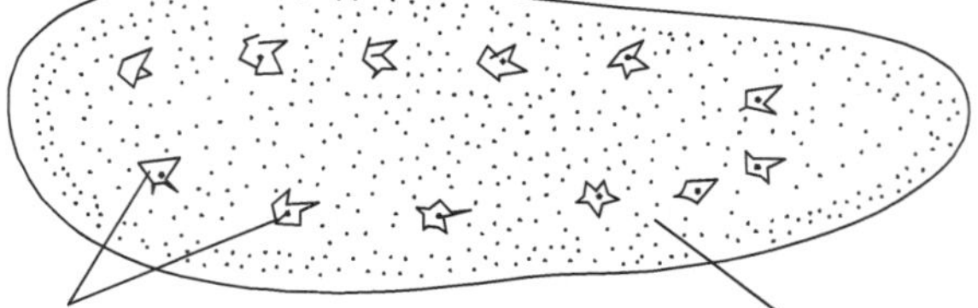

Figure 9.4 Separation of nuclei in the yolky egg of a beetle

Unequal, partial and superficial cleavages The most important examples of unequal cleavages are found in vertebrates. They exhibit a complete series of types ranging from those which show only a minor difference between the animal and vegetal cells to those with cleavage confined to a relatively tiny area at the animal pole. The amphibian (frogs and newts) eggs are best examples for slightly unequal cleavages, some of the cartilagenous fishes for the intermediate types (partial) and the teleosts, reptiles and birds for the classical superficial types. Roughly, the series, from the non-yolky, totally cleaving invertebrate eggs up to the very yolky superficially cleaving types, parallels the evolutionary pattern of the vertebrates. But this parellelism is entirely broken down in the case of mammals. The mammalian eggs need no large stores of yolk as the embryos mature in the uterus. In fact, these eggs are not provided with yolk, and so the cleavage is total and more or less equal but without well-defined symmetry.

CLEAVAGE IN MOSAIC AND REGULATIVE EGGS (DETERMINATE AND INDETERMINATE CLEAVAGE)

Depending upon the potency or the total range of developmental possibilities that an egg or blastomere possesses, cleavage has been divided into two types namely **determinate type** or **mosaic development** and **indeterminate type** or **regulative development**.

Determinate Type

In some invertebrates, especially in annelids and molluscs, the egg having undergone cleavage possesses a precise pattern and each part has its own characteristic position and fate. In Amphioxus, the early blastomeres are not totipotent and the role of the blastomeres has become fixed and determined from the very beginning. In 1888, **Wilhelm Roux** worked on the cleaving frog's egg. When one of the first blastomeres was killed, the other blastomere developed a half-embryo. The same results have also been noticed in the eggs of ascidians and in many of the spirally cleaving eggs. An isolated blastomere of the two-celled stage of a **dentalium egg** also develops into a half-larva while the destruction of even a part of a blastomere may result in a defective larva. From these experiments, embryologists began to speak of mosaic eggs which contain a mosaic of different cytoplasmic regions each of which would develop with some specific part of the embryo. The eggs of this type are called **mosaic eggs** and their development is called **mosaic development** or **determinate type**.

Indeterminate Type

Hans Driesch (1891) separated the first two blastomeres of an echinoderm egg and found that each gave rise to a complete embryo. He concluded that any part of the egg in early cleavage stages is capable of developing into a whole embryo. In vertebrates, the blastomeres possess more capabilities and their normal development exhibits a general relationship between the position and fate of blastomeres. In other words, all the cytoplasmic parts of these blastomeres in early stages are "**totipotent**" or "**equipotential**" and are capable of regulating so as to replace any part that has been damaged. For example, if the frog's egg is bisected through the grey crescent, then each half will develop into a full embryo. When a first cleavage blastomere of an amphibian or a mammal is isolated, it can alter its usual destiny and develop into a perfect embryo. Similarly, two frog's fertilized eggs develop into a single giant embryo when they are made to adhere to each other like a two-celled stage. Such eggs are described as **regulative eggs** and the process of this type of development is **regulative development** or **indeterminate type**. However, it is true that all types of eggs possess both characteristics with somewhat definite localization of parts having specific properties. Moreover, all the eggs have some capacity of adjusting themselves to injuries so that the differences are not so absolute.

CLEAVAGE IN EGGS WITH COMPLETE ABSENCE OF NUCLEI

Cleavage in the absence of nucleus was first observed by **Harvey** (1936) in sea urchin eggs. By strong centrifugation, he obtained non-nucleated halves of eggs which were subjected to parthenogenetic treatment. They underwent an irregular fragmentation of the cytoplasm and gave rise to morulae or blastulae which never formed cilia. More experiments have been conducted by **Lorch** (1953) who removed the nucleus in one of the blastomeres during early cleavage of sea urchin egg by micromanipulation. He found that the enucleated blastomere showed irregular and abortive cleavages only. Though these cells were in close contact with normal cells, they never take part in morphogenesis. In 1953, **Horstadius** tested the morphogenetic effects of enucleated cytoplasm of cells either from the animal pole or from the vegetal pole. From his experiments, he showed that the nucleated cytoplasm from the animal pole exerts a favourable effect on the morphogenesis of isolated vegetal halves while the enucleated cytoplasm of the vegetal half has no influence on the differentiation of the isolated animal half.

CHEMICAL TRANSFORMATIONS AT MOLECULAR LEVEL DURING CLEAVAGE

During cleavage, there is not much growth in the egg but many chemical transformations occur at the molecular level. Some of these chemical alterations are markedly intensified in the dividing eggs than in the unfertilized eggs. In these changes, the egg cytoplasm plays an important role in addition to the nuclear material. The nuclear material shows a steady increase at the expense of cytoplasm during the process of cleavage. The number of nuclei is doubled with every division of each blastomere so that there is an increase of nuclear substance, the DNA. Brachet (1950) has shown that the main source of DNA is the cytoplasm of the eggs in sea urchins. It is also found that some of the cytoplasmic DNA is traced in the mitochondria and some in the yolk platelets.

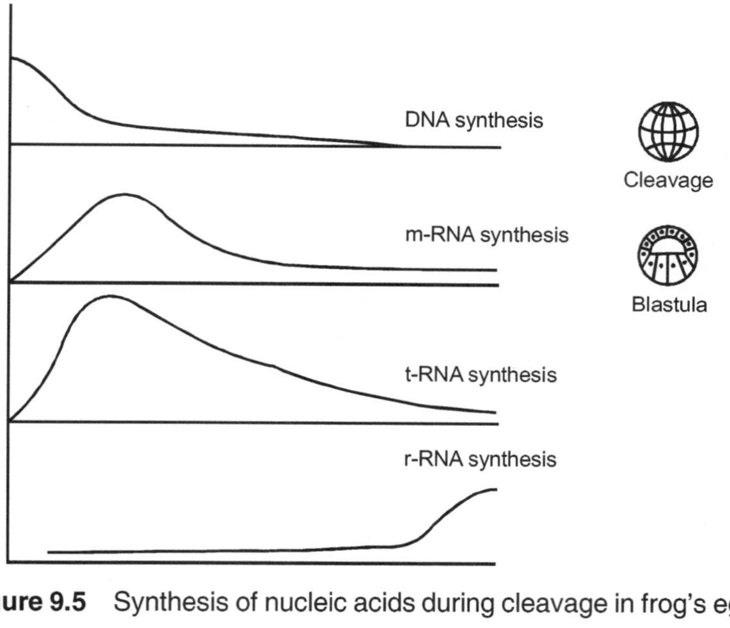

Figure 9.5 Synthesis of nucleic acids during cleavage in frog's egg

This cytoplasmic DNA is liberated and made available for building up of chromosomes. However, DNA is shown to be synthesised in the cleaving eggs from the low molecular weight precursors. The second important aspect at the time of cleavage is the synthesis of RNA. At cleavage or at least in the later stages of cleavage, mRNA and tRNA are synthesized. The synthesis of DNA and RNAs during cleavage are depicted in Figure 9.5. It is noticed that there is an enormous increase in protein synthesis which continues throughout the period of cleavage.

The importance of protein synthesis during cleavage is proved by many experiments. For example, when the cleaving eggs are treated with puromycin which inhibits protein synthesis, cleavage is immediately inhibited. The newly synthesized protein may be used for the formation of aster during cleavage, for the formation of new cell membrane or cortical cytoplasm and for the synthesis of an enzyme namely DNA Polymerase without which duplication of chromosomal DNA is not possible during cleavage.

TYPES OF EGGS AND CLEAVAGE

Based on the quantity and distribution of yolk, the eggs are highly variable and so also the cleavage patterns. The quantity of yolk may be lesser or greater, and may evenly or unevenly be distributed in the egg cytoplasm. Though the primary function of yolk is nutritional, yolk material determines the size and type of egg, the cleavage pattern and morphogenetic movement of cells during gastrulation. The eggs can be classified into the following types depending on the nature of the yolk present in them and are depicted in Figure 9.6.

Microlecithal or Homolecithal or Alecithal or Isolecithal or Oligolecithal Egg

Here the egg contains only very little yolk as in the eggs of Amphioxus and man.

Macrolecithal or Megalecithal Egg

Here, the egg contains too much yolk and this type can be divisible into two groups namely **centrolecithal** and **telolecithal eggs**. In centrolecithal egg, as in crustaceans, insects and arachnids, the yolk is found at the centre of the ooplasm. On the other hand, in telolecithal egg, the yolk is abundant and restricted to the posterior half of the egg or the vegetal hemisphere. In these eggs, the cytoplasm is restricted to a small region forming the animal hemisphere. Depending on the abundance of the yolk, the telolecithal eggs are of two types namely **moderately telolecithal** and **abundantly telolecithal eggs**. In moderately telolecithal eggs (e.g., frog's egg), the quantity of yolk is huge but is not too much while in abundantly telolecithal egg, the quantity of yolk is much more abundant as in the egg of chick.

Cleavage in different types of eggs

The eggs of various animals are found to undergo segmentation following certain basic principles and rules that control cleavage, and are given as laws **(Laws of cleavage)**.

I. *Sach's rule (1877)* According to this law, cells typically tend to divide into equal parts and each new plane of division tends to intersect the preceding one at right angles.

ii. *Hertwig's rule (1881)* This law states that the axis of the spindle typically lies in the longest axis of the protoplasmic mass and so the division cuts this axis transversely.

iii. *Balfour's rule (1885)* This law formulates that the rate of cleavage is inversely proportional to the amount of yolk present in the egg.

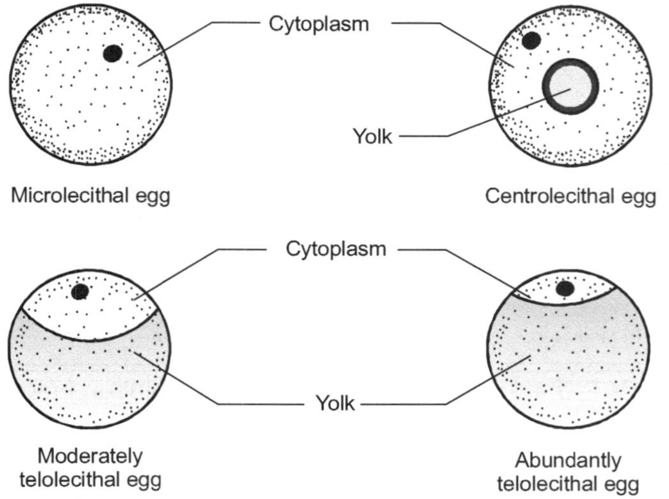

Figure 9.6 Types of eggs based on the nature of the yolk

Isolecithal Egg and Cleavage

In the egg of Amphioxus, the yolk material is very little and evenly distributed and so there is no obstacle for division. Thus the division is **total, complete, holoblastic** and **equal,** resulting in equal cells. The first cleavage is in the plane that runs through the animal pole and vegetal pole with the formation of two cells. The second cleavage is at right angles to the first and also meridional so that four blastomeres are formed. The third cleavage is latitudinal just above the equator and eight cells are formed, four upper and four lower. The fourth cleavage is longitudinal and sixteen cells are formed, eight upper and eight lower. Next two cleavages occur latitudinally and the embryo reaches the thirty-two-celled stage and then sixty-four-celled stage **(morula).** Now a cavity is developed at the centre of the cells forming the blastula called as the **coeloblastula.** This cavity is called as the **blastocoel** or **segmentation cavity** and the covering cells form the **blastoderm** (Figure 9.7). Thus the blastula is a creature with many cells forming the derm or skin which may be single- or many layered.

In the case of **man,** the first cleavage is holoblastic and the second one is also holoblastic, but after the first cleavage, the divisions are irregular and so odd number of cells (3, 5, 7 and so on) are formed. After a series of divisions, the structure becomes a morula, a solid mass of cells. Then the cells are arranged in such a way that they form a group called the **embryonic knob** which becomes surrounded by a covering layer namely **cyst.** Hence, the blastula is called as **cystoblastula** or **blastocyst** which has the blastocoel in between the embryonic knob and the cyst (Figure 9.8).

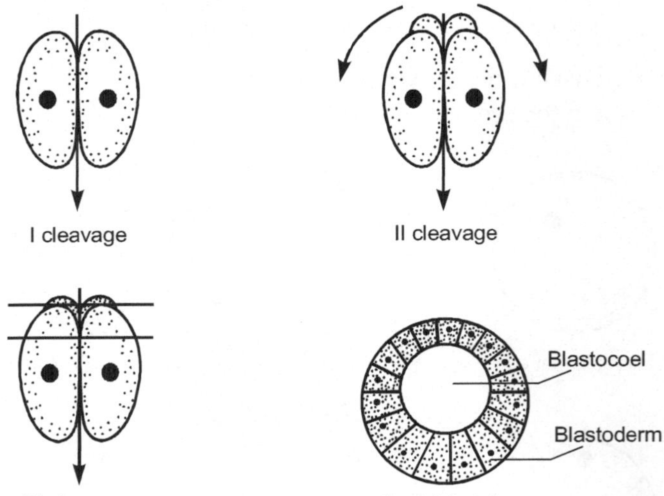

Figure 9.7 First three cleavages and coeloblastula in Amphioxus

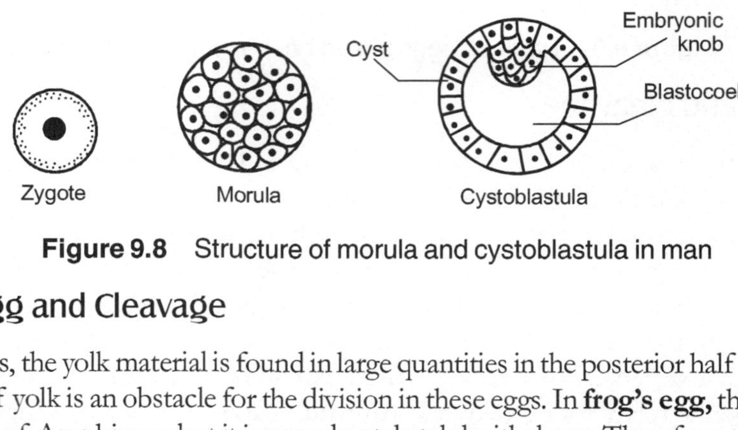

Figure 9.8 Structure of morula and cystoblastula in man

Telolecithal Egg and Cleavage

In telolecithal eggs, the yolk material is found in large quantities in the posterior half or vegetal pole and so the presence of yolk is an obstacle for the division in these eggs. In **frog's egg,** the cleavage patterns are similar to that of Amphioxus but it is a moderately telolecithal one. Therefore, the egg divides very vigorously in the animal pole whereas the division is very slow in the vegetal pole because of the yolk. In the resulting embryo, the micromeres are found in the animal pole while the macromeres are in the vegetal pole. Thus the cleavage is **holoblastic** but **unequal** and the blastula is **coeloblastula** in which the blastocoel is restricted only to the animal pole (Figure 9.9).

In the case of chick, the egg is abundantly telolecithal due to the presence of too much yolk. Therefore, the cleavage is restricted to only the animal pole, and the yolk region of the egg will never divide. Thus the cleavage is **incomplete** or **meroblastic** or **discoidal.** Here the first cleavage occurs longitudinally in the form of a small furrow in the middle of the blastodisc resulting in the formation of two cells. The second cleavage occurs at right angles to the first and four cells are formed over the egg. The third cleavage develops furrows whose direction is not regular, resulting in the eight-celled stage. By further cleavages, the number of cells at the centre increase. As a result, the inner cells are now separated from the outer cells and the embryo increases in diameter. At this stage, it is called as **blastoderm.**

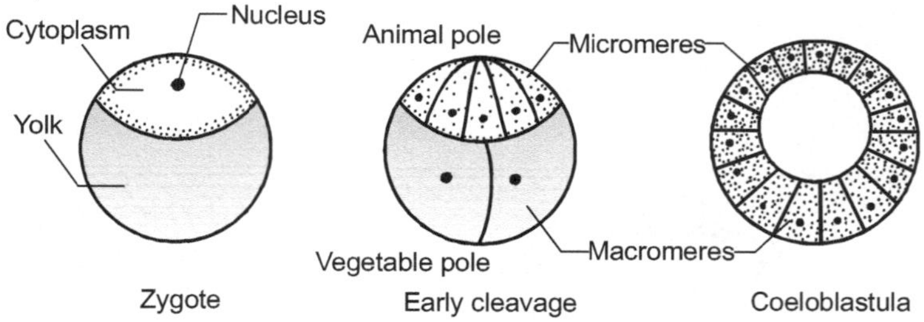

Figure 9.9 Early cleavage and coeloblastula in frog's egg

Cleavage also occurs parellel to the upper cells so that the blastomeres become separated off from the underlying yolk. Between this layer of cells and the yolk arises a space which represents the blastocoel. Now the structure is called blastula. Thus the result of cleavage is a disclike blastoderm called **blastodisc** and the blastula, a **coeloblastula** or **discoblastula.** In this way, the blastocoel is restricted only to the disclike region (Figure 9.10).

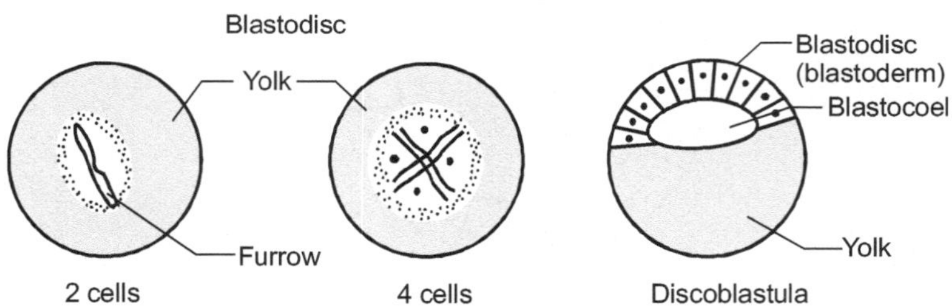

Figure 9.10 First two cleavages and discoblastula in chick.

In sponges, the cleavage of the egg exhibits the same condition as seen in the frog's egg. But the blastula develops flagella in the micromeres at the animal pole whereas the macromeres in the vegetal pole are non-flagellated. Therefore, the blastula is called as **amphiblastula** (Figure 9.11).

In crustaceans, arachnids and insects, the egg is **centrolecithal** in nature as the yolk is abundant at the centre of the egg. Here the egg divides only in the cytoplasmic region at the periphery. So cleavage is **meroblastic** because the division is restricted only to the periphery. Therefore, this type of cleavage is **superficial cleavage.** As the blastula has no blastocoel, it is also referred to as **solid blastula** or **steroblastula** (Figure 9.12).

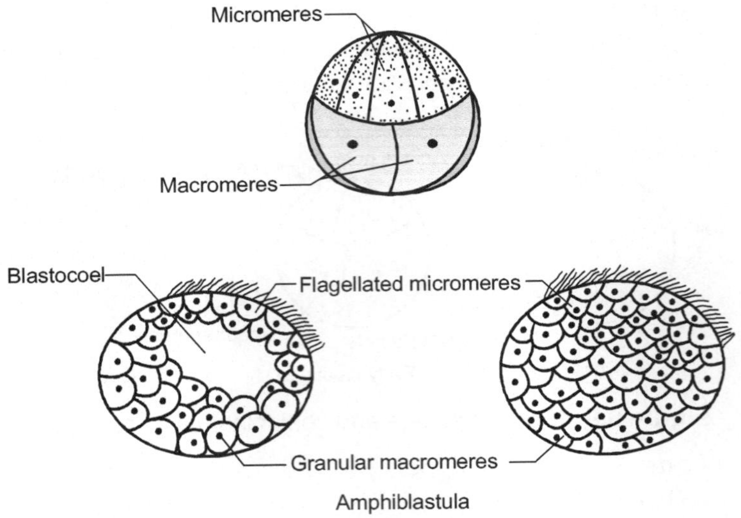

Figure 9.11 Early cleavage and amphiblastula in sponges

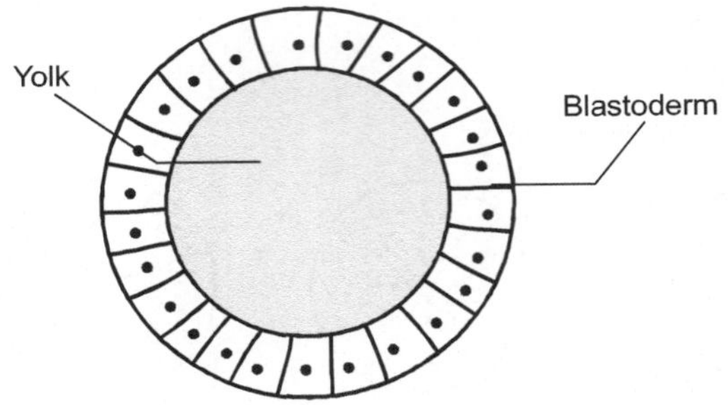

Figure 9.12 Structure of a steroblastula

SIGNIFICANCE OF CLEAVAGE, MORULATION AND BLASTULATION

The repeated division of the fertilized egg or the zygote results in the production of a ball of loosely arranged blastomeres. This structure superficially resembles a mulberry and so it is called as **morula** (L. *morum*-mulberry). As further divisions proceed, the blastomeres increase in number and arrange themselves to form a single layered or many layered blastoderm. As a result, a fluid-filled space called blastocoel is developed in the centre of the blastoderm. This spherical, hollow, fluid-filled embryonic stage with blastoderm is called **blastula**, the process of development of which is **blastulation.** It is believed that the hydrostatic pressure inside the blastocoel drives the blastomeres to the periphery and develops a hollow cavity filled up with fluid secreted by the dividing cells **(Hydrostatic pressure theory** of **Dan, 1960)**. It has also been shown that the development of blastoderm and blastocoel are due to the alterations in the surface tension of the membrane of the dividing cells and the adhesive nature of one cell with another **(Surface tension theory** of **Gustafson** and **Wolpert**, 1967). In short, it can be mentioned that the cleavage is the time dependent differentiation and the cell division establishes the fundamental conditions that are necessary for the next stage in embryonic development namely gastrulation. Cleavage and blastulation result in the seggregation of major presumptive and organ-forming areas of the future embryonic body into definite parts of the blastoderm. The blastocoel plays a key role during early embryonic development as it permits the migration and arrangement of the major presumptive organ-forming areas during gastrulation.

REVIEW QUESTIONS

1. What is cleavage? Explain the mechanism of cleavage.
2. Explain the various types of cleavage planes with suitable examples.
3. Classify and explain the cleavage types met within animal groups.
4. Write a note on metabolic transformations during the process of cleavage.
5. In what ways does cleavage help to classify the eggs?
6. Give a brief account of the rules or laws that govern the cleavage patterns.
7. Write an essay on cleavage patterns in different types of eggs.
8. What is the significance of cleavage?
9. Write brief notes on the following :
   i. Total and unequal cleavage
   ii. Blastulation
   iii. Determinate and indeterminate cleavage
   iv. Microlecithal and megalecithal eggs
   v. Morula
   vi. Coeloblastula
   vii. Cystoblastula
   viii. Discoblastula

10

FATE MAPS AND CELL LINEAGE—PRESUMPTIVE AREAS AND THEIR SIGNIFICANCE

Fate map is a chart which shows the fate of different parts of an early embryo, in particular a blastula. Without the knowledge of the position of the presumptive germinal areas in the blastula, the understanding of gastrulation is not possible and so the fate map is essential for the correct interpretation of gastrula in the developing eggs. In some animals, the cytoplasm of the fertilized eggs has natural colour differences in its various regions (natural markings). In others, the natural pigment differentiation of the egg cytoplasm does not occur and so some artificial methods are to be employed. Thus the fate maps can be constructed by natural and artificial markings.

NATURAL MARKINGS

A few eggs are provided with different colours in the cytoplasm so that some natural markings can be traced on the surface of these eggs. For example, the cytoplasm of the fertilized egg of an **Ascidian** (*Cynthia partita*) has natural colour differences in its various regions. The egg exhibits four different types of cytoplasmic areas due to the presence of different colours (Figure 10.1). The upper or the animal hemisphere has a clear transparent cytoplasm containing little yolk granules. The vegetative hemisphere is formed by dark grey yolky cytoplasm. Just below the equator, a pair of concentric areas are localized on opposite sides of the egg of which one area has a yellow crescent postero-ventrally and the other has a grey crescent antero-dorsally. During cleavage, these four kinds of cytoplasmic materials are found to be distributed to different blastomeres and the developmental fates of the above regions have been worked out by **Conklin** (1931). The blastomeres with clear cytoplasm give rise to the epidermal ectoderm, the yellow crescent to the mesoderm, the grey crescent to the neurectoderm and notochord and the dark grey yolky plasm to the endoderm. These presumptive areas actually possess biochemical differences for the parts to be produced and this can be proved by centrifuging the eggs prior to cleavage. Centrifugation causes shuffling of the presumptive areas so that they come to occupy abnormal positions. As a result, an embryo develops with irregular arrangements of its figures and rudiments of organs. Here each part of the embryo develops in the region where its cytoplasmic precursor comes to lie as a result of centrifugation.

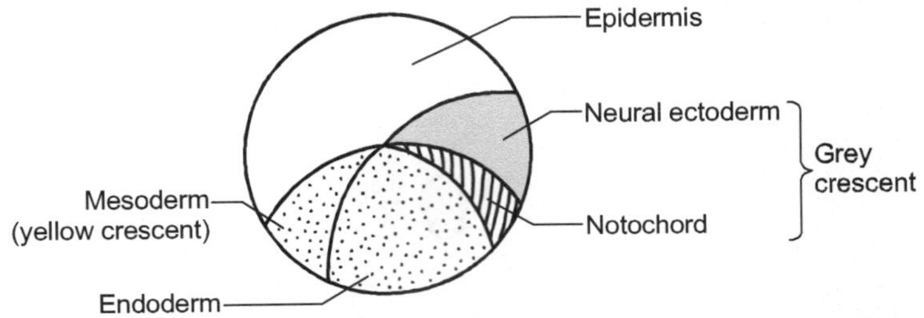

Figure 10.1 Fate map of a fertilized egg of an ascidian

The fertilized egg of **Dentalium** (an annelid) possesses three different cytoplasmic regions namely clear cytoplasm in both the animal and vegetal poles and granular cytoplasm in between the two poles. As the cleavage starts, the clear cytoplasm in the vegetal pole is pushed out as a **polar lobe**. When the egg divides into two blastomeres namely AB and CD, the polar lobe is absorbed by the cell CD which has all the three types of cytoplasm. But the cell AB contains only the clear cytoplasm of the animal pole and granular cytoplasm (Figure 10.2). When the two blastomeres are isolated and allowed to develop, the blastomere D develops into a complete normal larva and the blastomere B produces a larva without mesoderm. This is because of the absence of clear cytoplasm of the vegetal pole in the blastomere B. Again in the four-celled stage, the three blastomeres A, B and C have only two types of cytoplasm whereas the blastomere D contains all the three types of cytoplasm. When these four cells are separated and allowed to develop, then the blastomere D alone develops into a normal larva and the others develop into defective larvae without mesoderm. The removal of the polar lobe from the cell D makes it develop into a defective larva (Figure 10.2).

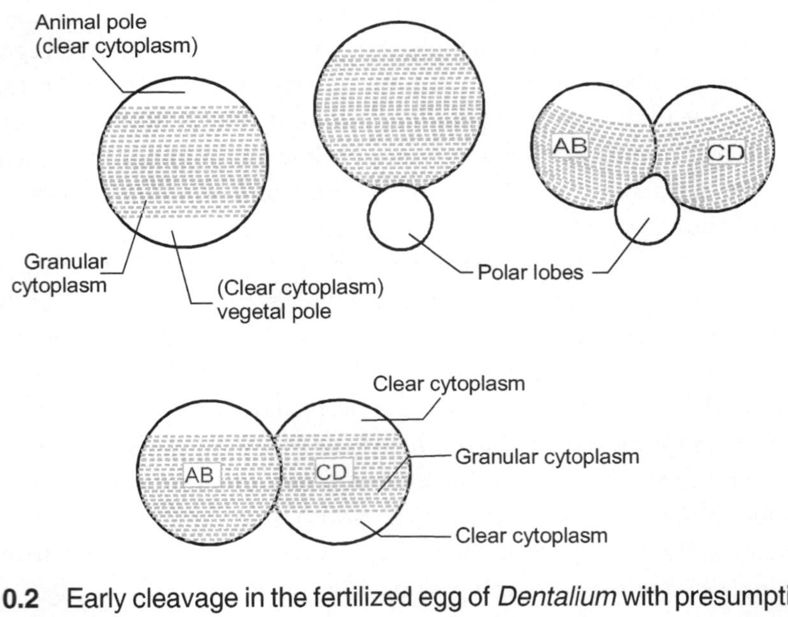

Figure 10.2 Early cleavage in the fertilized egg of *Dentalium* with presumptive areas

From the above experiments, it is clear that a particular area of the embryo develops into a specific organ and so the cells in that area are called '**presumptive organ forming areas**'. For example, the cells which develop into endoderm are said to be presumptive endoderm.

ARTIFICIAL MARKINGS

If natural colouration of the egg cytoplasm does not exist or if the pigment differentiation is not providing details for the construction of the fate maps, artificial marking of blastomeres by various methods have been used for the construction of the fate maps. Embryologists mark the blastomeres to study their fate by using vital stains, carbon particles and radioactive substances.

Vital Stain Method

This method was devised by **Vogt** (1925) and vital stains like Janus green, Nile blue sulphate, Bismarck brown, Neutral red, etc. are used to construct the fate maps. In this method, a piece of agar is soaked in a particular dye and placed on the surface of the embryo in the required place. At once, the dye diffuses into the blastomeres on which the agar is placed so that the cells are stained. As the descendants of the marked cells also get stained, the position of the stained cells shows the fate of the stained blastomere in the differentiated embryo. For example, if the stained cells are incorporated into the notochord, the marked blastomeres are destined to develop into the notochord. Several such stain marks can be used on the surface of the same embryo using several coloured dyes so that the fate map of an embryo can be prepared. Though this method was first employed to the amphibian embryos, it is now used for almost all embryos.

Carbon Particle Method

This method devised by **Spratt** (1946) uses carbon particles to mark the blastomeres. When the carbon particles are applied to the required area of the embryo, they stick on to the surface of the blastomeres. Therefore, it is possible to follow the movements of the marked cells in the embryo to construct the fate map.

Radioactive Method

In recent years, the fate maps of a number of eggs are constructed to study the fate of the blastomeres of various regions by labelling with radioactive substance like C^{14}, P^{32}, S^{35}, etc.

FATE MAPS OF CHORDATE EGGS

In **Amphioxus**, the substances of the egg cytoplasm get localized in definite areas after maturation. For example, the yolk-free superficial cytoplasm condenses in the form of a crescent at the posterior pole. Other regions of the cytoplasm namely the future ectodermal and endodermal areas also get separated. Experiments have proved that this determination of egg substance to form specific areas is almost final. These areas are the **organ-specific areas**. Therefore, the egg is a **mosaic egg** and the cleavage pattern is of **determinate type**. As a rule, the same organ-specific areas can be traced in the fully formed blastula as in Figure 10.3. Various organ-specific areas have been recognized in the fertilized egg of **Amphioxus** by **Conklin** (1932) and **Tungwu Tung** (1962). The micromeres in the animal pole with clear cytoplasm develop into skin epidermis and are called **presumptive epidermal ectoderm**. All the macromeres in the vegetal pole with granular yolky cytoplasm develop into endoderm and hence are called **presumptive endoderm**. The crescent-like area of one side of the blastula just below the equator develops into mesoderm (**presumptive mesoderm**). Opposite to mesoderm cells is another crescent-like area which develops into the notochord. A crescent of cells in between the notochordal cells and epidermal ectoderm develop into the nervous system (**Neurectoderm**). In this way, various substances of the ooplasm at the time of maturation in the egg of **Amphioxus** undergo no appreciable displacement during cleavage.

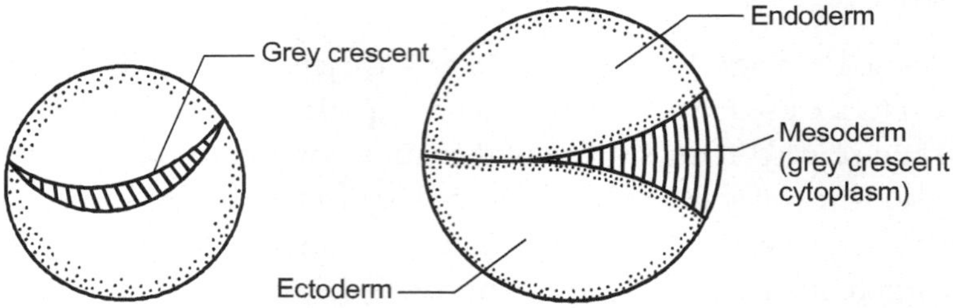

Figure 10.3 Fertilized egg of Amphioxus showing different organ specific areas.

In **frog**, the presumptive organ-forming areas in the blastula stage have been studied by **Vogt** (1925) using vital staining technique. In the egg of frog, the entry of sperm usually occurs near the equator. Opposite to the point of entry of the sperm, a crescent-like structure called **grey crescent** appears and causes a bilateral symmetry to the egg (Fig.10.4a). The significance of grey crescent may be shown by isolation of cells at the two-celled stage. If the two cells are separated in such a way that grey crescent passes into each of the cells, then each cell will develop into a complete embryo. If one of the cells contains the grey crescent, then the cell with grey crescent gives rise to a normal embryo. But the other cell without grey crescent when separated, fails to develop. It develops only a 'sac' of ectoderm around the endoderm. This clearly evidences the importance of grey crescent in normal development. Here the organ-forming areas are not differentiated even at this stage and the differentiation is delayed to the end of cleavage. Thus the fate of the blastomeres is not yet established as the frog's egg is a **regulative egg** which exhibits **indeterminate type of cleavage**. In other words, the organ-forming substances become established only after cleavage and so the organ-forming areas can be well-marked only towards the end of cleavage. These areas are known as **organ-presumptive areas** because the fate of these areas is changeable and are transversely arranged. Later on, the cells of different areas have become rearranged to occupy axial positions during gastrulation. Roughly, half of the blastula is marked to be the future ectoderm. The endoderm develops from the macromeres of the vegetal pole. Presumptive notochord lies just anterior to the endoderm on the dorsal lip. In between the endodermal and notochordal areas is the prechordal area. On either side of the notochordal materials lies the presumptive mesodermal cells. Above the notochordal area lie the neurectoderm and the epidermal ectoderm. When the blastula is seen from the front, these organ-presumptive areas are seen transversely as in the Figure 10.4b.

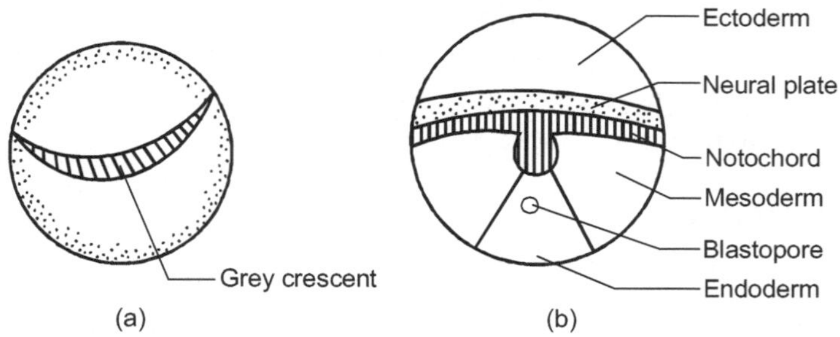

Figure 10.4 Frog's egg showing grey crescent (a) and organ presumptive areas (b) in the blastula

In chick, the egg is **abundantly telolecithal** and so cleavage is **meroblastic** affecting only the blastodisc. As a result of cleavage, the blastomeres become separated from the underlying yolk. The divisions occur only in the blastoderm so that a many layered structure is formed and up to this point, the future of the cells has not been fixed. By this time, the embryo is ready for gastrulation with the onset of differentiation so that the organ-presumptive areas can be marked. The blastomere in the **discoblastula** consists of two areas. A central area above the blastocoel is transluscent and is called **area pellucida**. The outer opaque area above the yolk is the **area opaca** which will not take part in the formation of organs. It is the **presumptive extra-embryonic ectoderm** which develops extra- embryonic membranes and blood vessels. Therefore the fate map of various areas are restricted to the area pellucida (Figure 10.5). Here, the blastoderm is a bilaminar structure namely **epiblast** and **hypoblast** and the fate maps have to be constructed for these layers. Various methods have been followed to trace the presumptive areas such as **vital staining method** (**Wetzel**, 1929 and **Pasteels,** 1940), **carbon particles method** (**Spratt,** 1946) and **radioactive method** (**Rosenquist**, 1966 and **Nicolet**, 1970). A small area is occupied by the **notochordal cells**, more or less in the centre of the area pellucida. Posterior to this area is an oval **presumptive endoderm** in the medium plane. On either side of the presumptive notochordal cells and endoderm lies the **lateral plate mesoderm** (**presumptive mesoderm**). The **presumptive somatic plate mesoderm** lies postero-lateral to the notochordal cells. The anterior part of the area pellucida is occupied by **presumptive ectoderm**. The **presumptive neural plate cells** are marked in the form of a semi-circular area anterior to the notochordal cells.

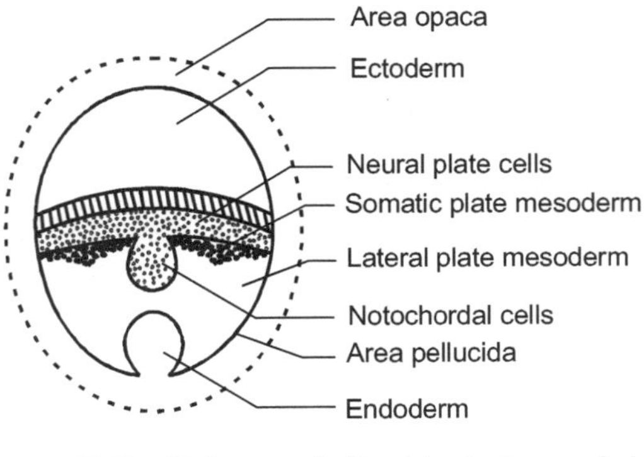

Figure 10.5 Fate map in the blastoderm of chick

In **mammalian egg**, the cleavage is **holoblastic** but the cells arrange to form a plate or a disc as in the egg of chick. Here also, the blastoderm is divisible into an **epiblast** and a **hypoblast**. The cells of the epiblast give rise to different presumptive areas as in chick and the hypoblast gives rise to endoderm. Therefore, the mammalian fate map is more or less similar to that of birds.

CELL LINEAGE OR CYTOGENY

During cleavage, the egg undergoes division for further development in which a particular blastomere or particular group of blastomeres give rise to the same type of derivatives in the adult. The fate or the end result of each blastomere can be studied by various methods. The observations of the developmental history of a cell in a cleaving egg is called **cell lineage**. In other words, it is the study to trace the fate of particular blastomeres and it can be achieved by **artificial marking** of blastomeres using **vital stains**, or by observation of cytoplasmic variations in different parts of the egg **(natural markings)** or by **naming of the blastomeres** with the alphabet. The study of cell lineage is significant in that it reveals the phylogenetic relationship between groups of animals which have a common body plan as in the case of flatworms, annelids and molluscs. It indicates that the differentiation of organogenesis is due to a number of divisions in each blastomere. The study clearly shows that the morphogenetic substances are predetermined in the egg cytoplasm and are separated into different cell lines. Wilson (1892) made his classical study on cell lineage in **Nereis** and the following account explains the cell lineage study by naming the blastomeres with alphabetic letters.

Naming of the blastomeres with alphabets is possible in the eggs which undergo **spiral cleavage** as in the eggs of polyclads, nemertines, annelids, molluscs and ascidians. In spiral cleavage, the spindle axes are oriented obliquely so that the blastomeres are arranged in a spiral manner. The turn of the spiral may be in a clockwise **(dextral)** or anticlockwise **(sinistral)** direction. In spiral cleavage, the egg (telolecithal egg) undergoes **holoblastic** and **unequal cleavage**. The first two cleavages are meridional and at right angles to each other. The resulting four blastomeres are named as A, B, C and D, usually in a clockwise direction (Figure 10.6). The third cleavage is latitudinal resulting in four micromeres in the animal pole and four macromeres in the vegetal pole. The micromeres are named as 1a, 1b, 1c and 1d and the macromeres as 1A, 1B, 1C and 1D in which the micromeres constitute the **first quartet of micromeres** (Figure 10.6). Then these macromeres and micromeres (first quartet) divide to produce 16 cells. That is, the four micromeres divide into eight micromeres and the four macromeres into four macromeres and four micromeres and are given names as shown in Table 10.1 and Figure 10.6. The micromeres 2a, 2b, 2c, 2d form the **second quartet** of micromeres. These cells divide into 32 cells where all the micromeres give rise to micromeres only and are given names as in the Table 10.2.

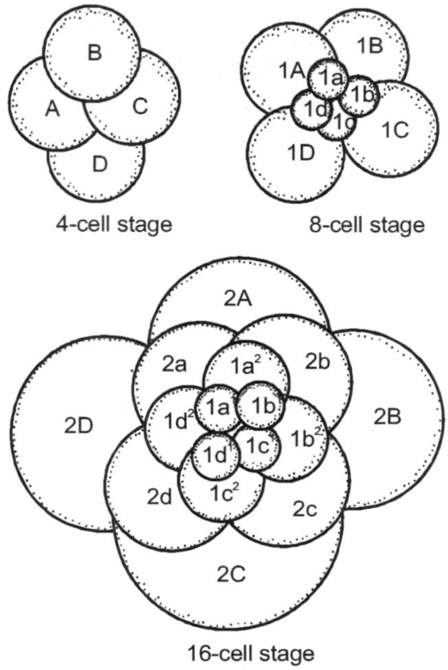

Figure 10.6 Cell lineage in the egg of polyclads at 4,8 and 16-celled stages

Table 10.1 Naming of the cells at 16-celled stage

Name of the parent cell		Name of Micromeres	Name of Macromeres
1a	First Quartet	$1a^1$ and $1a^2$	
1b		$1b^1$ and $1b^2$	
1c		$1c^1$ and $1c^2$	
1d		$1d^1$ and $1d^2$	
1A	Second Quartet	2a	2A
1B		2b	2B
1C		2c	2C
1D		2d	2D

Table 10.2 Naming of the micromeres at 32-celled stage

Name of the parent cell	Name of the divided cells	
$1a^1$	$1a^{11}$ and $1a^{12}$	Descendents of first quartet
$1b^1$	$1b^{11}$ and $1b^{12}$	
$1c^1$	$1c^{11}$ and $1c^{12}$	
$1d^1$	$1d^{11}$ and $1d^{12}$	
$1a^2$	$1a^{21}$ and $1a^{22}$	
$1b^2$	$1b^{21}$ and $1b^{22}$	
$1c^2$	$1c^{21}$ and $1c^{22}$	
$1d^2$	$1d^{21}$ and $1d^{22}$	
2a	$2a^1$ and $2a^2$	Descendants of second quartet
2b	$2b^1$ and $2b^2$	
2c	$2c^1$ and $2c_2$	
2d	$2d^1$ and $2d^2$	

The four macromeres namely 2A, 2B, 2C, and 2D divide into four macromeres namely 3A, 3B, 3C and 3D and the four micromeres into 3a, 3b, 3c and 3d. These micromeres form the **third quartet** of micromeres. By this time, the different germ layers are determined. As the first three quartets of micromeres and their derivatives give rise to the ectoderm, they are called **ectomeres**. They come to surround the entire embryo leaving an opening called **blastopore**. The four macromeres, 3A, 3B, 3C and 3D subsequently give rise to the **fourth quartet** of micromeres namely 4a, 4b, 4c and 4d and four macromeres give rise to the cells 4A, 4B, 4C and 4D. With the formation of the fourth quartet of micromeres, the egg has become a **blastula** and also the **germ layers** have become fixed. This can be illustrated as in Figure 10.7. Of these cells, 4a, 4b, 4c, 4A, 4B, 4C and 4D become divided into smaller cells forming the yolk which serves as the food. The cell 4d is much larger in size and it gives rise to the entire mesoderm and endoderm. Therefore it is known as **mesentoblast**. The cell $4d^1$ gives rise to the endoderm of the intestine whereas the cell $4d^2$ divides into $4d^{21}$ and $4d^{22}$, the cell $4d^{21}$ into $4d^{211}$ and $4d^{212}$, and the cell $4d^{22}$ into $4d^{221}$ and $4d^{222}$. The cells $4d^{211}$ and $4d^{221}$ give rise the **pharyngeal endoderm** and $4d^{212}$ and $4d^{222}$ give rise to **mesoderm** which develops into muscles, mesenchyme. reproductive system, etc. Figure 10.8 explains the derivatives of the cell A forming **quartet** A.

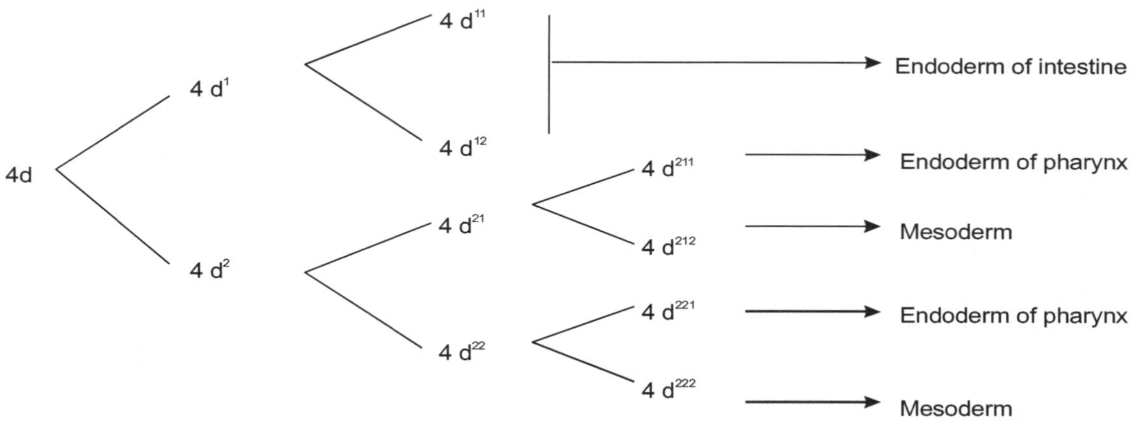

Figure 10.7 Derivatives of the cell 4d (mesentoblast)

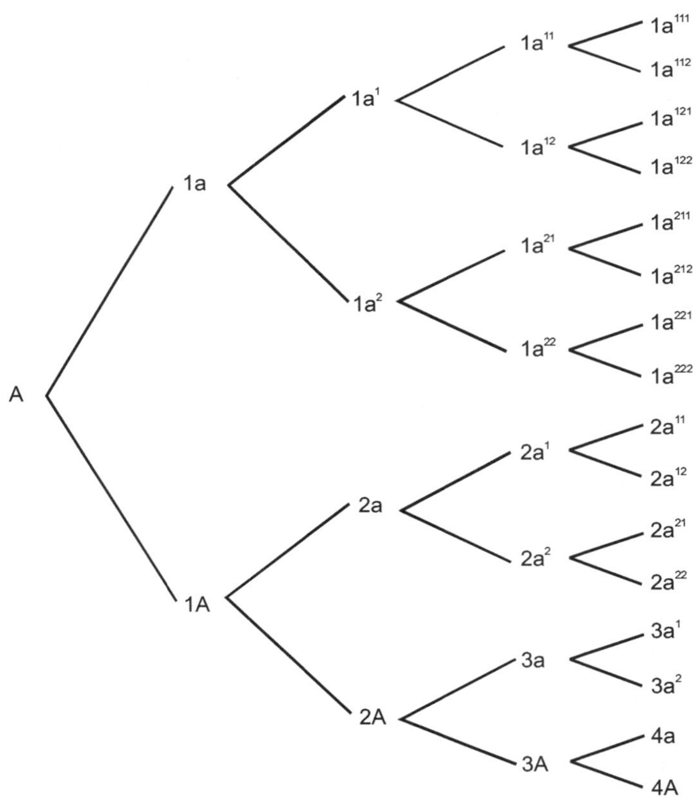

Figure 10.8 Derivatives of the cell A (Quartet A)

REVIEW QUESTIONS

1. Define fate map. Give a brief account of construction of fate maps with examples.
2. How could natural markings in eggs help to know the fate of the cells in the embryo?
3. Enumerate various artificial methods in the construction of fate maps.
4. Give an account of fate maps in different chordate representatives (Amphioxus, frog, chick, a mammal).
5. What is cell lineage? Describe its significance.
6. Explain cell lineage study with suitable examples.
7. Write notes on:
    i. Polar lobe
    ii. Presumptive organ-forming areas
    iii. First quartet
    iv. Second quartet
    v. Mesentoblast

11

MORPHOGENETIC MOVEMENTS AND GASTRULATION

Morphogenesis can be defined as the progressive formation of various tissues, organs and organ systems with changes in shape and organization during the development of an organism. It mainly includes the cell division resulting in multiplication and growth involving specific morphogenetic processes such as cell migration, cell aggregation, fusion, splitting, folding and local thickenings. These processes are relatively simple, occurring in an orderly and sequential manner. During the early development of an embryo, the initial major morphogenetic process is **gastrulation** by which the single-layered **blastula** is converted into a two-layered and then three-layered embryo called **gastrula** through the movement of cells and tissues. The three layers namely **ectoderm**, **endoderm** and **mesoderm** later differentiate morphologically and histologically to form definite new organs with characteristic form and shape.

The movement of cells results in many changes in the structure of the embryo due to the rearrangement of blastomeres. Characteristic cell movements are evident even at the stage of blastula. But in the gastula, the cell movements are very rapid. Cellular movements also occur in the later development of the embryo and even in adults. These movements are due to the integrated migration of cells and are irreversible in embryos and reversible in adults. As these cellular movements bring about new forms with new shapes in the embryo, they are referred to as **morphogenetic movements**.

TYPES OF MORPHOGENETIC MOVEMENTS

During development, the blastomeres of the embryo undergo one or more specific movements during the process of gastrulation in most animals. These morphogenetic movements can be studied under the following headings:

Epiboly or Evagination

It is the movement of presumptive neurectodermal cells which become rearranged as the inner layer after multiplication and flattening. It apparently begins with an increase in adhesiveness of cell surfaces as well as with an activation of locomotory mechanism. Here, all blastodermal cells move over each other to rearrange in fewer layers. The blastoderm cells are found to have an intrinsic capacity for spreading by using the periblast as the substratum. That is, the expanding periblast substratum is essential for the epibolic movement of blastoderm cells.

Emboly

It is otherwise known as **token invagination** in which the presumptive dermal, endodermal and chordamesodermal cells move inward by the inherent property present within a group of cells or due to the movement of other cell groups. This is accomplished by the following methods:

i. ***Invagination*** Here, a region of blastoderm is pushed into the blastocoel as the inner layer. It is the infolding or inpushing of blastodermal cells which may either be a process of passive infolding or active infolding. The first sign of invagination is the deformation of certain vegetal cells which become elongated and bottle-shaped in the perspective blastoporal region. These cells progressively move into the interior with their outer surfaces remaining in contact at the egg surface. The cavity due to the invagination of cells is the **archenteron** which opens to outside by the **blastopore**. The rims of the blastopore are called **blastoporal lips** (dorsal, ventral and lateral lips). Many factors such as increase in number of cells, and growth, change in shape, cellular lyophilic and lyophobic colloids, hydrocoel and external medium, differential cohesion of cells, alkalinity of the blastocoel, etc. are believed to be responsible for the inpushing of the blastodermal cells.

ii. ***Involution*** In this process, the blastodermal cells roll into the blastocoel, thus forming the inner layer. It is nothing but "**rolling in**" or "**turning in**" of cells which move and arrange along the inner margin of the blastopore on the inner side of the embryo. For example, in the gastrulation of frog's egg, the cells at the rim of the blastopore on the dorsal lip proliferate and get rearranged in transverse rows.

iii. ***Convergence*** This process involves active migration of cells from one region to another as seen in the movement of the chordamesodermal cells (blastodermal cells) from the outer surface of blastula to the outside margins of the dorsal blastoporal lips.

iv. ***Divergence*** It is the migration and spreading of cells as in the gastrulation of frog's egg where the lateral plate and ventral mesodermal cells enter the dorsal blastopore and start spreading out.

v. ***Infiltration or polyinvagination*** By this method, the blastodermal cells get detached and separated, forming an inner endodermal layer as noticed in the gastrulation of chick's egg.

vi. ***Delamination*** In this morphogenetic movement, a group of cells as a mass separate from other cell groups of the blastoderm as in the case of chick's egg.

GASTRULATION IN DIFFERENT GROUPS OF ANIMALS

Gastrulation is a process by which the single-layered embryo, the blastula, becomes changed into a double-layered embryo called the **gastrula** enclosing a cavity, the **gastrocoel** or **archenteron**, which opens out by an aperture known as **blastopore**. The outer layer of the gastrula is called as **ectoderm** or **epiblast** and the inner layer is called as the **endoderm** or **hypoblast**. Gastrulation is an active process in which there is realignment of different organ-forming areas into definite positions where they develop into different systems.

GASTRULATION IN AMPHIOXUS

In Amphioxus, gastrulation takes place by **invagination** in which a region of the blastoderm is pushed into the blastocoel and forms the inner layer.

Here, gastrulation starts by the flattening of macromeres (larger cells) in the vegetal hemisphere. These cells divide less frequently and become more columnar whereas the other cells (micromeses) divide more rapidly and become more cuboidal or spherical. This change in the shape and rate of cell division seem to be the principle cause of invagination, although it is shown to be due to other factors like exosmosis. Now the flattened larger cells become pushed into the blastocoel, thus forming the inner layer, the **hypoblast**. This inpushing continues towards the outer layer, the **epiblast**. At this stage, the embryo attains a cup-like structure where there is still existence of blastocoel as a small space. By this time, the inner layer begins to have a space called **gastrocoel** or **archenteron**. Finally, the inner layer touches the outer layer and the embryo becomes a double-layered **gastrula.** The blastocoel is completely lost and the only remaining space is the gastroceol which opens to outside by the aperture, the **blastopore.** By further development, the gastrula becomes elongated antero-posteriorly. The archenteron enlarges and the blastopore becomes very small. Now the cells actively migrate from the exterior over the rim of the blastopore to the interior by the process called **involution**. These cells are mainly notochordal and mesodermal cells. The entire process of gastrulation is depicted in Figure 11.1.

Thus, in Amphioxus, gastrulation involves two major processes namely **invagination** and **involution.** The roof of the archenteron is formed by **notochordal cells** and a narrow plate of **mesodermal cells** are seen on either side of these cells. The rest of the archenteron is made up of **endoderm.** The outer layer (epiblast) of the gastrula gives rise to the nervous system and the skin. From the hypoblast, the notochord and the alimentary canal with related structures develop.

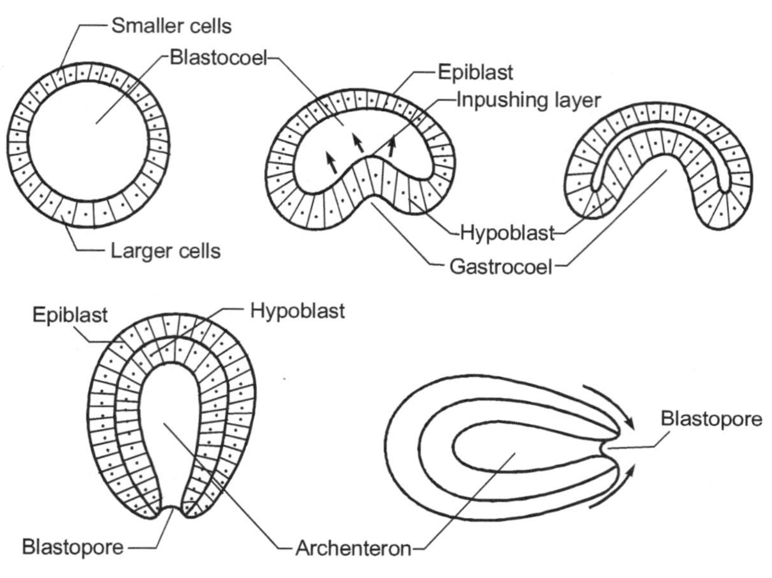

Figure 11.1 Events during the gastrulation in the egg of amphioxus.

GASTRULATION IN FROG

In frog, gastrulation occurs both by **involution** and **epiboly**. Involution causes the "rolling in" of blastodermal cells into the blastocoel, forming the inner layer. In epiboly, the blastodermal cells, usually the micromeres grow over the macromeres forming the macromeres as the inner layer.

The first indication of gastrulation is the formation of a small transverse notch in the grey crescent region. Crescently, the notch increases in size and tends to move down both ends becoming a small crescent. Thus the small cavity beneath the crescent-shaped knotch is the beginning of the archenteron. In this region, the blastodermal cells start rolling into the blastocoel, forming the inner layer. The appearance of the crescentric slit in the grey crescent region is supposed to be by **emboly**. **Invagination** takes place by the appearance of bottle-like cells whose necks will be at the surface as the bottom region goes on swelling. There will be an inpushing of this region, forming the slit (Figure 11.2). Factors like cell motility, contractility and selective adhesion are found to play a role in the formation of blastopore in frog's gastrulation.

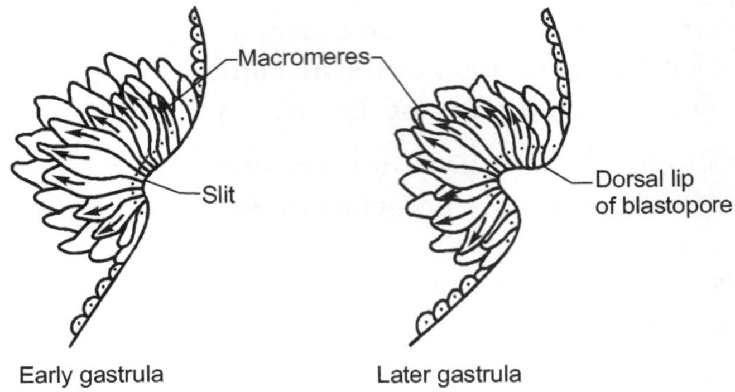

Figure 11.2 Formation of crescentric slit in early and late gastrula of frog

The micromeres or the pigmented cells now grow over the yolk cells (**Epiboly**). It begins slowly in the later blastula and increases with the advancing gastrulation. The cells of the animal hemisphere proliferate and grow down-wards on all sides except in the region of the blastopore where the cells roll inward, thus forming the inner layer (**chordamesoderm**). These involuted cells form the dorsal lip which continues to grow backwards as the inner layer towards the dorsal side pushing the blastocoel. When the crescent-shaped blastopore becomes ring-shaped, the cells that come from all directions take up the place in the archenteron as the roof and the sides. By this time, the lateral lips of the blastopore are formed. In the beginning, the archenteron is in the form of a small slit-like cavity and then expands dorsally and laterally with continued involution. By special staining techniques, **Vogt** (1926) showed that there is a streaming movement of cells of the dorsal and lateral surface towards the blastopore in the early gastrula (**convergence**). Most of these cells get involuted at the blastopore. When they enter in, they start spreading out (**divergence**). The floor of the archenteron is composed of a single layer of small endodermal cells which have derived from the yolk cells in the late gastrula. It is separated off from the archenteron only by a single layer of cells shortly before the entire blastocoel is eliminated.

The crescent-shaped dorsal lip continues to expand, assuming at first a semicircular structure and then a horse-shoe-shaped outline followed by the epiboly of the micromeres. Finally, it becomes circular when the ventral lip is formed. In this way, all the yolk cells are hidden by the pigmented cells except at the region of the blastopore where they can be seen from the outside as a mass called **yolk plug**. The ventral lip also undergoes involution forming a small archenteron, giving rise to the mesoderm. During this process, the dorsolateral wall of the archenteron differentiates into **chordamesoderm** which gives rise to the notochord in the middle, and the lateral portions as mesoderm. The innermost layer forms the **endoderm**. All these processes are believed to be due to **delamination**. Thus the mesoderm lies between the outer ectoderm and the inner endoderm. After the completion of gastrulation, the gastrula becomes elongated along with the archenteron which becomes the gut. The blastopore will be the posterior end as a highly reduced aperture.

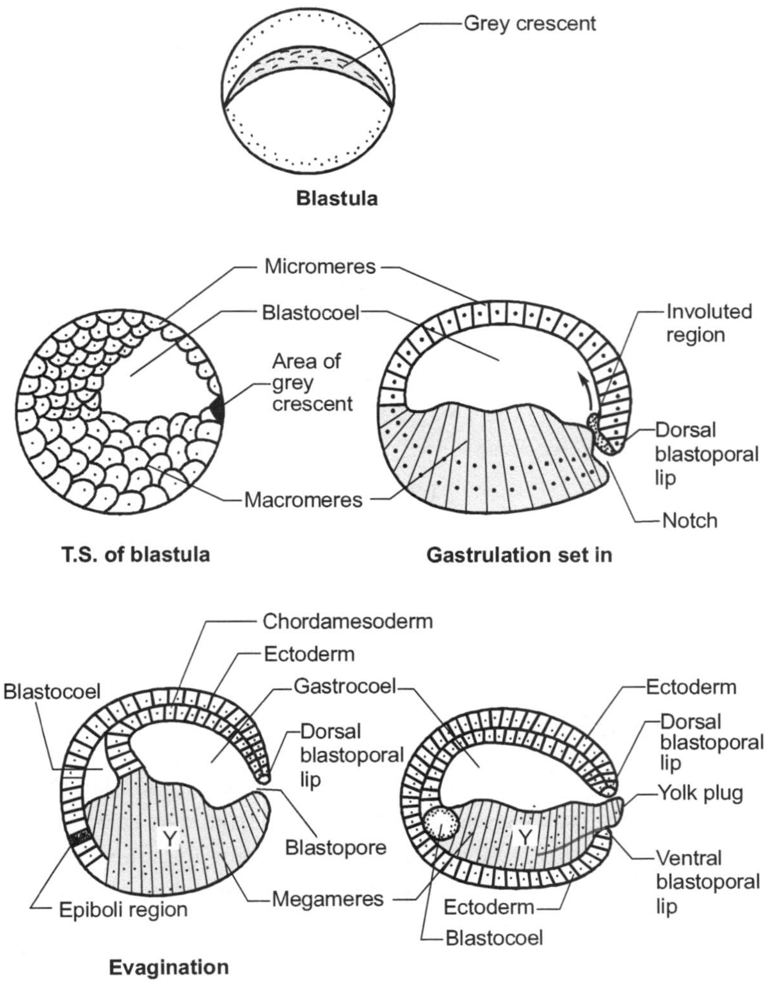

Figure 11.3 Process of gastrulation in frog's egg. (*Continued*)

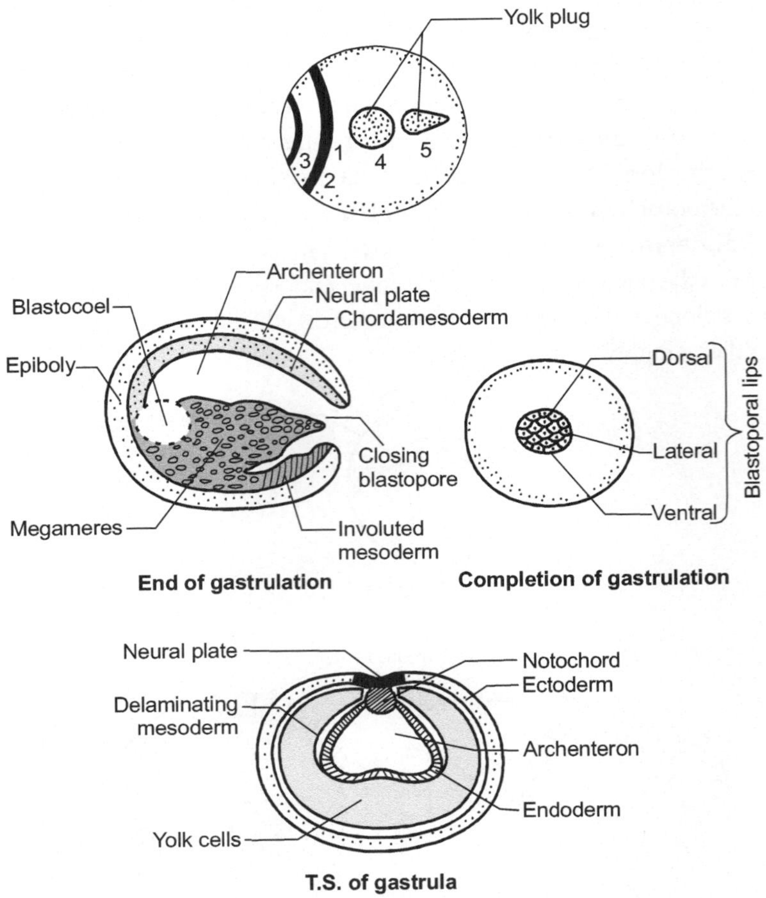

Figure 11.3 Process of gastrulation in frog's egg

Thus, gastrulation in frog's egg involves **epiboly, involution**, **emboly**, **convergence**, **divergence** and also **delamination** (Figure 11.3). These morphogenetic movements are necessary during the development of frog because of the presence of the inert yolk in the vegetal pole of the egg.

GASTRULATION IN CHICK

In chick, gastrulation is more prolonged and further modified compared to that in frog's egg because of the **meroblastic** nature of cleavage and presence of a **massive yolk**. Prior to gastrulation, the blastoderm is in the form of a tiny area with 2 mm in diameter and a few layers of cells in thickness. As in frog, gastrulation in chick involves **involution**, **convergence**, **divergence**, **streaming** and **delamination** and it can be studied under two headings namely separation of endoderm and formation of primitive streak.

Separation of Endoderm

There are different opinions with regard to the separation of endoderm during gastrulation. According to the view put forward by **Patterson** (1910), gastrulation in chick involves **involution** of cells along the posterior margin of the blastoderm, forming the endoderm. But according to **Pasteels** (1945), groups of blastoderm cells from the surface undergo multiple localized **invaginations** and produce an underlying sheet of endoderm (**infiltration** or **polyinvagination**). Here, the cells bodily migrate inwards and get arranged as the endoderm layer. These two explanations have been now mostly abandoned.

At present, the "**theory of delamination**" given by **Ollacher** (1869) has been universally accepted. By delamination, the cells become separated from the surface layer and spread out below as part of the endoderm (Figure 11.4). The beginning of the separation of the upper mesoectodermal layer is marked by the accumulation of large yolk- laden cells at the lower surface of the blastoderm. The cells of the upper surface are largely yolk-free and are aligned in a layer of one-celled thickness. Thus two distinct layers of cells are present even though they are still in contact. The delamination of the two layers might be due to the development and coalescence of scattered irregular slits between the two layers so that the endoderm is separated off beneath the mesoderm. In all probability, the endodermal layer spreads anteriorly by the addition of small groups of cells that are forced or squeezed out from the overlying layer. It was also demonstrated by **Spratt** (1946) that more endodermal cells are separated from the thickened area where the primitive streak will be formed and are added on to those set aside by delamination. It is apparent that the formation of archenteron in chick's gastrula is slightly different from that of Amphioxus or frog. This is because there is no true replacement of blastocoel by the gastrocoel in chick. The original blastocoel is directly transformed into the gastrocoel by the appearance of endoderm cells beneath the original blastoderm.

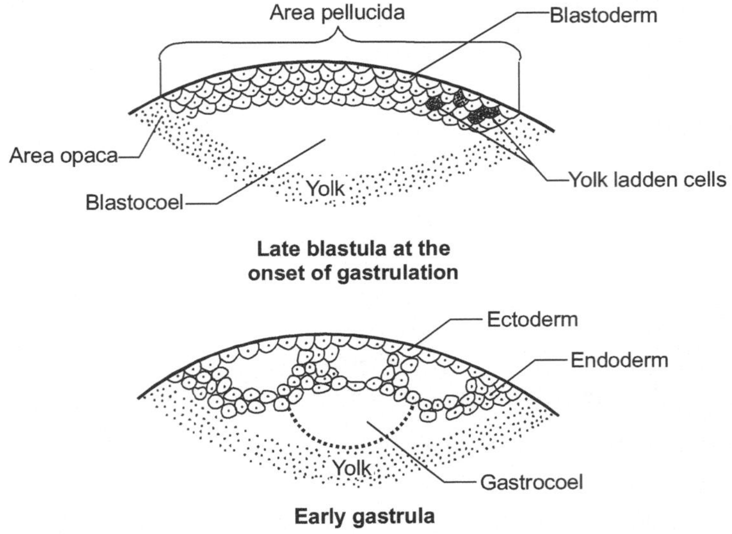

Figure 11.4 Separation of endoderm during gastrulation in the egg of chick

Development of Primitive Streak

By about 16 hours of incubation, a linear thickening called **primitive streak** is formed on the surface of the blastoderm. This is an area of rapid growth and proliferation of cells and is a conspicuous structure on the early blastodisc (Figure 11.5). Its groove, namely **primitive groove**, is flanked on both sides by two **primitive ridges**. Anteriorly, it ends in the **primitive pit** and posteriorly in the **primitive plate**. Immediately anterior to the primitive streak is an elevation called **Hensen's node**.

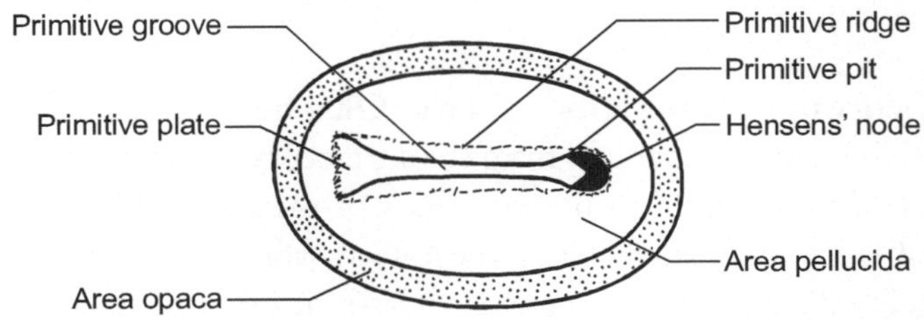

Figure 11.5 Chick's embryo (16 hours) showing the structure of primitive streak

Much uncertainty exists with regard to the mode of origin of primitive streak. According to the **theory of concrescence** put forward by **Patterson**, the primitive steak is probably homologous to the blastopore of lower vertebrate eggs. Due to the presence of abundant yolk, the ventral lip instead of growing over the yolk moves towards the presumptive dorsal lip in the animal pole itself. Both of them coalesce and then form the thick region, the **primitive streak** as shown in the figure 11.6.

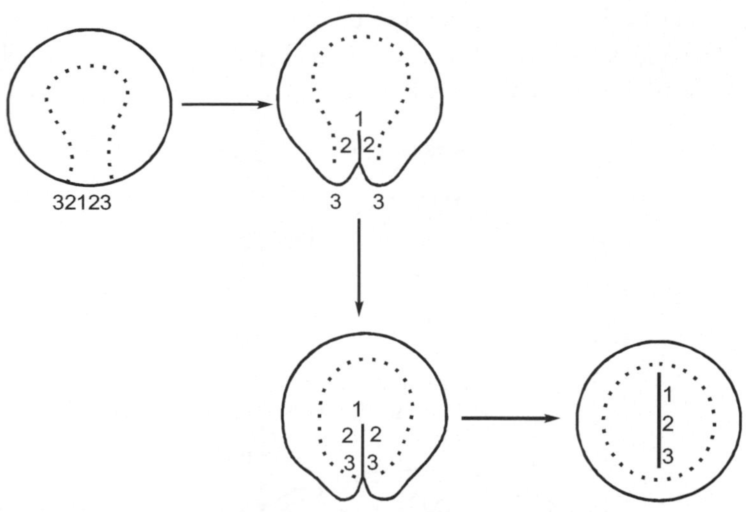

Figure 11.6 Formation of primitive streak as per 'Concrescence theory'

However, the work of **Spratt** gives reliable information concerning primitive streak formation. He followed the movement of blastodermal cells by marking them with carbon particles and observed that the primitive streak is formed by a posteromedial shifting or crowding of cells towards the midline so as to form a linear thickening (Figure 11.7).

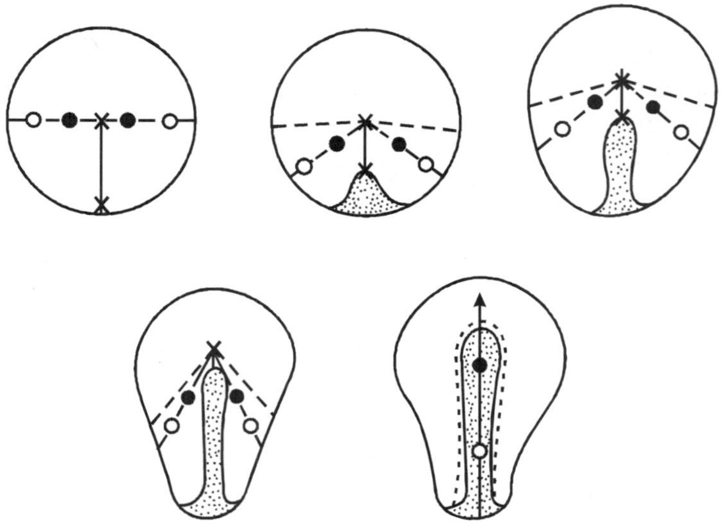

Figure 11.7 Formation of primitive streak as observed by Spratt

The Hensen's node is nothing but a thickening in close association with the notochordal cells in the anterior end of the primitive streak. The perspective notochordal cells converge on the node, sink through it and then move directly forward as a **head process**. The elongation of primitive streak completes as the head process is established. Then the primitive streak gradually shortens, ultimately becomes reduced to a fragment and finally disappears. The entire embryo develops anterior to the primitive streak. The head process consists of a thick central mass of cells from which notochord develops and more cells diffuse laterally contributing to the somatic mesoderm that comes to flang the notochord. After differentiation, the notochord becomes detached from the endoderm below except for a more persistent fusion at the extreme anterior end. The disappearance of the primitive streak is the end of gastrulation and the beginning of neurilation. The fully formed chick gastrula consists of three germ layers namely **ectoderm**, **chordamesoderm** and **endoderm** as in Figure 11.8.

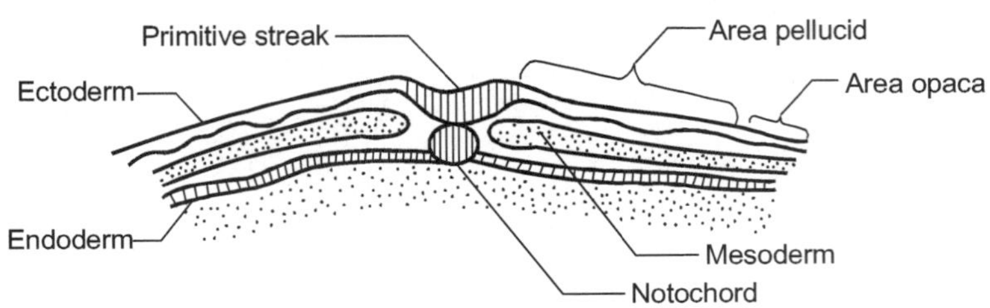

Figure 11.8 T.S. of late gastrula in chick

The primitive streak in chick is an important structure as it plays a prominent role in the formation of notochord and mesoderm. The groove and folds of the primitive streak correspond respectively to the blastopore and its lateral lips in frog's egg. The primitive node equals to the dorsal lip of the closed blastopore and the primitive pit represents the dorsal opening of the **neurenteric canal**. The posterior end of the primitive streak is comparable with the ventral region of the blastopore where the anus develops later.

GASTRULATION IN A MAMMAL

In the beginning of gastrulation, the mammalian embryo is in the stage of the **blastocyst** which contains a cavity corresponding to the blastocoel. The first step in the differentiation of the blastocyst is the appearance of a layer of flat cells below the embryonic knob or the inner cell mass. This layer is the **hypoblast** which corresponds to the endoderm of chick as it is the presumptive endoderm (Figure 11.9). Even though the hypoblast arises from the embryonic knob by a process of **delamination,** there is also evidence to suggest the formation of hypoblast from the outer layer of cells or **trophoblast.** The trophoblast corresponds to the chorion of bird's embryo. The hypoblast cells now spread along the inner surface of the trophoblast and so the cavity is now lined by the endodermal cells. Thus, there is no formation of separate gastrocoel and the originally existing blastocoel becomes gastrocoel. This represents the **yolk sac** of birds but there is no yolk. The inner cell mass now becomes thin and corresponds to the blastodisc of bird's egg. At this stage, the embryo resembles the bird embryo except for the absence of yolk. A primitive streak is also formed by the collection of mesodermal cells which migrate downward and sideways between the epiblast and hypoblast (Figure 11.10). These cells give rise to the mesoderm at the anterior end of the primitive streak and the notochordal cells collect to form **Hensen's node**. The notochordal cells move downwards and forward in the middle line and form the notochord. At the completion of gastrulation, the epiblast above the notochord represents the neural cells and the rest of the epiblast is ectoderm.

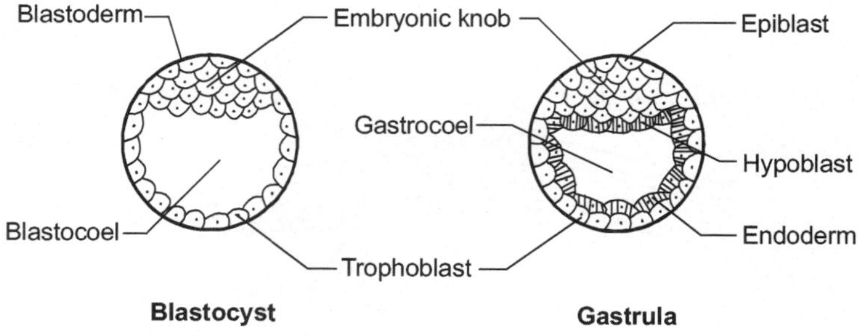

Figure 11.9 Formation of hypoblast in a mammalian egg

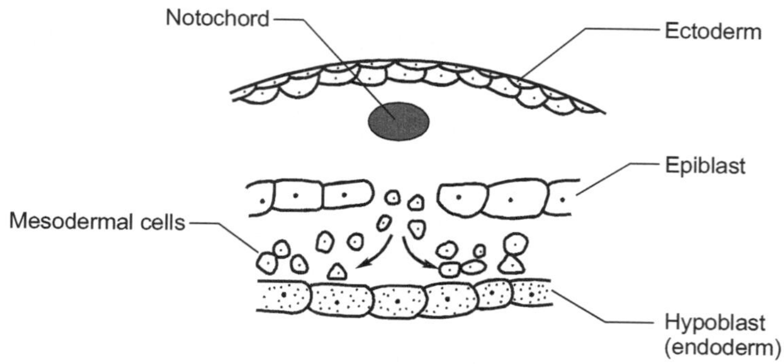

Figure 11.10 Structure of late gastrula in a mammal

EXOGASTRULATION

In animal eggs, there are two gradients namely **animal gradient** with the centre of activity at the animal pole and the **vegetal gradient** with the centre of activity at the vegetal pole. The normal development of the egg not only depends on the presence of both gradients but also on the equilibrium between them. If the animal gradient is weakened or suppressed, the vegetal gradient dominates and the embryo becomes **vegetalized**. If the vegetal gradient is weakened or suppressed, the animal gradient dominates and the embryo is **animalized**. This is well seen in the case of **exogastrula.**

If the blastomeres of sea urchin's egg are separated at the two- cell stage or four-cell stage, each blastomere develops into a complete but small sized larva. This is because the first two cleavage planes are meridional passing through the main axis of the egg. Therefore, each of all the blastomeres gets equal portions of three cytoplasmic regions namely **ectoderm, endoderm** and **mesoderm.** But if the egg is separated into the animal and vegetal halves after the third cleavage (equatorial), both halves produce deformed embryos. The animal half differentiates into an **ectodermal vesicle** without a gut and ciliary band but with the tuft of long cilia excessively in the animal pole. On the other hand, the vegetal half differentiates into an oval embryo with the large endodermal gut but without mouth, arms and ciliary bands (Figure 11.11).

In later cleavage stages, if the morula is cut transversely below the equator, the vegetal pole now produces a large endodermal gut and a small ecotodrmal vesicle. But the gut does not lie inside the ectodermal vesicle and is evaginated to the outside. This phenomenon is called **exogastrulation**.

When the fertilized sea urchin's egg is exposed to sea water containing lithium salts, an embryo is developed as in the case of isolated vegetal half. In this embryo, the gut is developed but is exogastrulated (evaginated) instead of invagination. Here the skeleton is absent and the ectoderm is in the form of vesicle and fails to develop further. The opposite effect is noticed when the egg is exposed to artificial sea water without calcium but with sodium thiocyanate. Here the embryo develops no gut and the ectoderm fails to develop the ciliary bands. But the animal pole develops long cilia with increased size. These experiments clearly indicate that each of the two halves lacks some parts contained in the other half and two mutually antagonistic principles interact with each other. Thus the normal development is due to equilibrium between the two principles or gradients and the activity of the two gradients declines in opposite directions.

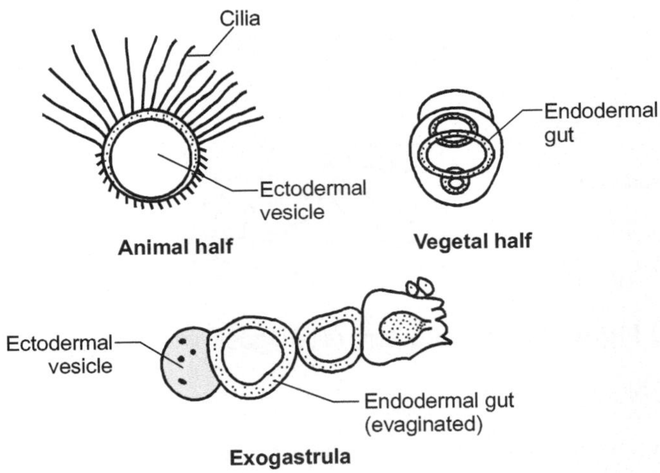

Figure 11.11 Development of animal and vegetal half cells and exogastrula in sea urchin's egg.

PHYSIOLOGY OF GASTRULATION

During gastrulation, the blastomeres are very active in morphogenetic processes which affect the metabolism of the cells to a large extent. In the cells, DNA synthesis is increased in relation to the duplication of chromosomes to facilitate cell division. mRNA and tRNA are produced in increased rate correlated with the synthesis of newer proteins. It is estimated that there is five-fold increase in protein synthesis in the early gastrula of amphibian eggs and three-fold increase in sea urchin's eggs. These proteins are produced from the protein yolk and are qualitatively different from the proteins formed in the blastula stage. There is an increased oxidation and oxygen uptake during gastrulation as the morphogenetic movements of the cells require an increased expenditure of energy in the form of ATP molecules. This required energy is obtained through the breakdown of reserve substances such as glycogen and yolk. Therefore, the quantity of glycogen and yolk granules diminish in the cells of gastrula.

REVIEW QUESTIONS

1. Define the terms morphogenesis, gastrula and gastrulation.
2. Give a brief account of the various types of morphogenetic movements met within animal groups.
3. Explain the process of gastrulation in Amphioxus, frog, chick and mammal.
4. Write a note on the physiology of gastrulation.

5. Give brief notes on the following:

i. Epiboly	ii. Emboly
iii. Invagination	iv. Involution
v. Infiltration	vi. Blastopore
vi. Chordamesoderm	vii. Primitive streak
viii. Exogastrula	

12

CELL DIFFERENTIATION

The differentiation of cell is one of the most important, interesting and universal phenomenon in living organisms during development. Cellular differentiation occurs in every developmental system but its mechanism has not been adequately investigated. Sooner or later, a few different kinds of cells from the fertilized egg undergo changes which can be explained through some facts and views. Various observations and experimental results of experimental embryologists are greatly useful to have an idea of the nature of some of the intra- and intercellular mechanisms which operate on cell differentiation. In general, differentiation is the modification or the progressive specialization in the structure and function of the cells. It is a process by which a cell becomes specialized in order to perform a specific function. It can be defined as a sort of transformation of more general homogeneous structure into a more specialized heterogeneous one during development. Cell differentiation occurs continuously and reaches its maximum at embryonic development. The fundamental properties of embryonic development are **growth**, **differentiation** and **metabolism**. Growth is due to multiplication of cells leading to an increase in the number and size of the cells whereas differentiation is characterized by **histogenesis** and **organogenesis**. Several investigations have made it clear that the first step in cell differentiation is **local accumulation of substances** that were previously distributed evenly throughout the egg. These accumulations have definite influence on the fate of those parts in which they occur. They are called as "**determining substances**". Experiments have also proved that the cells containing different types of protoplasm really do have different developmental potencies. Thus it is concluded that the **protoplasmic substances** are to be the determining substances for cell differentiation. Later, the **metabolic enzymes** are considered to be determining substances causing cell differentiation. In short, differentiation is a process that takes place inside an embryo and that determines which genes are to be expressed and hence what type of cell would result.

CHEMODIFFERENTIATION

The differentiation of a cell is not determined by a single substance. It is more likely that the direction for the development of any cell depends upon the natural qualitative relationships of great number of substances (**enzymes**) which together govern the cell metabolism. In other words, the originally more or less homogeneous egg cytoplasm, after the beginning of development, acquires a complicated spatial structure containing various concentrated structures in definite parts of the egg. These substances may be evenly distributed throughout the cytoplasm in the beginning. They accumulate at different parts of the cytoplasm under the influence of the coordinating system of chemical reactions that occur in the cells. These substances are not originally present in the egg but they arise as *de novo* as a consequence of chemical reactions that take place in the egg. i.e., the parts of the cell which were alike before, now begin to show differences in chemical composition. These accumulations have definite influence on the fate of the parts of the cell. It was believed that these accumulations supply materials for certain organs of the future embryo and so they have been named as **organ- forming substances** or **morphogenetic substances.** Though the accumulated substances exert determining influence on the future development of those parts, they cannot be simply recorded as building materials for the organs. Therefore, these substances are called as '**determining substances**'. Hence, following Huxley, this phenomenon may be referred to as '**chemodifferentiation**' which may set in at earlier or later stages of development.

In the development of the worm, **Tubifex**, special protoplasmic materials accumulate at both vegetal and animal poles of the egg immediately after fertilization. These protoplasmic masses are called as **poleplasm** which is considered to be due to the attraction of certain parts of the egg cortex. Even if the eggs are centrifuged, the poleplasm, in general, still accumulates at their original sites in the eggs. This poleplasm slightly differs from the rest of the protoplasm in the physiochemical composition and is very rich in enzymes. Soon, the two masses of the poleplasm unite at the centre of the egg and is found in one of the first four blastomeres during cleavage. Later it is distributed to two of the micromeres namely first and second **somatoblasts.** In later development, the first somatoblast divides to form **teloblasts,** which give rise to smaller cells forming the **ectodermal germ band.** The second somatoblast divides to form **mesoblasts** which bud off smaller cells constituting the **mesodermal germ band.** The nervous system and circular muscles arise from the ectodermal germ band and connective tissue, longitudinal muscles and nephridia from the mesodermal germ band. The skin and gut develop from the rest of the cells which are without poleplasm (Figure 12.1).

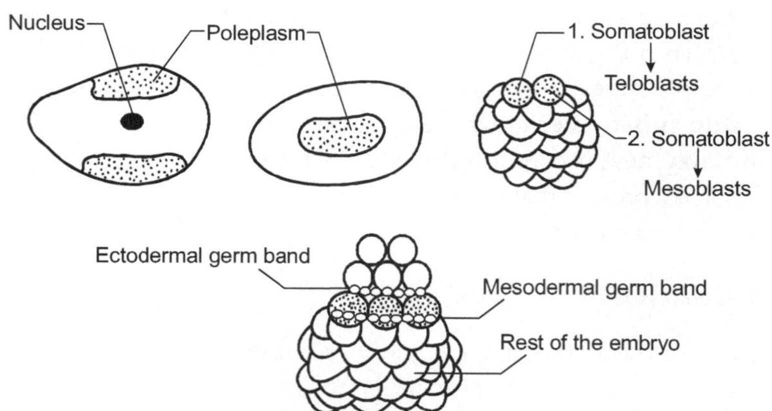

Figure 12.1 Fertilized egg of **Tubifex** showing poleplasm and development of ectodermal and mesodermal germ bands

When the cells containing the poleplasm are killed by ultraviolet irradiation, the remaining part of the egg is unable to produce an embryo. When a number of other cells without poleplasm are destroyed, a normal but small embryo is developed. The elimination of the first somatoblast results in the absence of ectodermal germ band and that of the second somatoblast in the absence of mesodermal germ band. These experiments clearly show that the poleplasm has the potency to form an embryo. But the **Tubifex** eggs exhibit a deviation of normal pattern of cleavage on centrifugation or on chemical treatment. From this, it is clear that the poleplasm exerts its determining influence only when it is present in the somatoblasts.

Similarly experiments on the development of ascidian egg also prove that the cells containing different types of cytoplasm really have different developmental potencies. It is also very clear that the localization of various cytoplasmic components after fertilization is probably due to the factors of influence in the egg cortex. The **mesoplasm** of asicidian is found to contain certain **enzymes** as in the poleplasm of Tubifex. These enzymes act as the determining substances that are found to be important for metabolic processes. Therefore, it is probable that these substances exert their influence through the metabolic processes which, in turn, may be the cause for differentiation. Chemodifferentiation may set in at earlier or later stages during development. The differences between the mosaic and regulative eggs is due to an earlier or later occurrence of chemodifferentiation. Once started, chemodifferentiation steadily proceeds until the intensive multiplicity is transformed into more and more intensive.

CELL DIFFERENTIATION AND NUCLEUS

As the cell also contains the nucleus apart from the cytoplasm, it is advocated that the complicated spatial structure is localized not in the cytoplasm but in the nucleus in some way or other. It is probable that there must be qualitative differences among the nuclei which are formed during cell division. The disturbance of the normal course of division must result in an abnormal distribution of the determinants on the cells leading to abnormal development. It is evidenced that there are no preformed structures in the nuclei that are differently distributed in different cells to give rise to different tissues and organs. Genetic and cytogenetic studies clearly indicate that the genes, the hereditary factors responsible for specific characteristics, are present in the nucleus where they are arranged in a linear order on the chromosomes. The nucleus conveys very specific instructions for a particular pattern of morphogenesis. Nuclear transplantation experiments reveal that the nucleus is the seat of chomosomes which are the bearers of genes that control the different activities of a cell in particular and the organism in general. The genes bring about a morphogenetic pattern by direct effect on specific biochemical reactions. In all organisms, the genetic material apparently determines the amino acid sequence of proteins and so cell differentiation is characterized by the changes in the amount, distribution and diversification of proteins.

To understand the **genetic control of development and differentiation**, it is necessary to know how the nucleus determines the orderly sequences of amino acids which form proteins. A segment of DNA coding for a particular protein transcribes the message or information in the form of code to the mRNA which reaches the ribosomes. The tRNAs found in the cytoplasm translate the message so that they pick up specific amino acids according to the sequences of codons in mRNA. Peptide bonds are formed and assembled to form a particular protein which is released from the ribosome. In higher organisms, the normal development involves a condition in which the cells engage for prolonged periods in protein synthesis. This has an advantage in that the messages remain for a long period and can be translated over and over again. For embryonic development, the stable differentiation in the cells should be marked by the presence of stable mRNA molecules. The phenomenon associated with fertilization provides ample evidence for the **delay of translation of message**. After fertilization or parthenogenetic activation in the egg, the amino acid uptake increases dramatically. This is not because of the increase in the permeability but because of the synthetic process that starts. The unfertilized eggs of sea urchin show an increased incorporation of radioactive elements immediately after fertilization or artificial activation. This suggests that the mRNA is present in the cytoplasm of the unfertilized egg in a masked or inactive form.

It is apparent that the cytoplasm provides the immediate material to bring about development whereas the genes act as directing and controlling agents. The normal development requires the presence of at least one gene of each kind. For example, the specialization within the cytoplasm of the egg becomes regionally different and becomes controlled by the **maternal genes** only. It is in this way that the cleavage cells acquire cytoplasm with diverse qualities. The influence of **paternal genes** may start shortly after fertilization in early cleavage. This shows that these elements by themselves are unable to initiate the process of morphogenesis, differentiation and growth. Hence a gene can produce differential effect only when it comes to lie in the cytoplasm. This is because the genes can interact with the cytoplasm. The opportunity for this reciprocal relationship is already operative when the cleavage subdivides the eggs into blastomeres with the cytoplasm of different qualities. Each newly formed cytoplasmic diversity sets up a fresh series of reactions between the genes and the local cytoplasmic substances and so differentiation unfolds progressively.

CELL DIFFERENTIATION AND GENES

Our present knowledge indicates that the properties of a differentiated cell are an ultimate reflection of the activity of its gene. During cell division, each daughter cell receives one identical set of chromosomes and thus an identical set of genes. Yet this cell differentiates into quite different cell types. It is not the genes or chromosomes that are distributed unequally but rather the chemical environment of the genes. The distinction among the differentiated cells can largely be due to the different proteins particularly enzymes. In this way, the cells within a single individual show conspicuous differences in protein content and therefore in gene function. It has been proved beyond doubt that different cells possess different capacities to synthesize materials specific to the production of specific molecules by some cells, thus leading to differentiation **(Microenvironment)**. Experiments have proved that the microenvironment of the cell is also influenced by the surroundings. The local environment of the inner cells would be different from that of the outer cells because the inner cells would not be directly exposed to the environment. In addition, the products produced by one group of cells may also influence or control the differentiation of other cells **(Cellular interactions)**. Thus the environmental changes are effective in modifying or directing the course of differentiation or gene function. For instance, **cytoplasmic heterogeneity** is built up in the egg at the beginning so that the nuclei come to lie in different cytoplasm during early cleavage. The different kinds of cytoplasm can induce changes in the nuclei of the cells and their chromosomes. So the cell differentiation is due to the reciprocal interactions of genome and environment leading to **differential gene function**. Experimental embryology, genetics and biochemistry also support that the differential gene function characterizes diverse cells in metazoans.

The events of progressive differentiation of a cell can be explained through a model as shown in Figure 12.2. Specific molecules 'N' from the environment enter the cell and pass through the cytoplasm into the nucleus. One or more "N" molecules stimulate a specific gene, DN, to direct the synthesis of the corresponding RN molecule, probably mRNA. Some other N molecules suppress the activity of another gene DS responsible for the differentiation of skin cell. The RN molecule with a copy of DN gene code now comes out of the nucleus and directs the synthesis of specific protein molecule PN responsible for the differentiation of nerve cell. The PN molecules thus formed may either initiate an endogenous cell-stabilizing mechanism or bring out a change in the quality of the products. In other words, these molecules would promote further activation of DN gene indirectly or aid in suppressing the DS gene. This environment, thus formed, could interact with other cells bringing about the differentiation. Similar mechanism might also operate in differential gene activation, the products of which would lead to differentiation in an another line.

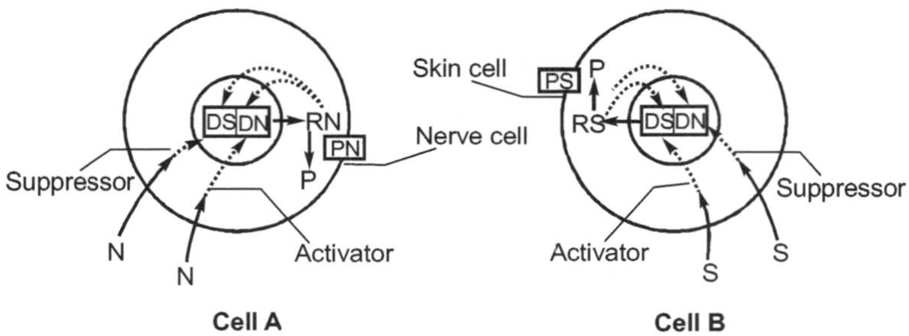

Figure 12.2 Influence of microenvironment in the progressive differentiation of a cell.

FUNCTIONAL MECHANISMS OF DIFFERENTIATION

In a broader sense, differentiation is a process in which the cells become differentiated from one another and also from their original condition. Strictly speaking, differentiation is nothing but a process in which the cells or groups of cells acquire the ability to do special functions. This phenomenon can be called as **histological differentiation**. The differentiated cells are capable of performing special functions other than the basic functions such as metabolism, ability of amoeboid movement, irritability and so on which are found both in undifferentiated and differentiated cells. The special functions of differentiated cells mainly depend on the specific mechanisms which may either be visible sometimes in the cells or not. The functional mechanisms in histologically differentiated cells are cytoplasmic in nature so that they bring alterations in the relative volume of the nucleus and cytoplasm. In differentiated cells, the nuclei do not undergo changes during development and so they possess the same chromosomes and genes. The mass of cytoplasm increases in the cells during differentiation whereas no change or little change occurs in the nuclear mass in comparison with cytoplasm. The ratio of mass of cytoplasm to that of nucleus increases in differentiating cells and this ratio is indicative of the degree of differentiation. As far as chemical substances are concerned, the nucleus possesses DNA whereas the cytoplasmic structures contain proteins. Again the enzymes which are involved in functional mechanisms of a cell are formed by proteins. Therefore the relationship between the altered quantity of DNA and proteins in the cell could also indicate the degree of differentiation.

REVERSIBILITY OF DIFFERENTIATION

Differentiation is **reversible** to some extent as morphological and physiological processes of the cells depend on their surrounding environment. It is seen that there is an increase in quantity of proteins in differentiating cells when compared to nucleic acids. The reverse is the case in **dedifferentiation** in which there is breakdown of the protein part of the cells. As a result, the quantity of protein is decreased in the cells in comparison with the amount of nuclear substance. Experiments have shown that the dedifferentiation in embryonic cells occurs due to the changes in the environment in which the cells lie and every type of cell differentiates only after disaggregation in relation to its previous differentiation. Moreover, the dedifferentiated cells are incapable of reverting to the embryonic cells. That is, they do not acquire new competencies.

REVIEW QUESTIONS

1. What you mean by cell differentiation?
2. Write an essay on chemodifferentiation.
3. Explain the role of nucleus in cell differentiation.
4. Describe the mechanism by which the microenvironment influences the differentiation of a cell.
5. Explain the phenomenon of histological differentiation
6. Write notes on:
   i. Poleplasm
   ii. Microenvironment and differentiation
   iii. Cytoplasm heterogeneity
   iv. Chemodifferentiation and histological differentiation
   v. Reversible differentiation

13

GERM LAYERS AND ORGANOGENESIS

During development, fertilization leads to the formation of a zygote that undergoes cleavage by many mitotic cell divisions resulting in a tiny ball of cells called **blastula**. This early embryonic form goes through **gastrulation** forming a **gastrula** in which the cells undergo prominent morphogenetic movements giving rise to the **germ layers**. A germ layer is a group of cells that are developed during animal embryogenesis especially in vertebrates.

All animals produce two or three primary tissue layers called **primary germ layers**. The diploblastic animals with radial symmetry produce two germ layers whereas the triploblastic animals with bilateral symmetry produce a third layer between these two layers. Thus the gastrula possesses all the materials for the development of adult organs in the form of three germ layers namely an outer **ectoderm**, a middle **mesoderm** and an inner **endoderm**.

DERIVATIVES OF GERM LAYERS

After the establishment of the three major germ layers during gastrulation, various cell lineages are derived from these germ layers. The formation of ectoderm is the begining in the formation of the body tissues and the ectoderm is the tissue that covers the body surface and develops from the outermost of the germ layers. It forms the central nervous system, the lens of the eye, cranial and sensory ganglia and nerves, pigment cells, head connective tissue, epidermis, hair, mammary glands, etc. The endoderm is formed by the inward migration of cells along the archenteron and it forms the digestive system, lining of digestive, respiratory and urinogenital systems and also glands like thyroid gland, parathyroid gland, liver, pancreas, etc.

During gastrulation, some inwardly migrating cells contribute to the mesoderm which is an additional layer between the ectoderm and endoderm. It forms the coelom, skeletal muscles, skeleton, dermis of the skin, connective tissue, urinogenital system, heart, blood, lymph cells, spleen and so on. Thus gastrulation rearranges the blastula to form the three embryonic germ layers which eventually develop into all parts of the adult animals through **organogenesis**. The derivatives of the germ layers can be summarized as given below.

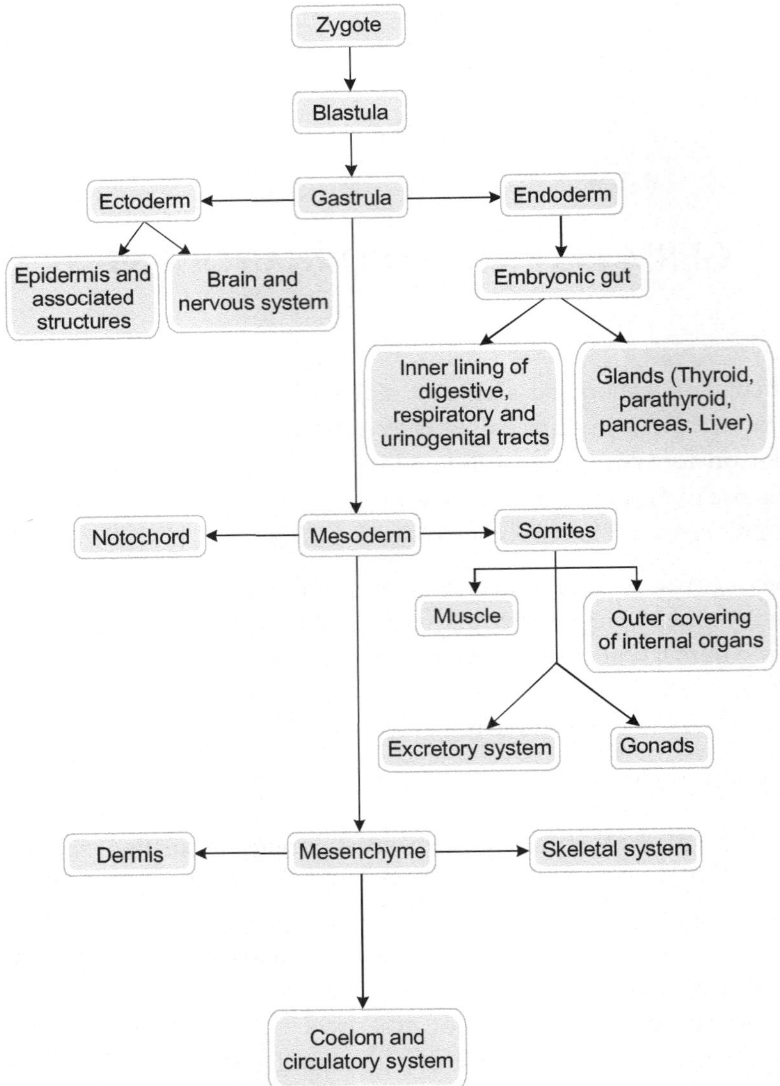

ORGANOGENESIS (FORMATION OF ORGANS AND ORGAN SYSTEMS)

The process of the formation of organs from the three germ layers is **organogenesis** (organ formation). Organogenesis involves an initial stage in which the continuous mass of cells of the germinal layers split up into smaller groups of cells called **primary organ rudiments,** each of which is destined to produce a certain organ or a part of the adult animal body. These primary organ rudiments subdivide into **secondary organ rudiments** which further differentiate and develop into the organs of adults.

ORGANOGENESIS IN AMPHIOXUS

The period of development in Amphioxus can be divided into the **embryonic period**, the **larval period** and the **adolescent period**. The embryonic period begins with fertilization and ends with mouth formation. This period includes two phases—the first phase starts with fertilization and ends with hatching (embryo comes out of the egg and freely swims but cannot feed as there is no mouth) and the second stage includes hatching and development of mouth. During the embryonic period, the development is rapid but it is slow during the larval period. Metamorphosis is extensive at the end of the larval stage and the larva becomes an adult becoming sexually mature.

Neurulation or formation of nerve cord or development of dorsal tubular nerve cord

In Amphioxus, the first system to develop is the nervous system. The **neurula** is the stage in which the neural plate appears in the embryo and **neurulation** is the process of transformation of the neural plate into the neural tube.

The beginning of the central nervous system is foreshadowed by flattening and cellular thickening of the dorsal region of the elongated gastrula. So, the central region of this flat ectodermal surface becomes slightly depressed forming the **neural** or **medullary plate**. At the same time, the ectodermal cells on either side of the neural plate become raised and are called as **neural ridges**. Now the neural plates sink down and the neural ridges come together to form a roof over the neural plate. This fusion begins just in front of the blastopore and extends in both ways. Then the neural plate begins to roll upwards and the two edges of the plate rise up and ultimately fuse. In this way, the neural tube is formed enclosing a longitudinal canal called **neural canal** or **neurocoel**. At the posterior end, the blastopore comes to open into the neural tube. The neurocoel is ciliated along its length and opens to the outside by the **neuropore**. The archenteron is connected to the neurocoel by a short canal called **neurenteric canal**. Thus the archenteron is connected to the outside through the neurenteric canal and neurocoel. The entire process of neurulation is shown in Figure13.1.

The anterior end of the neural tube becomes dialated to form the **brain** or the **cerebral vesicle**. As the neural tube sinks down, the brain also becomes deeper. Later the neuropore closes leaving behind a pit called the **olfactory pit** in the adult. At the same time, the neurenteric canal also disappears and the neural tube becomes a completely closed tube. The adult nervous system of Amphioxus is more or less in this condition.

Mesoderm and Coelom Formation

At the time when the neural plate begins its transformation into neural tube, the dorsolateral walls of the archenteron appear to be folded to form shallow grooves on either sides. Each groove on its concavity facing the archenteron is shallower near the blastopore than it is anteriorly. Immediately, these two lateral grooves become divided by transverse partitions into smaller units called the **archentric** or **enterocoelic pouches**. These pouches continue to grow both outwards and downwards between the ectoderm and endoderm. These are the primordia or the beginning of the first mesodermal **somites**.

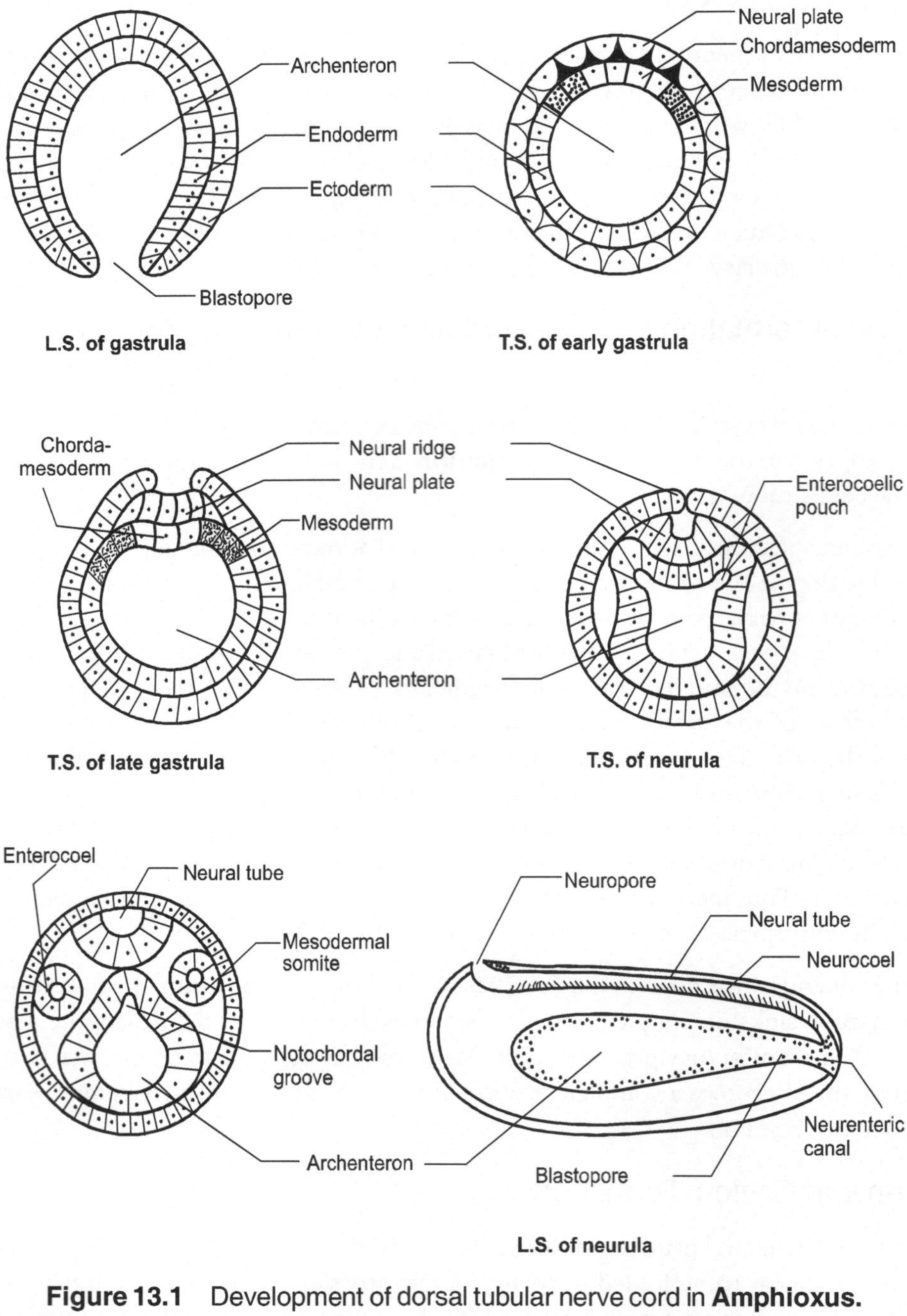

Figure 13.1 Development of dorsal tubular nerve cord in **Amphioxus.**

For a while, their cavities remain connected with the archenteron but later they are separated off from it (*Refer* Figure13.1). This method of mesoderm formation occurs only in the first two pairs of somites. Posterior to the second pair, the enterocoelic pouches lose their cavities before they are separated from the archenteron. Here, they are pinched off as solid blocks of cells within which a new coelomic cavity is formed. From the fifteenth pair of somites, the formation of enterocoelic pouches stops and the two halves of the original fold become opposed to each other to form a solid band of cells extending to the blastopore. The remaining mesodermal somites are developed from these lateral bands.

Thus, the mesoderm in Amphioxus can be divided into two types based on the differential origin namely the **gastral mesoderm** and the **peristomial mesoderm**. The gastral mesoderm is derived from the archenteron whereas the peristomial mesoderm is derived from the solid band of cells extending from the blastoporal region and are added in the posterior region of the growing gastrula.

Differentiation of mesoderm, and coelom formation The mesodermal differentiation in the development of Amphioxus occurs first in the anterior region of the embryo and then proceeds further progressively behind in an orderly sequence. After the mesodermal somites have become detached from the primitive gut, differentiation of mesoderm takes place. The upper part of the mesoderm is the **myotome**. Each myotome buds off cells dorsally to form a thin outer sheath called **dermatome** which is a thin sheath underlying the ectoderm of the skin. At the lower end of the myotome, another plate develops from the inner side. This is called as **sclerotome** which gives rise to the supporting sheath around the notochord. The mesoderm continues ventrally as the **lateral mesoderm** which consists of two sheaths, the outer **somatic mesoderm** and the inner **visceral** or **splanchnic mesoderm**. The cavity located between these two sheaths is the **coelom**. More specifically, the somatic mesoderm lines the outer coelomic wall forming the **parietal peritoneum** and the splanchnic mesoderm found around the alimentary canal forms the **visceral** or **splanchnic peritoneum**. By the union of the paired sheaths of the lateral mesoderm beneath the alimentary canal, the coelomic cavities unite and become continuous. These differentiations in the mesoderm and the formation of coelom are illustrated in Figure13.2.

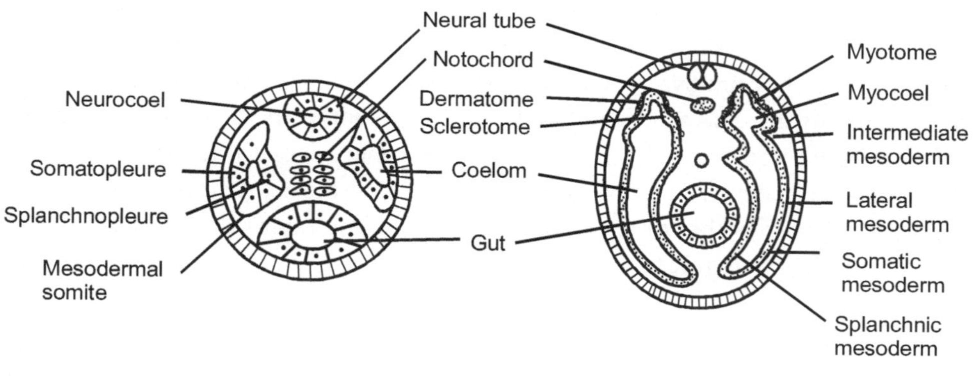

Figure 13.2 Differentiation of mesoderm and development of coelom in **Amphioxus.**

In Amphioxus, the coelom is originally the space from the enteron which is enclosed by the entrocoelic pouches. In other words, the coelom develops from the archenteron of the developing embryo and so the coelom is **enterocoelic** in nature. The coelom is then greatly restricted in the adult animal because of the formation of the bronchial clefts and the atrium.

Formation of Notochord

The notochord takes its origin from a narrow strip of cells located in the dorso-median region of the archenteron between the two mesodermal grooves. The notochordal cells will also form a groove with its concavity towards the floor of the archenteron. In the meantime, the embryo increases in length and the notochordal cells are continuously formed by rapid proliferation from the region near the median dorsal lip of the blastopore. Other cells are also added by the division of the cells in the wall of the notochordal groove. At the time when some of the first archenteric pouches are constricted off, the notochordal groove becomes obliterated by the approach and fusion of the two sides forming the notochordal rod (Figure 13.2). This begins anteriorly in the region of the first pairs of archenteric pouches and extends backwards as well as forwards from this point. The separation of the notochord from the endoderm takes place after the formation of the ninth and tenth mesodermal somites. Up to this time, the notochordal cells have more or less the appearance of the mesodermal cells. Later, they develop many vacuoles which contain a jelly-like supporting substance. After the complete separation of the notochord from the archenteron, the endodermal cells grow together to close the gap established by the separation of the notochordal cells forming the gut wall.

Development of Alimentary Canal and Gills

After the separation of the notochord and mesoderm from the wall of the primitive gut, the dorsal ends come together and the gut comes to have a lining of endoderm. The gut is connected to the outside through the neurenteric canal, neurocoel and neuropore (Figure13.3.). Soon after hatching, the embryo becomes elongated and the gut also becomes long.

The anterior region remains wide and forms the pharyngeal region and the posterior narrow region forms the stomach–intestine region. By this time, the anterior gut diverticula become separated. Behind this region, two structures develop on the floor of the pharynx. One is a club-shaped gland which becomes tubular and disappears later. At its left end, it opens to the outside. The other structure is the **endostyle**. Now the primitive gut comes to have three openings, namely the mouth, anus and the first gill slit. The mouth arises as an opening at the meeting point of the outwardly growing endoderm and inwardly growing ectoderm at the anterior end of the pharynx on the left side. Similarly, the anus is formed at the posterior end of the alimentary canal just below the neurenteric canal. The first gill slits develop in the same way as that of the mouth but it is on the right side as shown in dotted lines opposite to the mouth as in Figure13.4.

When these openings are formed, the larva becomes elongated and the two openings and the gut are ciliated. Now the larva leads a free-living habit feeding on small organisms near the surface waters. This stage lasts for three months.

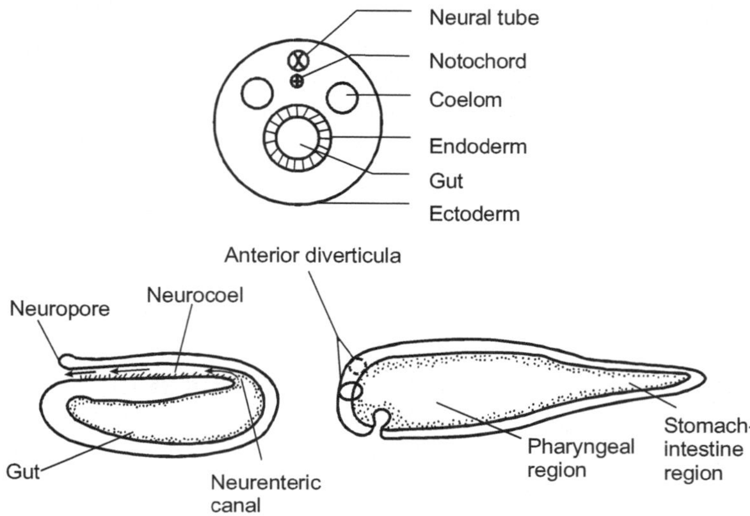

Figure 13.3 Formation of gut in **Amphioxus**

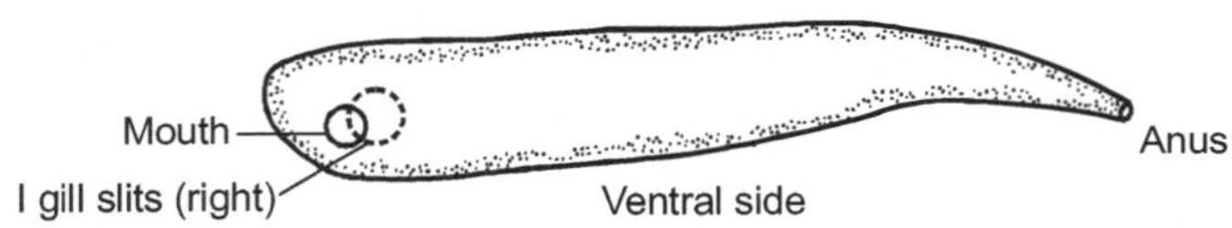

Figure 13.4 **Amphioxus** larva showing mouth, first gill slits and anus.

The most important event during the larval life of Amphioxus is the formation of gills. A series of fourteen gill slits develop ventrally and move to the right side of the larva. The first gill slit is the highest in position and the last slit is still ventral in position. These gill slits are called **primary gill slits**. A second set of gill slits develop on the right side dorsal to the primary gill slits. These are called **secondary gill slits** which appear at first as a thickening dorsal to the primary gill slits. Then it cuts up into eight sections forming eight gills slits. As they enlarge, they push the primary gill slits to the ventral side and finally to the left side (Figure13.5).

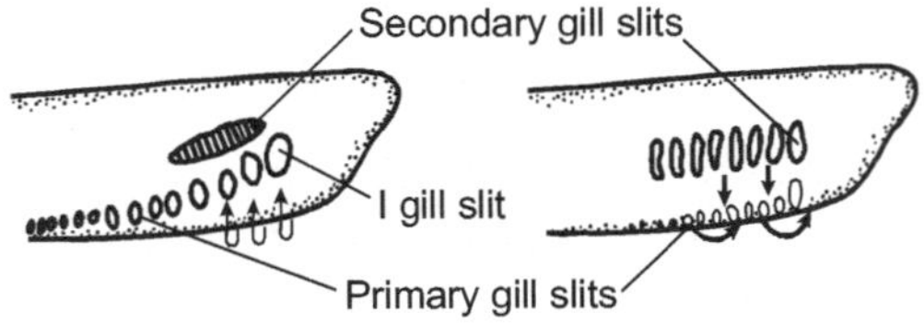

Figure 13.5 Formation of gill slits and their shifting in the larval **Amphioxus.**

Thus the primary gill slits are shifted to the left side so that they are found opposite to the secondary gill slits found on the right side. During shifting, each gill slit becomes divided into two by the growth of a tongue bar. In the secondary gill slits, the tongue bar also grows from the dorsal edge but in the primary gill slits, it grows from the ventral edge. When the gill slits have shifted, the tongue bar grows from the dorsal side in the primary gill slits (Figure13.6) and fuses with the opposite edge of the gill slit, dividing it into two. The first and the last five gill slits disappear so that there are eight primary gill slits corresponding to the eight secondary gill slits on the right side. By this time the **atrium** develops and so the gill slits come to open into it.

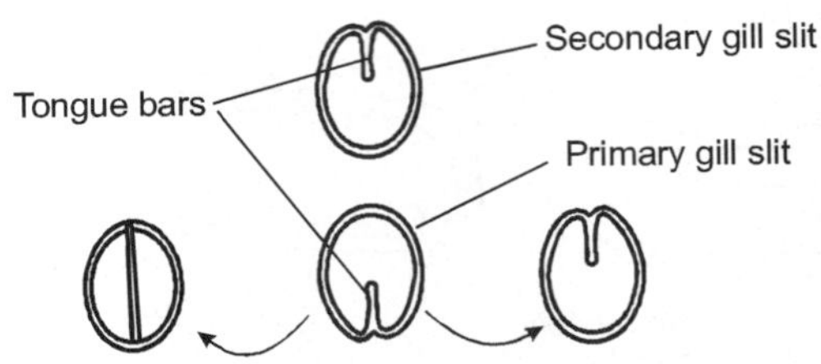

Figure 13.6 Development of tongue bars in the gill slits of **Amphioxus.**

In Amphioxus, the larval period extends for about three months. At the end of the larval stage, the asymmetry of the larva is corrected and the body becomes symmetrical. Now the mouth is shifted to the anterior end and structures on the right side of the pharynx are also shifted to the adult position. With the development of gonads, it attains the adult stage.

ORGANOGENESIS IN FROG

Mesoderm and Coelom Formation

The dorsal and lateral sheet of cells formed by involution at the roof of the archenteron is several cells in thickness. It appears that the cells that are involuted represent more than the endoderm. As a matter of fact, these cells contain mesodermal material including that of notochord so that they form the so-called **chordamesoderm**. When the simple sheet of endoderm has separated itself dorsally and laterally, a second sheet, the **mesoderm**, is formed between the ectoderm and endoderm. It begins its delamination anteriorly and proceeds slowly backwards ending in the undifferentiated cells of blastopore. Subsequently, the sheet is divided into two halves by the delamination of the narrow band of cells which is destined to become the **notochord** in its midline. Laterally, the two separated sheets extend down the yolk cells. However, with the advancing development, they continue their delamination in the ventral side and separate from the yolk cells also. Finally, the right and left mesodermal sheets meet on the midventral line and become continuous with each other.

The most anterior portion of the late gastrula is filled up with loose cells which are produced anteriorly from paired mesodermal sheets instead of well-defined mesodermal layers. Though there are no archenteric pouches, the same dorsolateral mesoderm of the archenteron gives rise to the mesoderm as in Amphioxus. In later stages of development at the time when the tail bud is forming, the mesodermal sheets devide into mesodermal somites. At the time when the neural folds are united to form the neural tube, each mesodermal sheet thickens into the dorsal part posterior to the pharyngeal region. In this way, a heavy band of cells called **dorsal mesoderm** becomes differentiated along with a ventrolateral band referred to as **lateral mesoderm**. The space in the developing mesoderm is the beginning of the coelom. As the coelom develops by splitting of the mesodermal cells, the origin of coelom in frog is considered as **schizocoelic coelom.** The lateral mesoderm is separated into two layers, an outer **somatic mesoderm** and an inner **splanchnic mesoderm.** The cavity between the two layers is the **coelom.** Then the two lateral mesodermal plates unite in the midventral line and the lateral coelomic cavities become fused thus forming a single continuous coelom (Figure13.7).

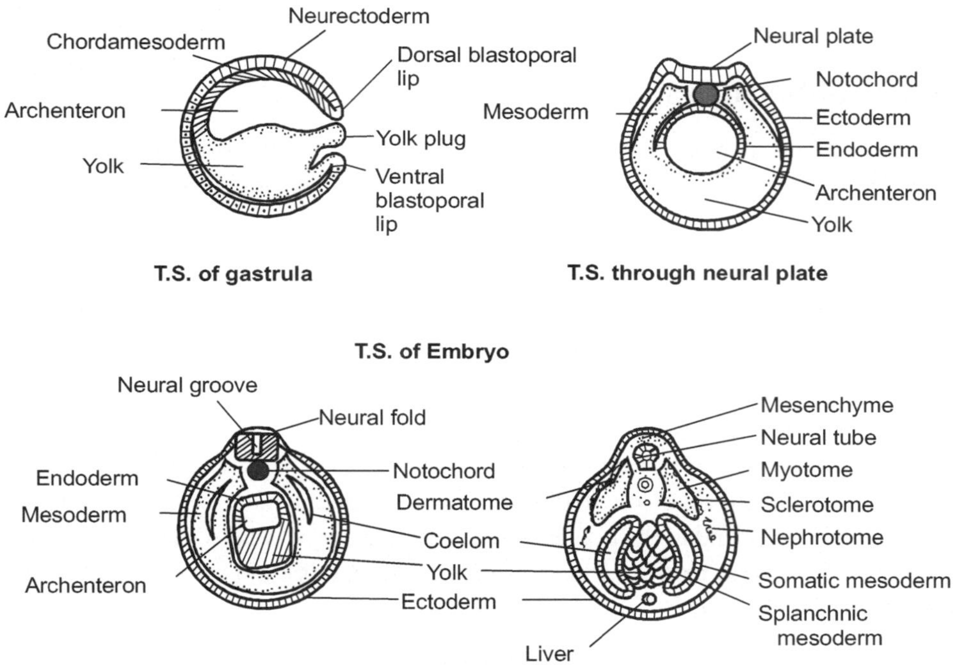

Figure 13.7 Development of mesoderm and coelom in frog.

Immediately after its differentiation, the dorsal mesoderm (myotome) divides into segments or metameres called **mesodermal somites** which increase in number as the embryo grows. Being continuous with the lateral mesoderm at first, they separate off from it later. Each somite contains a small cavity, the **myocoel** which disappears shortly after hatching. In the head region and in the extreme posterior portion of the embryo, the mesoderm is in the form of loose cells called **mesenchyme.** These cells are budded off from the somites and they have the power of differentiating into various mesodermal organs and systems like urinogenital and circulatory systems. The **sclerotome** forms loose mesenchymal cells which are budded off from the lowermost inner region of the myotome and give rise to the vertebral element. The **dermatome** are formed by the mesenchymal cells from the uppermost outer region of the myotome and gives rise to the connective tissue and dermis. Shortly before the separation of the dorsal mesoderm from the lateral mesoderm, rapid proliferation of cells occurs in the upper region of the somatic layer of the mesoderm. These cells arise as separate units called **nephrotome** which give rise to the kidney tubules.

The somatic mesoderm becomes a thin sheet forming the outer lining of the body cavity called **parietal peritoneum.** On the other hand, the splanchnic mesoderm forms the outer covering of the gut called **visceral peritoneum** which divides the coelomic space into different regions. The coelomic space covering the heart is the **pericardial space** and the separating membrane is **pericardium.** The cavity surrounding the lungs is the **pleural cavity** and the separating membrane is the **pleural membrane**. The rest of the cavity is called as the **general body cavity** or **abdominal body cavity** which is lined externally by the parietal peritoneum and internally by the visceral peritoneum.

Development of Nervous System or Brain

The vertebrate animals such as frog, chick and mammal show similarities in their organogenesis. Though there are differences in development, the nervous system is the first to develop in all vertebrate types.

At the end of gastrulation, the rudiment of the nervous system is seen in the mid-dorsal region of the gastrula extending from the anterior end to the posterior end. This is called as **neural plate** or **medullary plate** which is thicker than the rest of the ectoderm.

The edges of the neural plate is called **neural ridges** which become more thicker. These ridges grow up so that the neural plate forms a neural **groove**. Now the neural ridges converge, meet dorsally and fuse. This fusion takes place at the level of the junction of the brain and spinal cord in frog whereas in chick, the fusion is at the level of the midbrain. The fused neural plate is now in the form of a tube extending from the anterior end to the posterior end. At this stage, it is called **neural tube** which opens to the outside anteriorly as **neuropore** which disappears soon. It is connected posteriorly to the gut by means of the **neurenteric canal** (Figure 13.8).

When the neural tube becomes completely separated, a strand of nerve cells is left behind on either side of the neural tube dorsolaterally. These are the **neural crests** which are the rudiments of the ganglia of cranial and spinal nerves. Thus the nervous system is now in the form of a tube with broader anterior end and narrower posterior end. The broader anterior end is to become the future brain and the more uniform posterior end is to become the spinal cord.

The first step in the differentiation of the brain is the anterior dialation of neural tube which gives rise to the brain. The differentiation that occurs in the neural tube during the formation of the brain can be studied under the following headings namely constrictions, unequal thickenings of walls, invagination and evagination and bendings or curvatures.

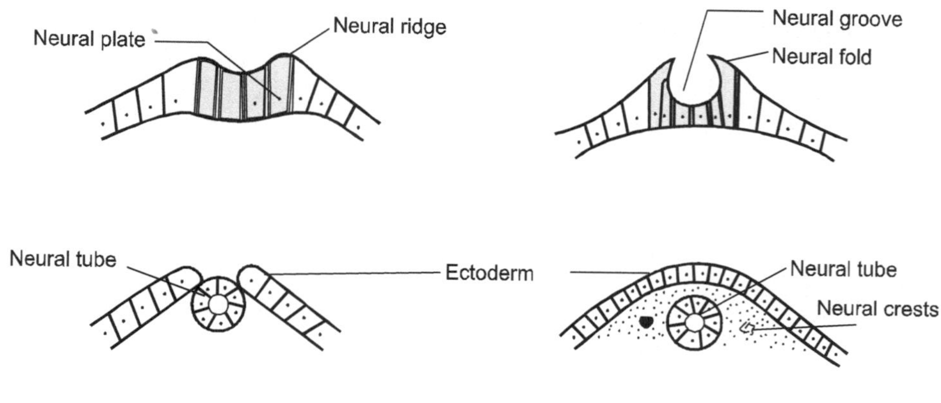

Figure 13.8 Formation of neural tube in frog.

Constrictions The anterior region of the neural tube that differentiates into brain is called **encephalon.** It becomes marked off into three regions in very early embryonic development by two constrictions. These primitive regions are called as **prosencephalon** or **forebrain, mesencephalon** or **midbrain** and **rhombencephalon** or **hind brain.** A little later, the prosencephalon becomes further constricted into two subregions namely **telencephalon** and **diencephalon.** Similarly, the rhombencephalon is subdivided into **mesencephalon** and **myelencephalon** (Figure13.9.). Thus the brain is now marked off into five definite areas.

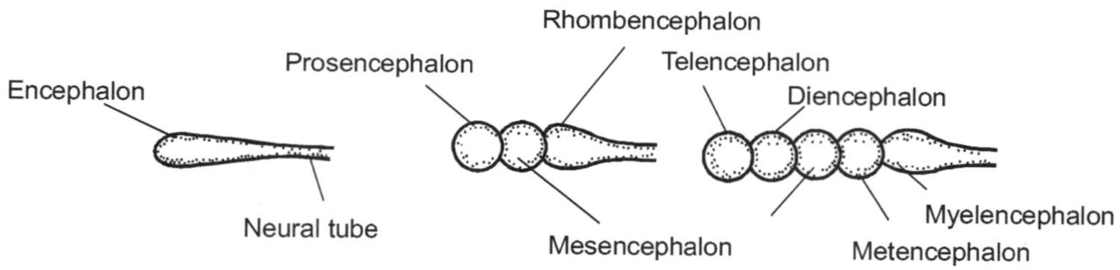

Figure 13.9 Constrictions of neural tube in frog's development.

From these five divisions various parts of the brain are developed. The anteriormost region gives rise to the **cerebral hemispheres** and **olfactory lobes**. The olfactory lobes arise as outgrowths of the cerebral hemispheres. Because of the growth of the cerebral hemispheres, the forebrain seems to point forward. The diencephalon shows invaginations and evaginations. The mesencephalon gives rise to a pair of **optic lobes**. The metencephalon is the place where the **cerebellum** develops and the myelencephalon gives rise to the **medulla oblongata.**

Unequal thickenings of wall The wall of the primitive encephalon at first seems to have more or less equal thickness. But, as the neurons develop and collect into centres, different thickenings appear in different parts of the brain as shown in Figure13.10.

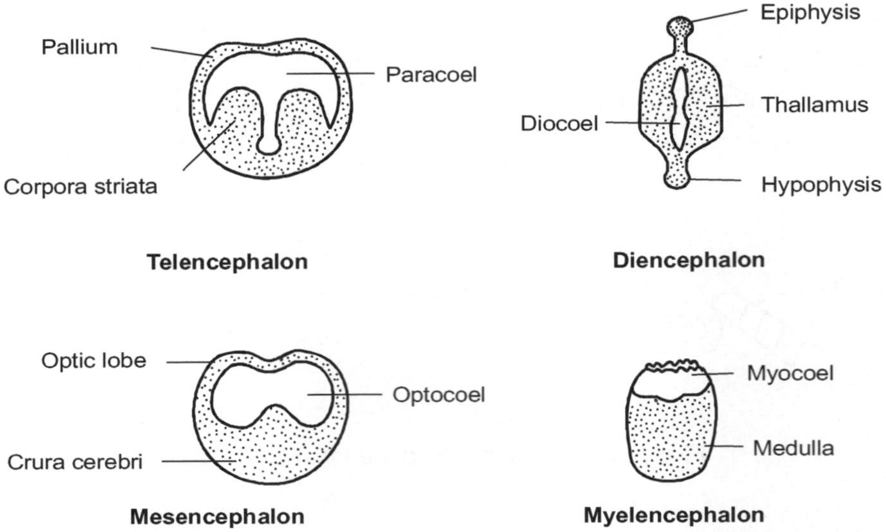

Figure 13.10 Different thickenings in various parts of the brain during development in frog.

The thinnest regions are seen at two regions namely the roofs of diencephalon and myelencephalon. On the other hand, the cerebellum that develops from the dorsal part of the metencephalon possesses thickest wall. The wall of the cerebral hemispheres and the paired anterolateral outgrowths of the telencephalon are thick.

Invaginations and evaginations The telencephalon gives rise to an outgrowth by evagination to form the **olfactory lobe**. The roof of the diencephalon becomes pushed in, non-nervous and vascularized to form the **anterior choroid plexes**. Similarly, the roof of the mylencephalon also becomes pushed in, non-nervous and vascular forming the **posterior choroid plexus**. These capillary networks are formed by the invaginations of the wall to provide blood supply to the inside of the brain. From the walls of the diencephalon also, various evaginations occur. A finger-like outpushing develops on the dorsal side just behind the anterior choroid plexus. This is the **pineal body** or **epiphysis** which is reduced in adults. An outgrowth arises from the floor of the diencephalon and is called **infundibulum** (Figure13.11). It becomes joined with a glandular structure namely **pituitary gland** or **hypophysis** which arises as an outgrowth of the roof of the gut.

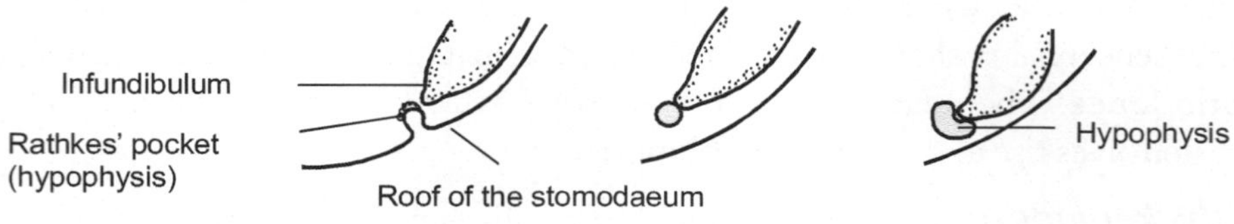

Figure 13.11 Invaginations and evaginations during development of brain in frog

Bendings or curvatures Different curvatures that arise during the development of brain are shown in Figure 13.12.

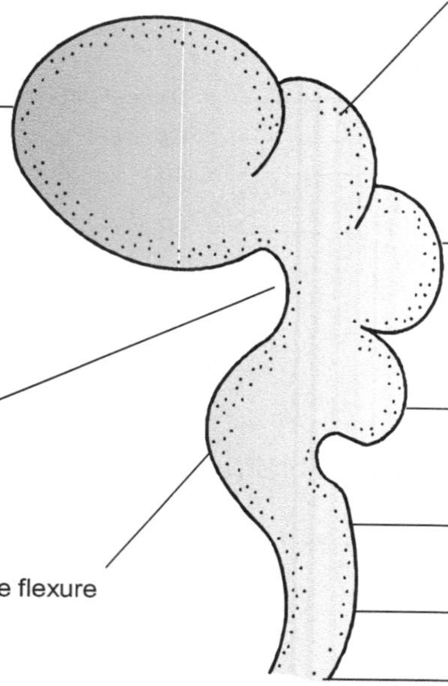

Figure 13.12 Curvatures during the development of brain in frog

The anterior end of the brain becomes bent around the tip of the notochord at the region of the midbrain so that the forebrain points backwards. This curvature is called as **cranial flexure** which is a permanent one. In addition, two more curvatures appear in the developing brain namely **Pontine plexure** between the midbrain and medulla oblongata and **cervical plexure** at the junction of medulla oblongata and the spinal cord.

Behind the region of the medulla oblongata, the spinal cord begins without any demarcation. Moreover, the cavity of the developing neural tube becomes differentiated into various **chambers** or **ventricles** of the embryonic brain as shown in the Figures 13.13 and 13.14. The cavity in the olfactory lobe is called as **olfactory ventricle** or **rhinocoel**. A mid-dorsal septum, **lamina terminalis** divides the telencephalon into two chambers, the cavities of which are called **paracoel** or **lateral ventricles**. These represent the first two major ventricles. The cavity in the diencephalon is **diocoel** which forms the third ventricle. The cavity in the optic lobe is **optocoel** and in the metencephalon is **metacoel** which is the fourth ventricle. The two lateral ventricles open into the third one (diocoel) through an opening called **foramen of Manro**. The diocoel opens into the metacoel (fourth ventricle) via a tubular opening called **Iter**.

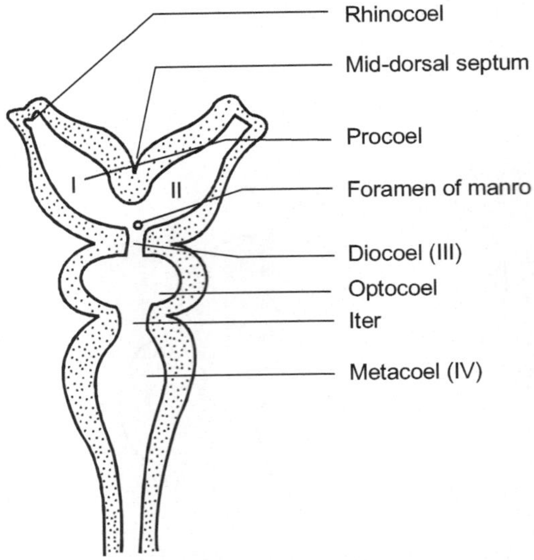

Figure 13.13 T.S of embryonic brain showing various ventricles in frog

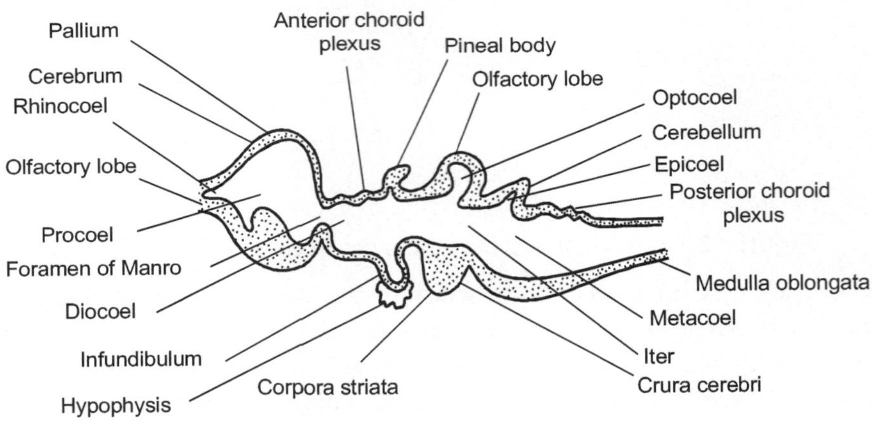

Figure 13.14 L.S. of brain of frog.

The brain during development becomes enclosed by two **membranes** or **meninges** namely an outer tough **duramater** and an inner delicate, vascular **piamater** in frog. But in higher vertebrates, a third spongy layer called **arachnoid membrane** develops between the duramater and piamater.

Induction The development of neural plate depends on the stimuli from the chordal cells. In other words, the development of neural tube is due to the induction of the underlying **presumptive chordamesoderm**. The anterior archenteric roof induces the development of forebrain and eye, the posterior archenteric roof, the development of hind brain and associated structures and the more posterior roof, the spinal cord. This has been shown by transplantation experiments. The transplantation of a graft consisting of neural plate cells alone resulted in the differentiation of graft into similar cells like that of its surrounding. On the other hand, the graft containing neural plate cells together with the underlying archenteric roof was found to differentiate in agreement with its original presumptive structure. It is also shown that in the absence of the **olfactory rudiments**, the corresponding lobe of the forebrain remains undeveloped.

Development of Eye

In vertebrates, the eyes develop at a very early period as lateral outgrowths of the forebrain (diencephalon). The region of the forebrain which develops into the eye, evaginates ventro-laterally to form an **optic vesicle.** At the point where the optic vesicle touches the ectoderm, two reactions occur. One is the formation of **lens placode** and the other one is the invagination of the outer surface of the optic vesicle developing into the **optic cup**.

The optic vesicle continues its evagination until it touches the inner surface of the ectoderm. Now the outer wall of the optic vesicle which is in contact with the ectoderm becomes flattened and invaginates. As a result, the optic vesicle is transformed into a double-walled **optic cup**. The proximal region of the optic vesicle becomes constricted and remains connected with the brain by a narrow **optic stalk.** The outer thin layer of the optic cup forms the **pigment layer** and the invaginated thick layer becomes the **neurosensory layer** or **retina.** At the rim of the optic cup, these two layers are continuous, thus forming the edges of the **pupil.** In the pigment layer, **melanine** is secreted. The outer layer of the sensory region contains layers of cells which differentiate into **rods** and **cones.** Below these, several intermediate layers of cells develop into nerve fibres with large ganglia thus forming the **nuclear layer** (**outer nuclear layer** and **inner nuclear layer**) as well as **ganglion layer.** The axons of the ganglia form the **fibrous layer** which lines the cavity of the optic cup. The axons of the ganglionic cells of the retina converge at the optic stalk forming the **optic nerve.**

In the meantime, the ectoderm in the head region opposite to the optic vesicle thickens, differentiating into the **lens placode.** On each side, the lens placode invaginates to form the **lens pit.** By gradual deepening, the lens pit forms a closed **lens vesicle** which gets pinched off from the ectoderm, thus forming the functional **lens** within the optic cup. Around the optic cup and optic stalk, a layer of mesenchyme cells accumulate and give rise to an inner delicate **choroid coat** (a network of blood vessels) and an outer fibrous layer called as **sclerotic coat** outer to the pigment layer. The choroid coat in front of the lens forms the **iris** of the eye and the sclerotic coat is transformed into the transparent **cornea.** At the corneal region, the ectoderm forms the **conjunctiva** which becomes fused with the cornea. The space between the lens and the cornea contains the **aqueous humour** and the cavity of the optic cup is filled with **vitreous humour.**

The events during the development of eye in frog are given in Figures 13.15, 13.16 and 13.17.

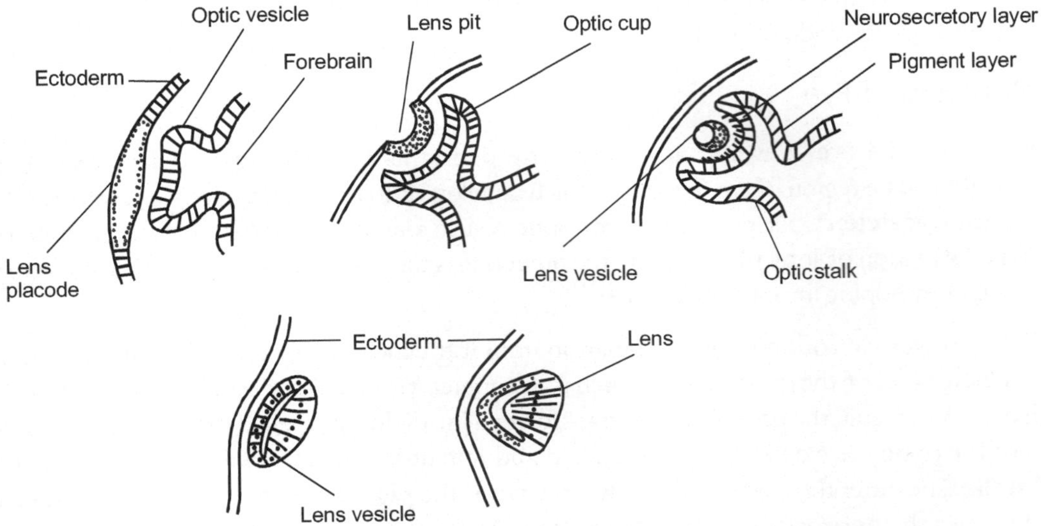

Figure 13.15 Diagrams to show stages ofdevelopment of eye in frog

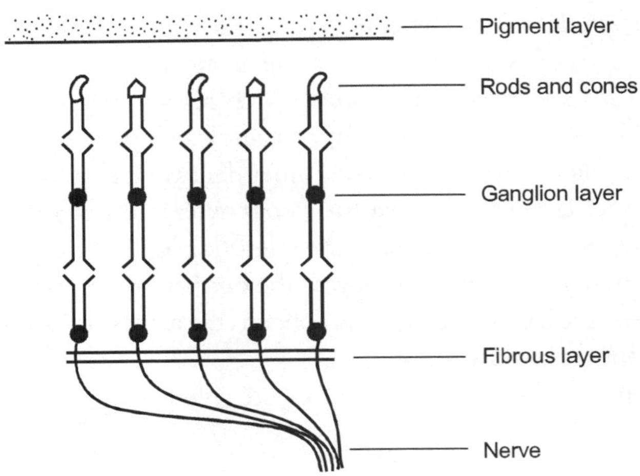

Figure 13.16 Differentiation of optic cup into different layers

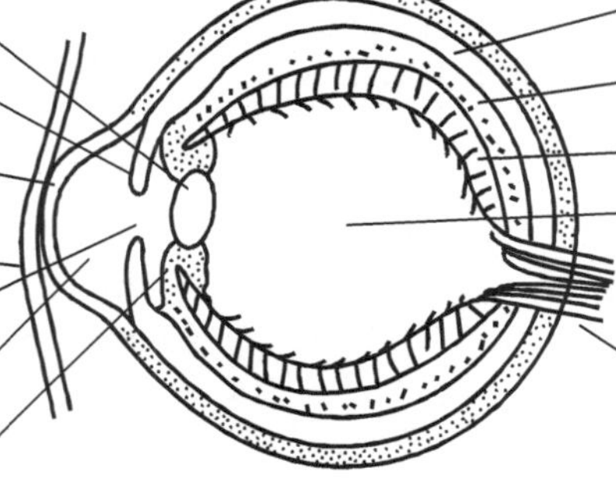

Figure 13.17 T.S of eye of frog

Induction It is found that the development of eye is under the influence of a number of inductors. The rudiment of the optic cup which is a part of the neural plate is induced by the action of the underlying **roof of the archenteron** (**Primary inductor**). It is shown that the transplanted eye rudiment is not capable of developing into the normal eye in the absence of the surrounding mesechyme cells. When the presumptive epithelium of the optic cup of an embryo is transplanted at the vicinity of the eye of another embryo, it developed into the normal eye. The **optic vesicle** acts as the **secondary inductor** as it induces the development of the lens placode. The removal of eye rudiment before it touches the epidermis or prevention of contact between the optic vesicle and outer epidermis by inserting cellophane resulted in the absence of lens development. On the other hand, when a porous membrane is placed between them, there was normal development of eye. If the opidermis in the region of the eye is removed and the epidermis from another part of the embryo is transplanted, the grafted epidermis developed into a lens. Again, the **lens placode** serves as a **tertiary inductor** which influences the development of cornea, choroid coat and sclera from the epidermis and mesenchyme.

Development of Ear or Auditory Organ

In frog, the ear conists of three regions namely an **internal ear**, a **middle ear** and an **external ear**.

The **internal ear** develops from the **epidermis** at the sides of the hind brain. The head epidermis becomes thickened on either side of the hind brain to form the **auditory placode**. This thickened epidermal layer invaginates forming a cavity called **auditory pit** which is transformed into an **otic vesicle** or **auditory vesicle** by deepening of the invagination. The otic vesicle is the most important part of the internal ear and becomes a closed vesicle. The closed otic vesicle gets pinched off from the epidermis and attains a pear-shaped structure with its pointed end directed upwards. Later this pointed end develops into the **endolymphatic duct**. Now the otic vesicle expands unequally by bulgings at some regions and constrictions in some other regions, thus forming a **membranous labyrinth**. The lower part of the vesicle differentiates into the **sacculus** and the upper part, the **utriculus**.

The utriculus is drawn into three **semicircular canals** and the sacculus gives rise to a hollow outgrowth differentiating into **lagena** (in birds) or **cochlea** (in mammals). The sacculus is connected to the brain the through the **auditory nerve**. Now the surrounding mesodermal cells give rise to cartilage which protects the internal ear. Later the cartilaginous membranous labyrinth becomes bony. The development of internal ear in frog is shown in Figure13.18.

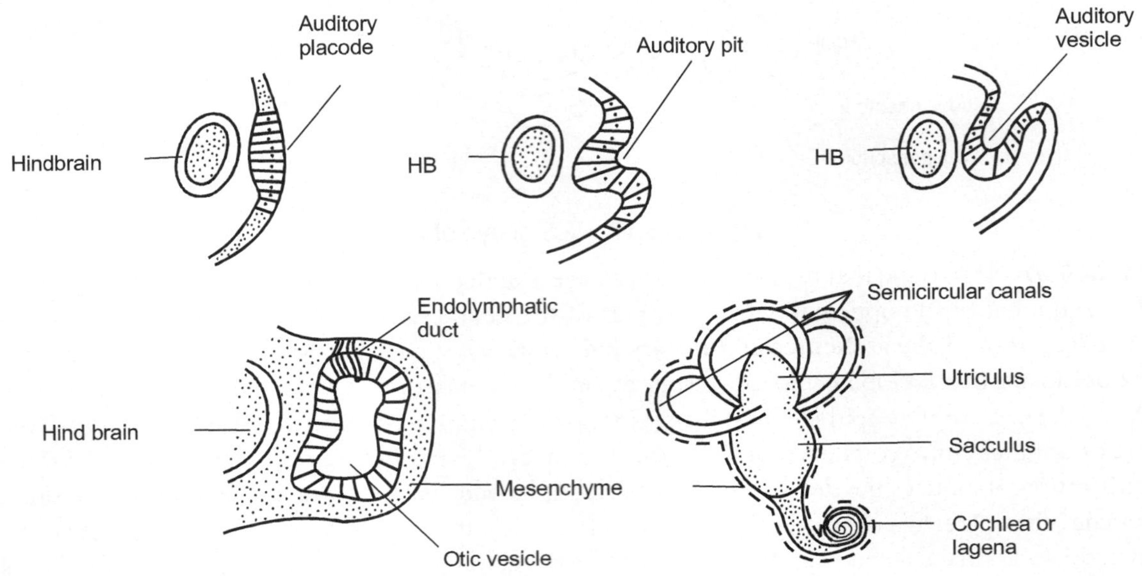

Figure 13.18 Development of internal ear in frog

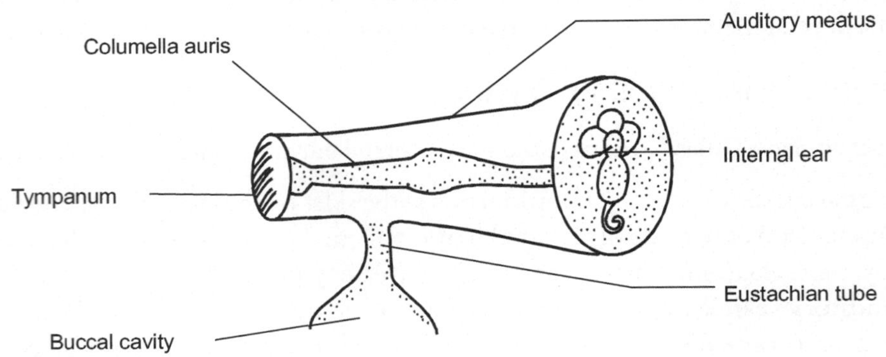

Figure 13.19 Structure of middle ear in frog.

Structure of the middle ear is given in Figure13.19. After the development of the internal ear, the middle ear differentiates as a space between the internal ear and the outer skin. This is the **tympanic cavity** or **auditory meatus** which is occupied by the **columella auris** (the modified cartilaginous hyomandibular piece of the branchial skeleton) which connects the internal ear and the outer skin (tympanum). The skin touching the outer end of the columella auris gets circular shape and vibratile forming the **tympanum** (external ear). At the same time, the buccal cavity of the alimentary canal evaginates into a tube which meets and opens in the middle ear. This is the **eustachian tube** which equalizes the pressure both in the inner and outer sides of the ear.

Induction As in the development of the eye, the formation of the ear in embryos is also influenced by successive embryonic inductions. The **roof of the archenteron** (**chordamesodermal cells**) is the primary inductor as it stimulates the development of the **hindbrain**. The hindbrain, in turn, is the secondary inductor and causes the formation of the **auditory vesicle** which subsequently acts as the tertiary inductor and induces the development of the **ear capsule** from the mesenchyme cells.

Development of Heart

The most dramatic event, during the development of vertebrates, is the formation of the heart. It originates from the **splanchnic layer** of the mesoderm as a simple tube ventral to the pharynx in a space between the ventral ends of the mesoderm. Below the pharynx, the splanchnic mesoderm separates from the endoderm leaving behind a few mesenchymal cells. These cells organize into a delicate tube on each side and are called as **endocardial tubes**. These two tubes are thus situated between the endoderm and the splanchnic mesoderm. Now the splanchnic mesoderm grows around these tubes. In the meantime, the two endocardial tubes unite to form a single tube. Within the embryo, folding movements of the ectoderm and endoderm in the formation of the foregut bring the two heart rudiments together to form a single median tube. The mesoderm surrounds the heart tube and covers it to form the **epimyocardium** which gives rise to the cardiac muscles. The mesoderm of the two sides meet and they form the **dorsal mesocardium** dorsal to the heart and the **ventral mesocardium** ventral to the heart. The ventral mesocardium disappears soon and the heart tube becomes suspended by the dorsal mesocardium which also later disappears. In the beginning, the pericardial space is continuous with the coelomic space and becomes separated from the body cavity later. The events during the development of heart tube is shown in Figure13.20.

The epimyocardium forms a thick muscular layer of the heart called **myocardium** and a thin, non-muscular outer covering layer called **epicardium**. The endocardial tube becomes the inner lining or **endothelium** of the heart. Thus the heart begins as a simple free tube after the disappearance of the dorsal mesocardium. As in Figure 13.21, the primary coiling of the heart tube is towards the right so that the heart which is in the form of a straight tube becomes C-shaped. By further growth, the heart becomes twisted into an 'S' shaped structure. Then the original posterior part of the heart is pushed forward dorsally so that it comes to lie dorsal to the morphologically anterior end. The original chambers of the heart are produced by local dilations which, from posterior to anterior, are **sinus venosus**, **atrium**, **ventricle** and **bulbous arteriosus**. The sinus venosus is the chamber into which the primitive veins enter. The atrium is thin-walled whereas the ventricle is thick-walled. The bulbous is a pulsating chamber from which blood passes into the primitive arteries.

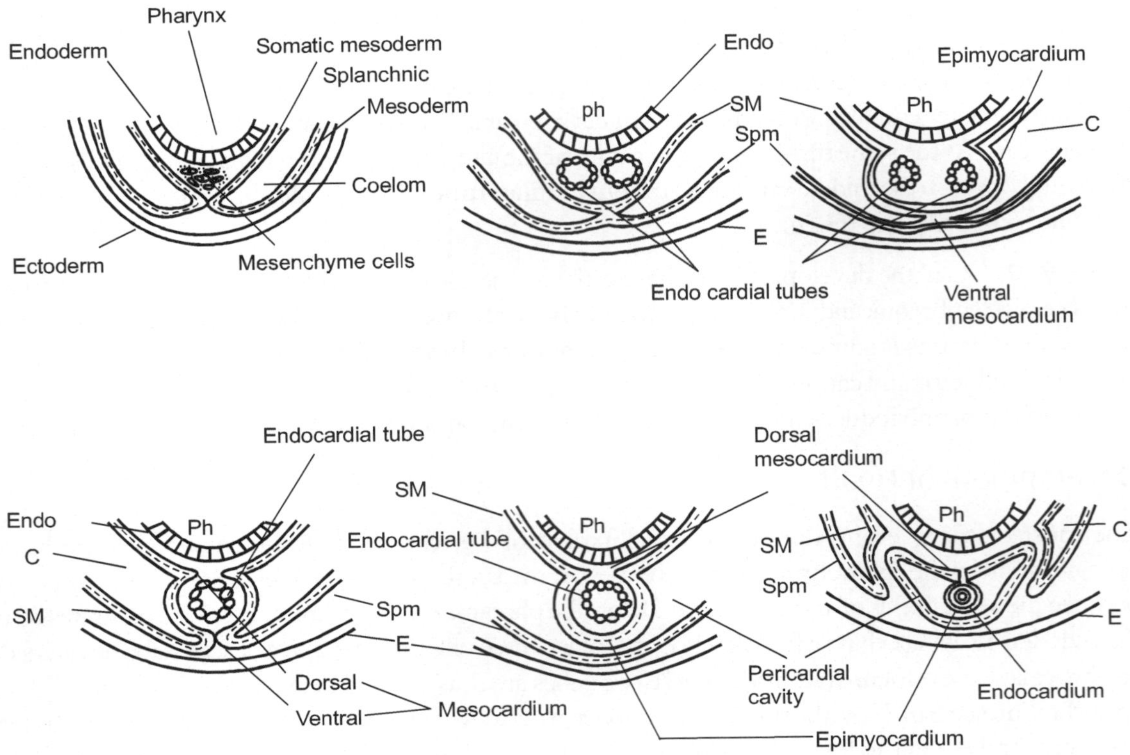

Figure 13.20 Diagrams showing the development of heart tube in frog—Ph-Pharynx, C—Coelom, SM—Somatic mesoderm, Spm—Splanchnic mesoderm, E—Ectoderm, Endo—Endoderm

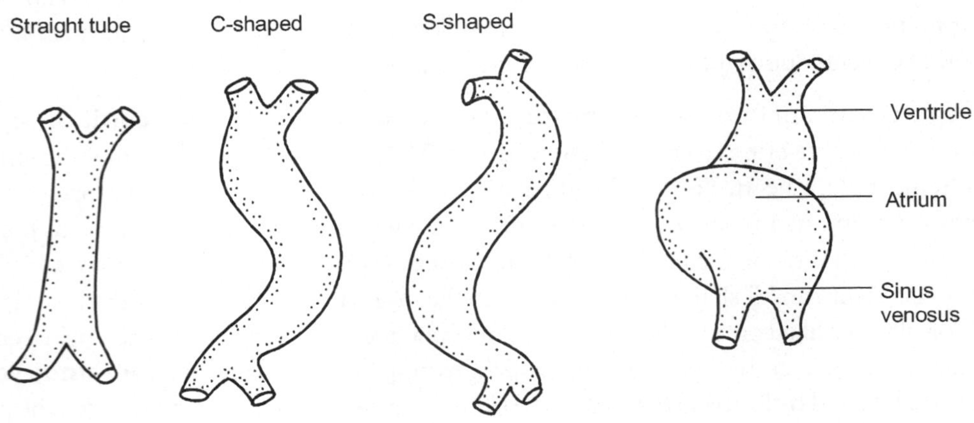

Figure 13.21 Coiling of the heart tube and development of chambers in frog.

Induction The development of heart is in some way dependent on the **endoderm**. By cutting and removing the whole of the endoderm, it is possible to produce **Newt embryos** in which there is a complete absence of heart (Mangold, 1936; Balinsky, 1939). By vital staining in the neurula stage, it has been shown that the **presumptive area of heart** is located in the **edge of the mesoderm.** It is observed that this mesoderm shifts in later stages to the ventral region and eventually comes to lie mid-ventrally (Figure 13.22). This stained rudiment on each side gives rise to one-half of the heart rudiment and the other half is being derived from a similar area on the other side.

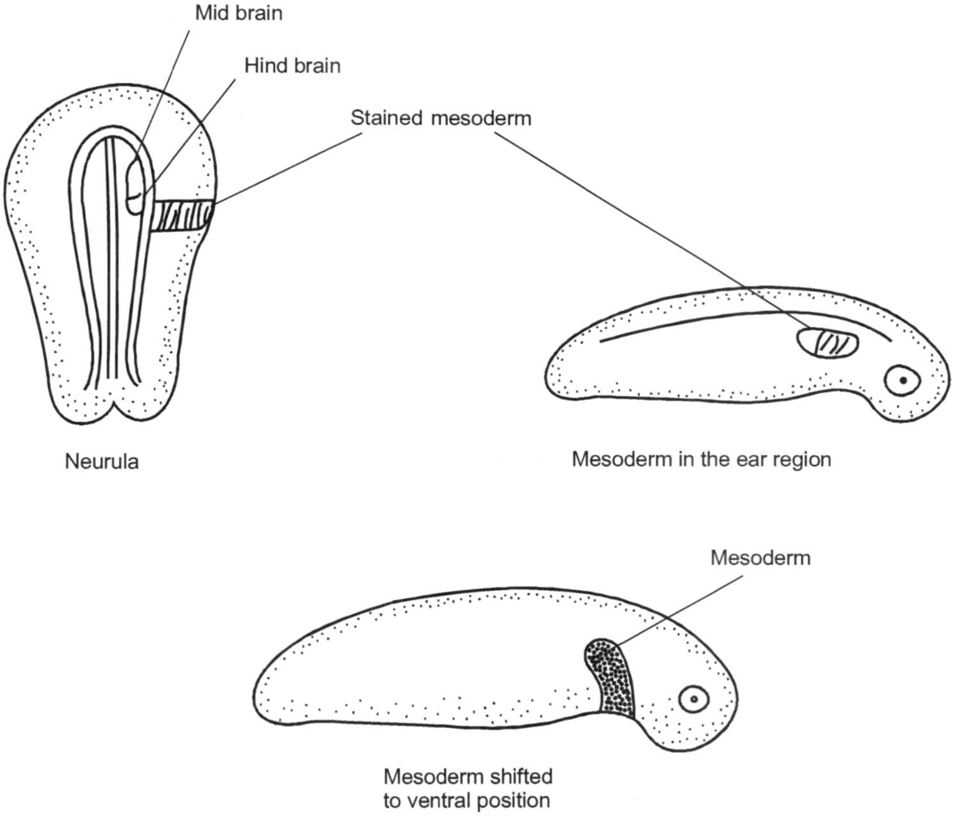

Figure 13.22 Shifting of mesoderm to the ventral region in amphibian neurula.

The dependence of heart development on the endoderm has been tested by hanging-drop cultures. When pieces of mesoderm in Newt embryos were explanted during gastrula stage, there was no differentiation of heart. But in neurula, the differentiation occured to the maximum level. The addition of bits of endodermal tissue increased the percentage of differentiation. However, the rudiment of the heart at the end of neurulation is not strictly determined. The right or left half of the heart rudiment can be removed and the remaining half then develops into a complete heart.

It may be possible to produce two hearts in the same embryo by cutting the heart rudiment lengthwise prior to the union of the two halves of the heart in the middle. Insertion of a somite may prevent the two halves of the heart rudiment from coming together. Under these conditions, two complete pulsating hearts develop.

In addition, it is also found that the **anterior epidermis** is capable of stimulating heart development. But this effect can be considered as only a **supporting factor** because the heart failed to develop in endoderm-free embryos when the epidermis is present.

Modifications of the heart chambers in various vertebrates The heart chambers undergo different changes during development among various vertebrates (Figure 13.23).

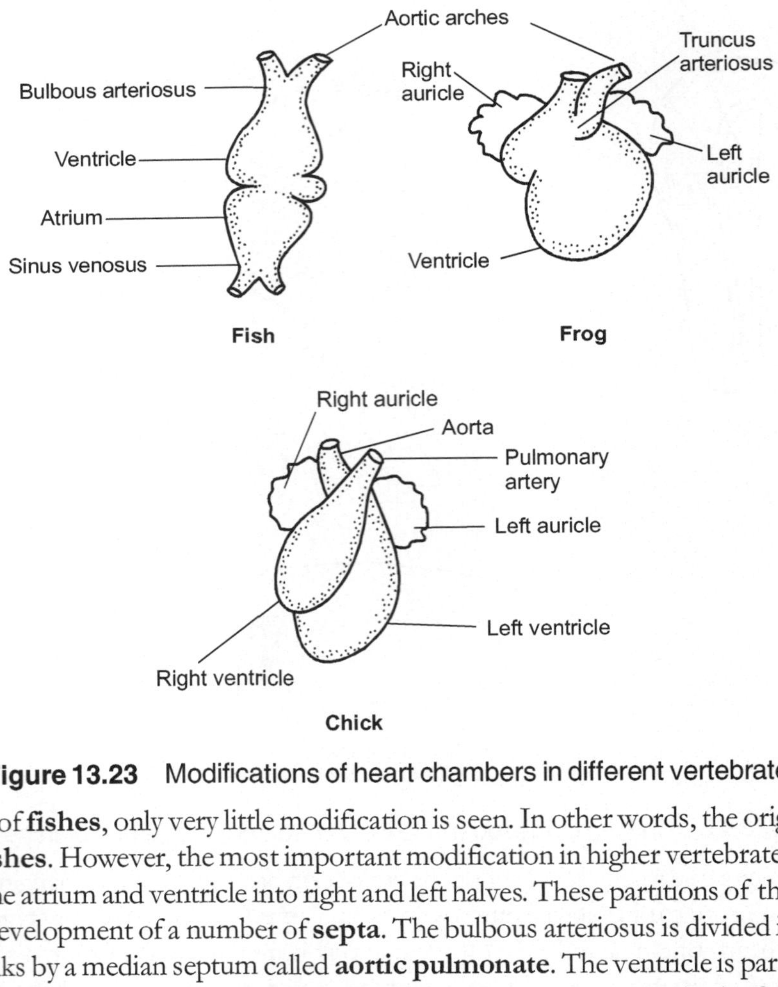

Figure 13.23 Modifications of heart chambers in different vertebrates.

In the case of **fishes**, only very little modification is seen. In other words, the original tubular plan is retained in **fishes**. However, the most important modification in higher vertebrates is a progressive separation of the atrium and ventricle into right and left halves. These partitions of the heart chambers are due to the development of a number of **septa**. The bulbous arteriosus is divided into systemic and pulmonary trunks by a median septum called **aortic pulmonate**. The ventricle is partitioned into right and left ventricles by the **interventricluar septum** in birds and mammals. As far as the atrium is concerned, a single septum namely **interauricular septum** develops in tetrapods. However, in birds and mammals, the partition is not complete in embryonic condition because an aperture namely **foramen ovale** persists until hatching or birth respectively.

Development of Arterial System

When the heart develops as a simple tube, it bifurcates into two large vessels called **omphalomesenteric veins** at the posterior end just in front of the developing liver. They enter into the yolk on the floor of the gut and help to bring the digested yolk. Numerous groups of mesenchyme cells appear in the mesoderm surrounding the gut. These are **blood islands** some of which become blood cells and others form the capillary tubes. The capillaries unite to form larger veins which ultimately open into the omphalomesenteric vein as the **vitelline vein.** This is the venous part of the **vitelline circulation**. At this stage, there is no circulation as the arteries are not yet formed. From the bulbous arteriosus arise two branches each of which gives rise to **four aortic arches** upwards around the pharynx. These aortic arches are at first continuous from the ventral end to the dorsal end. The main ventral vessel is called **ventral aortic roots** (ventral aorta). Dorsal to the pharynx, these vessels form the **dorsal aortic roots** which unite to form a common dorsal aorta behind the pharynx. The **dorsal aorta** is continued as the caudal artery in the tail region.

In frog, the four aortic arches run through third, fourth, fifth and sixth visceral arches. As the first two visceral arches are vestigial, the first and second aortic arches do not function in these visceral arches. In the head region, the ventral aorta continues as the **external carotid artery**. Similarly, the dorsal aortic root is continued in the head region as the **internal carolid artery**. From the common dorsal aorta, a pair of vessels namely **vitelline arteries** arise and break into capillaries in the yolk mass. These capillaries unite with the capillaries of the vitelline vein, thus completing the **vitelline circulation**.

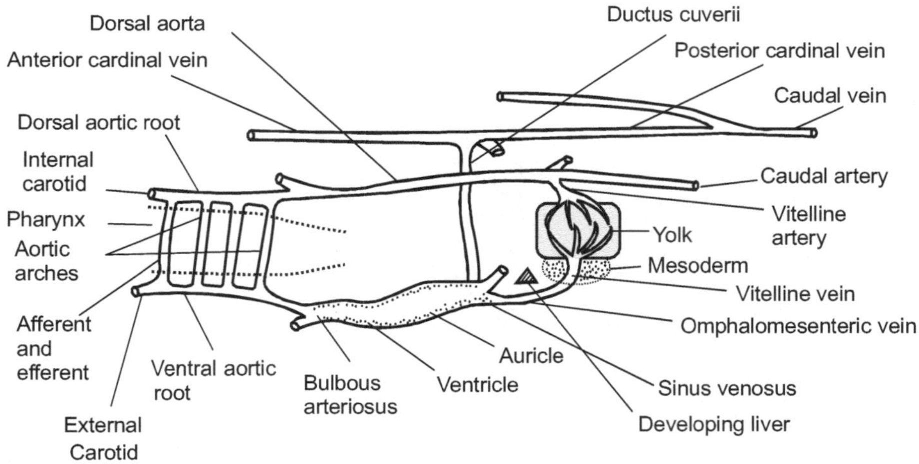

Figure 13.24 Development of circulatory system showing the basic plan before hatching of the tadpole in frog.

By this time, the heart begins to beat and circulation begins. The blood that goes to the head is collected by a pair of veins called **anterior cardinal veins** that appear in the mesenchyme. These veins join with the transverse vessels called **ductus cuverii** which open into the sinus venosis. Similarly, the blood from the posterior part is returned by the **posterior cardinal veins**. These cardinal veins are the principal veins and they bring back blood to the heart. The two posterior cardinal veins unite posteriorly to form the **caudal vein**. Thus the basic plan of the circulatory system as shown in Figure 13.24 is completed even before the tadpole hatches.

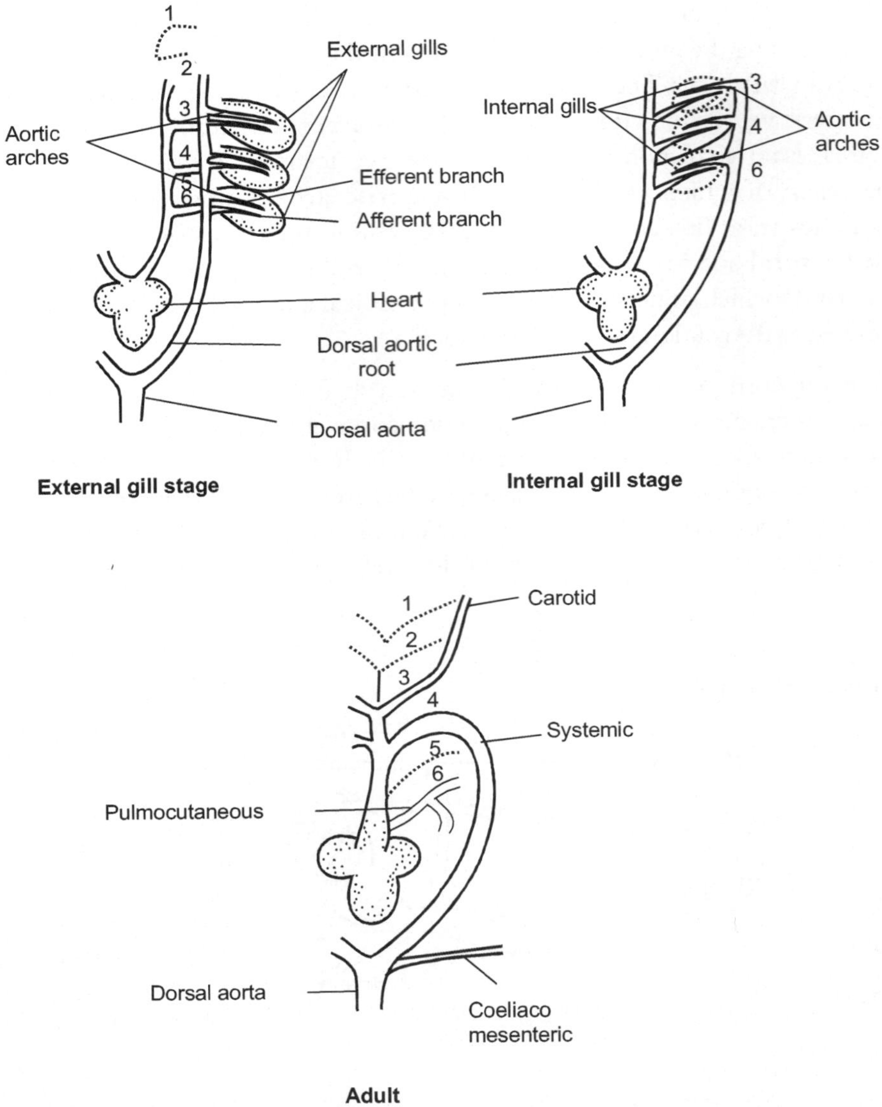

Figure 13.25 Changes in the embryonic circulation at different stages of development in frog.

In frog, many changes occur in the embryonic circulation during larval period and these changes are related to the development of the respiratory organs as well as the kidneys as shown in Figure13.25. When the gills develop on the visceral arches, the aortic arches lose their continuity and become broken. Now the blood passes through the capillaries of the gills. Thus each aortic arch shows the **afferent** and **efferent** sections at the stage when the external and internal gills develop. But at metamorphosis, the afferent and efferent parts in this region once again become continuous. This is because of the disappearance of gills and development of lungs as respiratory organs. The dorsal aortic root between the first and second arches now undergo breakdown. As a result, the blood from the ventral aorta passes through the third arch and then flows forward to the head. This arch becomes the **carotid artery** of the adult. The next aortic arch which passes through the fourth visceral arch becomes prominent and forms the **systemic artery** of the adult. The aortic arch, which is small right from the beginning and passes through the fifth visceral arch, is lost. The aortic arch which passes through the sixth visceral arch develops a new blood vessel and becomes the **pulmocutaneous artery**. The connection of this artery with the dorsal aortic root is lost. Now the vitelline arteries fuse to form the **coeliacomesenteric artery** of the adult. At the time when the tail is lost, the caudal artery is lost.

Changes are also prominent in the part of the venous system during its development. Of the two omphalomesenteric veins, the right one disappears and the left one becomes conspicuous forming the **hepatic vein**. The vitelline vein now opens into the liver thus becoming the **hepatic portal vein** of the adult (Figure13.26.). The cardinal system also undergoes changes. The anterior cardinal veins remain as **internal jugular veins** of the adult and the **external jugular** veins are new formation. These two jugular veins combine to form the **precaval vein** of the adult after the separation from the postcardinal vein. The **postcaval vein** arises as a new formation and its development is complicated and related to the development of successive kidneys. Along with the development of the postcaval vein, there are changes in the postcardinal veins. The **anterior abdominal vein** is a new formation on the ventral body wall. With the formation of the **renal portal system**, the adult condition of circulatory system is reached.

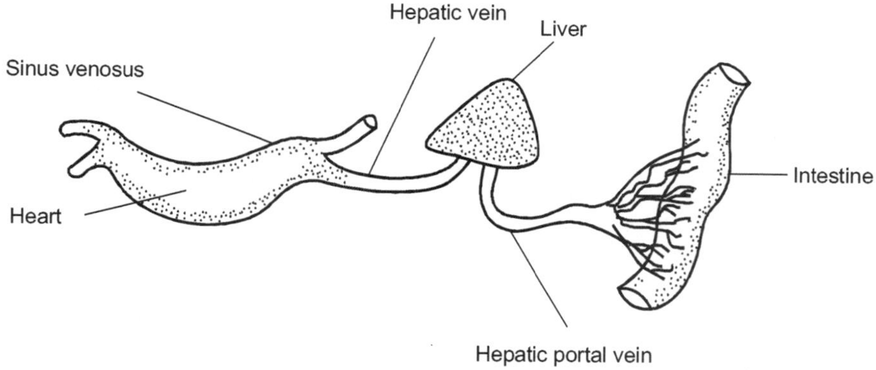

Figure 13.26 Development of hepatic portal system in frog.

ORGANOGENESIS IN CHICK

Development of Arterial System

In chick, the heart becomes chambered as in the case of frog with the omphalomesenteric vein opening into the sinus venosus and the bulbous arteriosus continues as the ventral aortic roots. The two **ventral aortic roots** run forward and bend anteriorly around the pharynx as the dorsal aortic root. As it bends, it runs through the mandibular arch of that side forming the first aortic arch. Then a second arch develops at about the second day of incubation and these two arches disappear on the fourth day of incubation. Later, the third, fourth, fifth and sixth aortic arches appear. The fifth one is very weak from the beginning and it finally disappears. The **dorsal aortic root** of the two sides unite to form the **dorsal aorta** which remains separated in the posterior end and continues in the tail region. A pair of **vitelline arteries** arise from the dorsal aorta and enter the yolk sac (extra-embryonic region). The capillaries of the vitelline arteries and of the vitelline veins become connected, thus completing the vitelline circulation (Figure13.27).

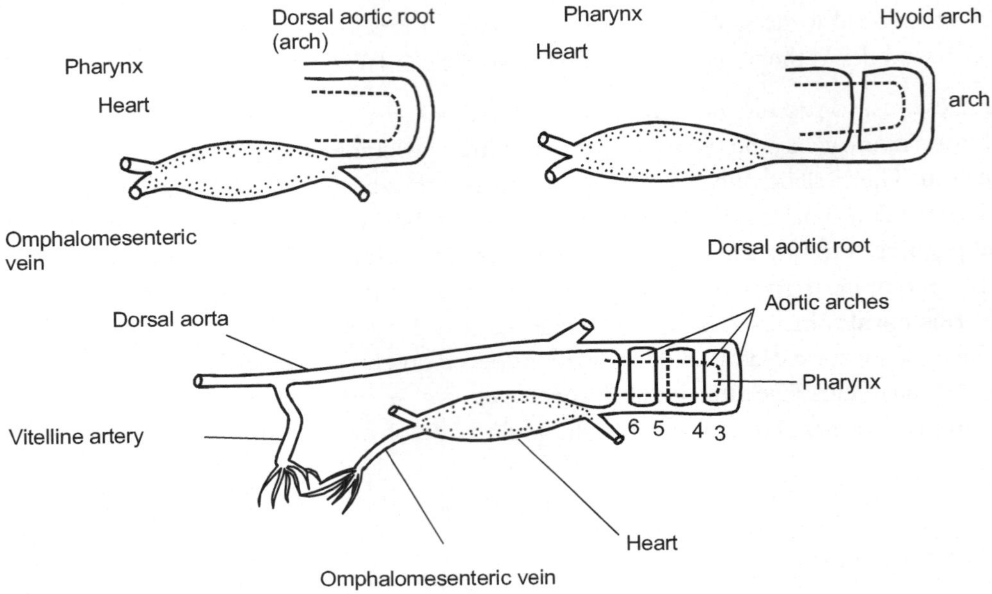

Figure 13.27 Development of aortic arches and vitelline arteries in chick.

As the yolk lies outside the embryo, this is an extra-embryonic circulation. As in the case of frog, in chick also, the anterior and posterior cardinal systems develop to bring the blood back to the heart. At a later stage, the **allantois** develops from the hindgut and receives the **allantoic artery** from the iliac branch of the dorsal aorta. The blood from the allantois is returned by the **allantoic vein** which runs straight to the heart opening into the sinus venosus, thus completing the **allantoic circulation**. This is the **second extra-embryonic circulation** in chick. Figure 13.28 explains the formation of blood vessels during the development of chick embryo. The embryonic circulation described above becomes gradually transformed into the adult condition through the occurrence of the following changes:

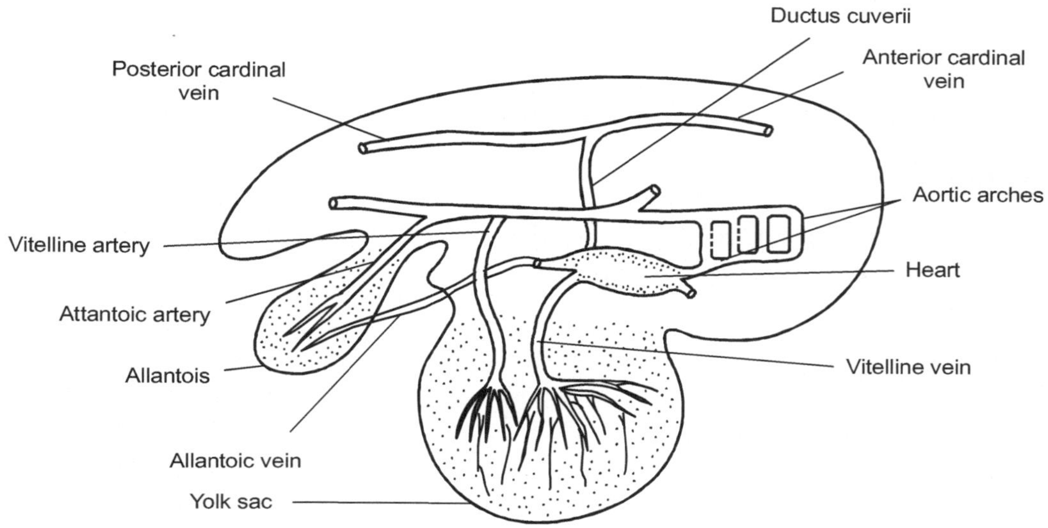

Figure13.28 Development of blood vessels exhibiting extra-embryonic circulation in chick embryo.

1. Of the remaining aortic arches, the first one (the original third one) becomes the **carotid artery** of the adult.
2. The continuation of the dorsal aortic root becomes the **internal carotid artery**. Similarly, the **external carotid artery** is formed as a continuation of the ventral aortic root.
3. The next aortic arch (the fourth one) on the right side becomes the **right systemic artery** whereas the **left systemic artery** disappears. (But in mammals, the right one disappears and the left one is retained).
4. The original fifth arch completely disappears and the sixth one develops a new artery, the **pulmonary artery** which goes to the lungs. The dorsal aortic root now breaks its connection with the pulmonary artery.
5. Behind the pharynx, there is a single **dorsal aorta** which is continued as the **caudal artery.**
6. The vitelline arteries become the **anterior mesenteric** artery of the adult.
7. When the **yolk sac** is absorbed, most of the vitelline circulation disappears. The newly formed liver now surrounds the omphalomesenteric veins. The posterior part of the vitelline veins open into the liver to become the **hepatic portal vein** of the adult.
8. The anterior cardinals become the **precaval veins** whereas the posterior cardinals undergo extensive changes in relation to the development of successive kidneys. Likewise, the development of the **postcaval vein** occurs in relation to the development of the kidneys.

DEVELOPMENT OF KIDNEYS IN VERTEBRATES

In vertebrates, kidneys develop from the **intermediate mesoderm** or **nephrotome**. During embryonic stages of all vertebrates, certain tubes make their appearance in the anterior region of the embryo at the upper part of the lateral plate mesoderm. These are called as **pronephric tubules**.

Pronephros or Head Kidney

Pronephros appears during the development of all vertebrates but disappears in adults. However, this kidney remains as a functional one in ammocoetus larva, some larval fishes and amphibians. In adult Myxine, there is an indication of pronephros.

The development of pronephoros is shown in Figure13.29. In the anterior region of the embryo, the nephrotome differentiates as the nephridial tubules called **pronephridial tubules**. A pair of tubules develop in each segment. Each tubule opens into the coelom by a ciliated funnel called the **nephrotome**. The other ends of these tubules will join together to form a common duct called **pronephric duct** or **segmental duct** which runs posteriorly and opens into the cloaca.

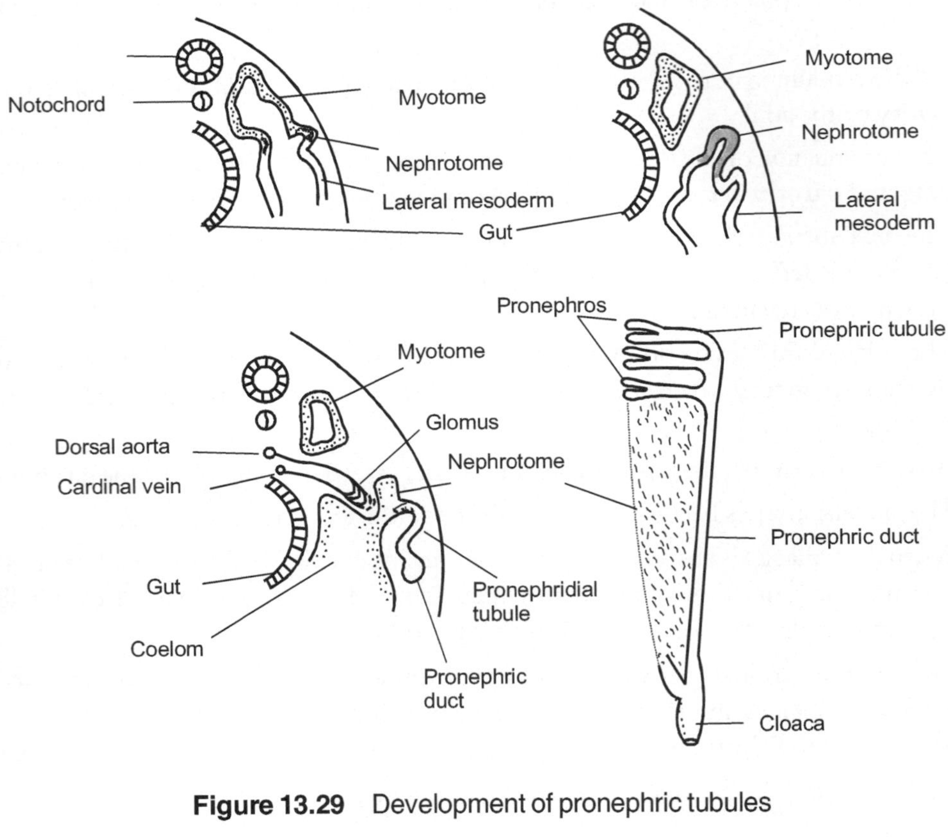

Figure 13.29 Development of pronephric tubules

These tubules do not have direct connection with the blood vessels. However, the blood vessels form a network called **glomus** in the coelomic epithelium. It is this region where the nitrogenous wastes are separated and passed on into the coelom. From the coelom, the wastes are collected and passed on to the cloaca through the nephridial tubules and segmental duct. The pronephros usually disappears when the embryo is about to hatch and then the next kidney called the **mesonephros** is formed.

Mesonephros or Trunk Kidney

It is the adult functional kidney in all the **anamniotes**. In frog, the kidney is highly advanced.

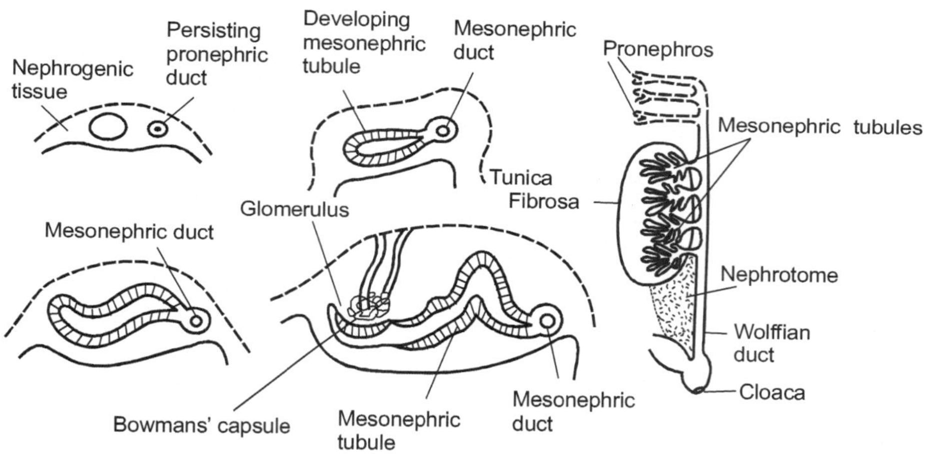

Figure 13.30 Development of mesonephros

This kidney is formed posterior to the region of the pronephros and the development of mesonephros is shown in Figure 13.30. From the nephrotome, mesonephric tubules develop, i.e., the nephrogenic tissue becomes tubular and establishes connection with the already existing pronephric duct which is now called as **mesonephric duct** or **Wolffian duct**. The tubules divide and subdivide so that many nephridial tubules are formed. Each tubule has two structures in its free end. One opens into the coelom as the **nephrotome** and the other one becomes cup-like and is called **Bowmann's capsule** enclosing a network of blood vessels called **glomerulus**. These two structures together constitute the **malpighian body**. All the tubules of each side become enclosed by a membrane called **tunica fibrosa**, thus forming a compact body. In frog, the nephrotomes are few in number and they do not open into the coelom but are found enclosed within the kidney.

Metanephros or Tail Kidney

It is the adult functional kidney in the amniotes and is found in the posterior region of the body.

It also develops from the nephrotomes of the posterior region and its developmental processes are shown in Figure 13.31. The nephrogenic tissue forms a large number of tubules which are highly coiled in each segment. These tubules develop only the malpighian bodies and the nephrotomes never appear. From the base of the mesonephric duct, a projection is formed. This continues as a duct towards the group of metanephric tubules. All these tubules open in a common place called **pelvis** which in turn establishes connection with the newly formed duct, the **ureter**. All the tubules become enclosed by the **tunica fibrosa** forming a compact body.

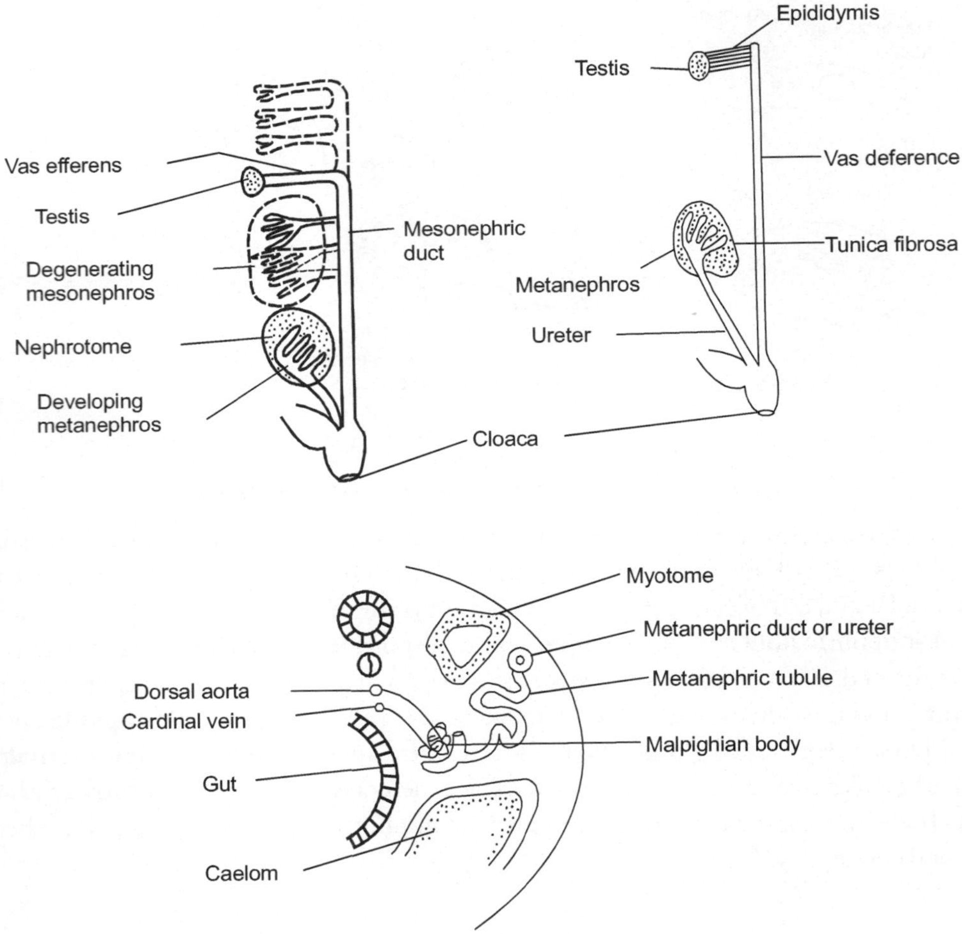

Figure 13.31 Development of metanephros.

REVIEW QUESTIONS

1. Write on essay on the germ layers and their derivatives.
2. Describe the development of dorsal tubular nerve cord/notochord/alimentary canal and gills in amphioxus.
3. Explain the formation of coelom and differentiation of mesoderm in Amphioxus.
4. Describe the development of brain/eye/ear/heart/in frog.
5. Describe the development of coelom and mesoderm in frog.
6. Write explanatory note on the development of circulatory system with the basic plan in the embryogenesis of frog.
7. Enumerate the changes in the embryonic circulation at different stages of development in frog.
8. In what ways does the development of arterial system in chick differs from that of frog?
9. Give an account of extra-embryonic circulation in chick.
10. Describe the role of induction on the development of brain/eye/ear/heart.
11. Write an essay on the development of kidneys in vertebrates.
12. Give notes on the following:
    i. Primary germ layers
    ii. Neurula
    iii. Medullary plate
    iv. Neurenteric canal
    v. Somatic and splanchnic mesoderm
    vi. Enterocoelic coelom
    vii. Schizocoelic coelom
    viii. Encephalon
    ix. Optic cup
    x. Auditory placode
    xi. Endocardial tubes
    xii. Vitelline circulation
    xiii. Extra-embryonic circulation

14

INDUCTION (ORGANIZER CONCEPT)

In multicellular organisms, the normal development involves interacting systems in which some embryonic cells are capable of stimulating the differentiation of specific tissues or organs. In other words, the embryonic cells and tissues get some kind of stimulus from the neighbouring tissues so that the recipient tissues develop into particular organs. This stimulus is called as **induction** or **embryonic induction** or **induction interactions**. Here a stimulus of chemical nature is transmitted by an embryonic tissue which influences the formation of a specific organ in the adjacent region. The tissue which produces the induction on another tissue is called **inductor**. Some more efficient cells or tissues that induce the entire process of development are known as **organizers**. The chemical substances produced by the inductors are called **evocators**.

If the organizer is removed from early embryos, they normally fail to develop. **Spemann** (1935) made experiments in newt's egg to emphasize this concept. When the fertilized egg of newt was constricted into equal halves passing through the grey crescent by ligature, each half developed into a compete larva. If the ligature was made on the egg in such a way that one half contained the grey crescent and the other one without the grey crescent, the half with the grey crescent developed into a complete larva and the other half without the grey crescent was transformed into an unorganized mass (Figure14.1). From these experiments, he concluded that the greycrescent is important for the normal development of the embryo.

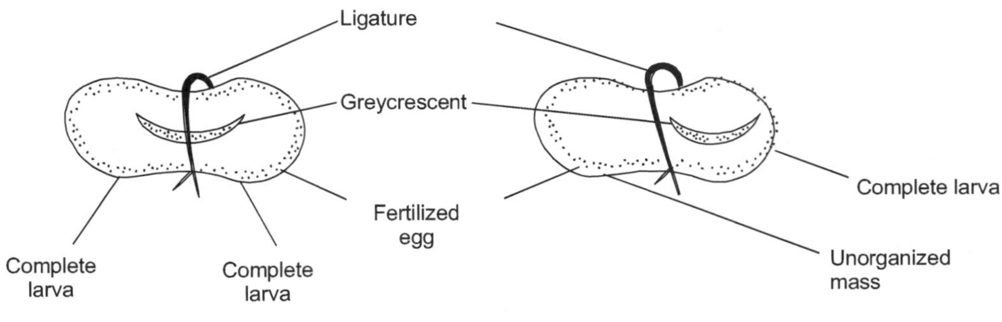

Figure 14.1 Ligature experiments in Newt's eggs.

In an early gastrula, the grey crescent represents the dorsal lip of the blastopore which is formed by involution, developing into chordamesoderm. If this dorsal lip is removed from an early gastrula, no further development was noticed in the embryo. On the other hand, if a dorsal lip from an early gastrula is grafted into another one, the embryonic tissue was influenced by the grafted dorsal lip to develop into the secondary embryo (Figure 14.2). Thus the, dorsal lip is undoubtedly an organizer which causes the development of a complete embryo. **Spemann** and **Mangold** (1924) considered the dorsal lip as the **primary organizer** as it serves as the first embryonic induction during development. In this way, the grey crescent in the fertilized egg, the dorsal lip in the early embryo and the chordamesoderm in the gastrula have the properties of organizers.

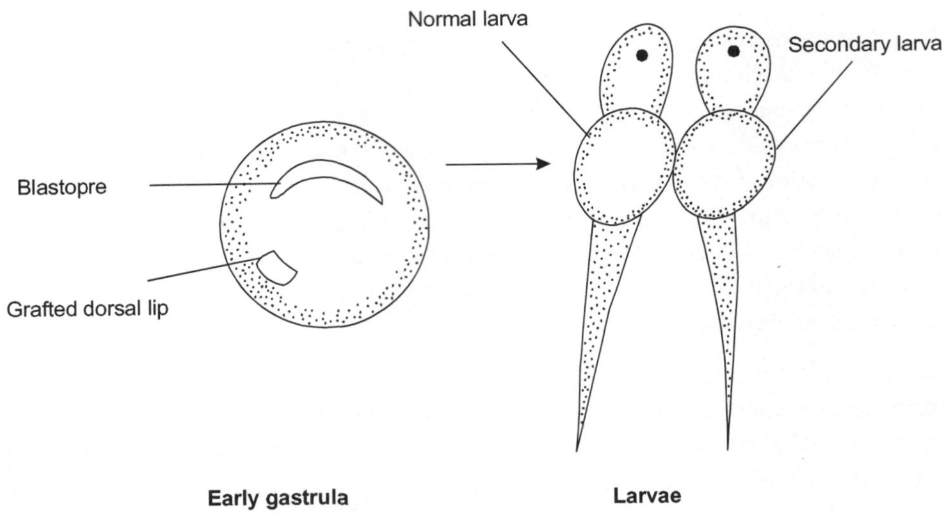

Figure 14.2 Grafting of dorsal lip to an early gastrula of Newt

TYPES OF ORGANIZERS

According to Lovtrup (1974), the embryonic inductions basically include two major types namely **endogenous induction** and **exogenous induction.**

Endogenous Induction

Here the embryonic cells like the dorsal lip of the amphibian blastopore possess endogenous evocators and so they undergo gradual diversification involving self-differentiation or self-transformation.

Exogenous Induction

In this type of induction, a cell or a tissue exerts certain external influence on the neighbouring cells. If the influence of the inductor produces its own kinds of cells, then it is known as **homotypic**

induction. On the other hand, if the inductor influences the formation of different kinds of tissues, it is **heterotypic induction**. The development of an adjacent tissue only in presence of inducer depending on its presumptive fate is known as **permissive induction**. The stimulation of the development of the same cells with different presumptive fates by the inductor is **instructive induction.**

Based on the specific influences exerted by the induction on the receptor sites, the inductors are distinguished into various types. The dorsal lip or the anterior part of the roof of the archenteron influences the development of head organs and so is called as **head inductor** which may induce the development of forebrain, eyes and rudimentary nose. Therefore, it can also be referred to as **archencephalic inductor**. The dorsal lip, at a later stage of development, stimulates the development of midbrain and hindbrain along with the ear vesicles and so it is **deuterencephalic inductor**. As the posterior part of the roof of the archenteron at the end of gastrulation exerts influence on the development of trunk organs and tail somites, it is the **trunk** or **spinocaudal** inductor.

Sequential induction During embryonic development, one kind of tissue, in general, influences the neighbouring tissue to develop into a particular organ which simultaneously gets the ability to induce the adjacent one. This tissue, in turn, may induce the development of successive organs. For example, the chordamesoderm influences the development of the forebrain and optic region at the anterior end of the embryo and so is called as **primary organizer**. During the development of the eye, the optic vesicle (optic cup) induces the development of the lens from the overlying ectoderm and so that is called **secondary organizer**. Again, the developing lens causes the formation of cornea, constituting the **tertiary organizer**. Thus, the induction of a series of organizers resulting in the progressive development of embryonic organs is called **sequential induction**. Here, if one step is disturbed, the next steps of development fail to occur.

Mutual or Synergistic Induction

In this type of induction, two different tissues mutually interact with each other so that each causes the other to develop. If the two inductors are separated, they will not undergo development. In tissue culture experiments, the uretery bud and the nephrogenic cord of mouse embryo interact with each other and develop into kidney tubules as in the embryo. When these two embryonic tissues are separated by a porous membrane, they are found to develop kidney tubules.

Neural Induction and its Mechanism

The roof of the archenteron induces the differentiation and development of the nervous system and this phenomenon is called **neural induction**. The mechanism of neural induction is not fully known. It is believed that the movement of the cells generates a dynamic effect which induces differentiation. But this view has been proved to be wrong. When the organizer tissues were subjected to crushing, freezing, heating or other injuries and explanted to the embryos, they were found to induce the differentiation of the neural tube. Therefore, it was concluded that induction is a chemical effect caused by the chemical substances called **evocators**. The evocators probably originate as products of cell metabolism, especially as diffusible substances of protein nature and diffuse into the environment.

Moreover, the cells in the environment must be sensitive to the action of these substances. It was thought that the appearance of organizing power was somewhat linked to the metabolism of glycogen. But it is shown that the evocator substances are soluble in solvents like ether but not in water and so they could not be glycogen in nature. Some embryologists have opined that the evocators could be sterol derivatives. It was also claimed that they are nucleic acids as the dorsal lip contains numerous granules with nucleic acids. But recent studies indicate that the substance may not be a single entity but a group of nucleoproteins, each specific to the induction of a particular tissue. In addition, a number of inorganic and organic substances have been found to be neural inductors. Therefore, many theories are put forward with regard to the mechanism of neural induction and are as follows :

***Gradient theory (Toivonen,* 1955 *and Yamada,* 1961)** According to this theory, two chemical factors namely **"neuralizing agent"** and **"mesodermalizing agent"** are involved in the process of neural induction. The neuralizing agent occurs in highest concentration on the dorsal side of the embryo and diminishes laterally. But the "mesodermalizing agent" is an antero-posterior gradient with highest concentration in the posterior region. Thus, the neural agent induces the development of forebrain behind which the mesodermalizing agent stimulates the formation of mid and hindbrains.

One-factor hypothesis (Nieukoop, 1996) This theory postulates that the inductor is nothing but only one factor which induces different organs at different times.

Ionic theory (Barth and Barth, 1968) This theory points out that the release of ions in bound forms causes induction by altering the ratio of free and bound ions in the cells.

Protein denaturation theory (Ranzi, 1963) According to this theory, the centres which possess greater metabolic activity are the sites of protein denaturation. For example, the grey crescent of frog's egg stimulating the development of notochord and neural tube is shown to be the centre of high metabolic activity. Therefore, it is presumable that protein denaturation in inductors is the main cause for the embryonic induction.

PROPERTIES OF ORGANIZERS

1. Organizers are capable of self-differentiation and self-organization.
2. They possess the power to induce changes within and in the surrounding cells.
3. They have the ability to induce even after crushing, freezing or killing.
4. Induction occurs not only in the tissues of the same or closely related species but also in the tissues of animals belonging to different groups.
5. More acidic and alkaline solutions are shown to have the ability of induction.

It is clearly evident that any part of the presumptive ectoderm of gastrula can induce the development of nervous system. This reaction is the highest in early gastrula and midgastrula, diminishes in late gastrula and completely disappears at the beginning of neurilation. Moreover the reacting cells must be in a particular state to differentiate into a specific organ by the induction. For example, if the inductor is transplanted in the blastula stage of frog's egg, the ectoderm reacts only after gastrulation. This is the

competence of the embryonic tissue which is the ability of a specific tissue to react with a particular inductor. The competence of cells can be related with the transcription of RNA molecules as these molecules are transcribed only during the process of gastrulation. Further, the transplantation experiments conclude that while the organizers determine what organs are to be formed, the genes control the details of those organs.

REVIEW QUESTIONS

1. Write an essay on induction or organizer concept.
2. Classify the different types of organizers with examples.
3. Give an account of neural induction and its mechanism.
4. Explain the various theories with regard to neural induction.
5. Write brief notes on:
    i. Spemann's work on induction
    ii. Sequential induction
    iii. Important properties of organizers
    iv. Evocators

15

FOETAL MEMBRANES OR EXTRA-EMBRYONIC MEMBRANES IN AMNIOTES (CHICK AND PIG)

In the development of amniotes, a few important embryonic structures are formed. However, they do not remain in adults as such and these structures have evolved to meet out the needs of development on land. In other words, they develop as an adaptation for land development. In amniotes, the young ones hatch out or are born at a comparatively late stage as small adult forms. Therefore, there is need for the provision of food during this long period in terrestrial eggs. In the eggs of birds, there is plenty of yolk whereas in typical placental mammals, nourishment is absorbed by the embryo from the mother through the **placenta**. In vertebrates, only a portion of the fertilized egg develops into an embryo while the other parts around the embryo constitute the extra-embryonic regions. These areas give rise to various foetal membranes such as **yolk sac**, **amnion**, **chorion** or **serosa** and **allantois** which are collectively called **extra–embryonic membranes**. In the embryo, these foetal membranes play a major role in nutrition, respiration and excretion as well as in providing protection.

TYPES OF FOETAL MEMBRANES

i. Yolk Sac

In chick, a structure develops to digest the yolk and pass it on to the embryo. This membrane is called as **yolk sac** which is made up of **splanchnopleure** (endoderm and splanchnic mesoderm). In other words, a part of the wall of the gut extends out of the embryo and envelops the yolk. The yolk sac becomes vascular and folds into the yolk to facilitate the digestion and absorption of the yolk. The absorbed yolk is passed on to the embryo through the vitelline circulation. In mammals, the yolk sac is formed as an ancestral memory from the reptilian ancestors and remains functionless.

ii. Amnion

This is another foetal membrane which seems to have developed as a protective structure arising from the **somatopleure** (ectoderm and mesoderm) to prevent desiccation. The amnion encloses a cavity called **amniotic cavity** containing a fluid namely **amniotic fluid** which prevents the drying up of the embryo inside the egg during development. In mammals, the amniotic fluid is slightly alkaline in nature and it can be detected at the 8th week of gestation. It is in continuous circulation inside the amniotic cavity and its content is replaced at an interval of 2–9 hours through the foetal and maternal circulation at a rate of 300–400 ml/h. But in the case of mammals, protective function is not necessary as the foetus develops inside the body of the mother. However, the ammion still develops in mammals and acts as a shock absorber preventing mechanical shocks.

iii. Serosa or Chorion

The third embryonic membrane is the serosa in the case of birds and chorion in mammals. Like that of amnion, this membrane also develops from the **somatopleure** (ectoderm and somatic mesoderm). In chick, the serosa is very close to the egg shell and so helps in respiration. In mammals, the chorion and its villi play an important role in the formation of placenta.

iv. Allantois

It is the another embryonic membrane formed from the **splanchnopleure** as an extension of the hindgut. It helps in respiration and in storing the excretory products in birds. In mammals, the allantois participates in the formation of placenta. The extra-embryonic membranes of chick are depicted in Figure 15.1.

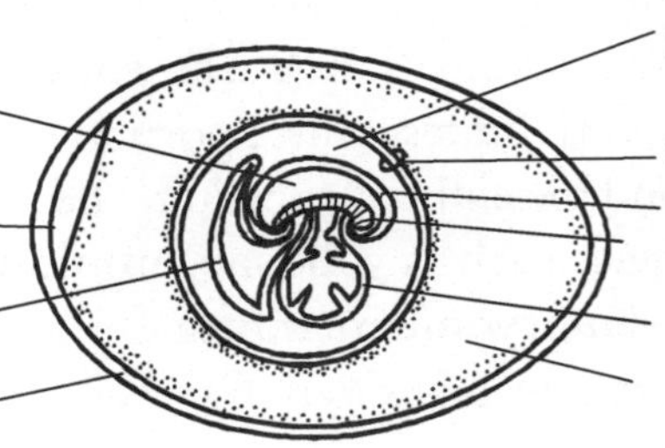

Figure 15.1 Chick's egg showing the extra-embryonic membranes (5–6 days of incubation).

DEVELOPMENT OF FOETAL MEMBRANES IN CHICK

Yolk Sac

Earlier than 20 hours of incubation, the embryo is not separated from the rest of the blastoderm. At About 20 hours of incubation, a groove appears in front of the head. As a result, the head becomes lifted up from the rest of the blastoderm. This groove develops into the head and the fold consists of all the three germ layers namely ectoderm, endoderm and mesoderm. The space under the head is called **subcephalic pocket**. When the fold is formed, the foregut comes to have a floor and extends backwards so that the fold becomes deeper (Figure 15.2a and 15.2b). A similar fold arises at the tail end of the embryo with the resultant formation of the floor of the hindgut. As the hindgut extends forwards, the midgut becomes reduced. When these two folds are formed, the mesoderm splits into two layers namely somatic and splanchnic layers (Figure15.2 c). The ectoderm and the somatic mesoderm are together called as **somatopleure** and the endoderm and the splanchnic mesoderm are collectively called as **splanchnopleure.** Now the splanchnopleure surrounds the yolk forming the **yolk sac** which becomes vascular and folds into the yolk, thus penetrating the whole yolk (Figure 15.2d).

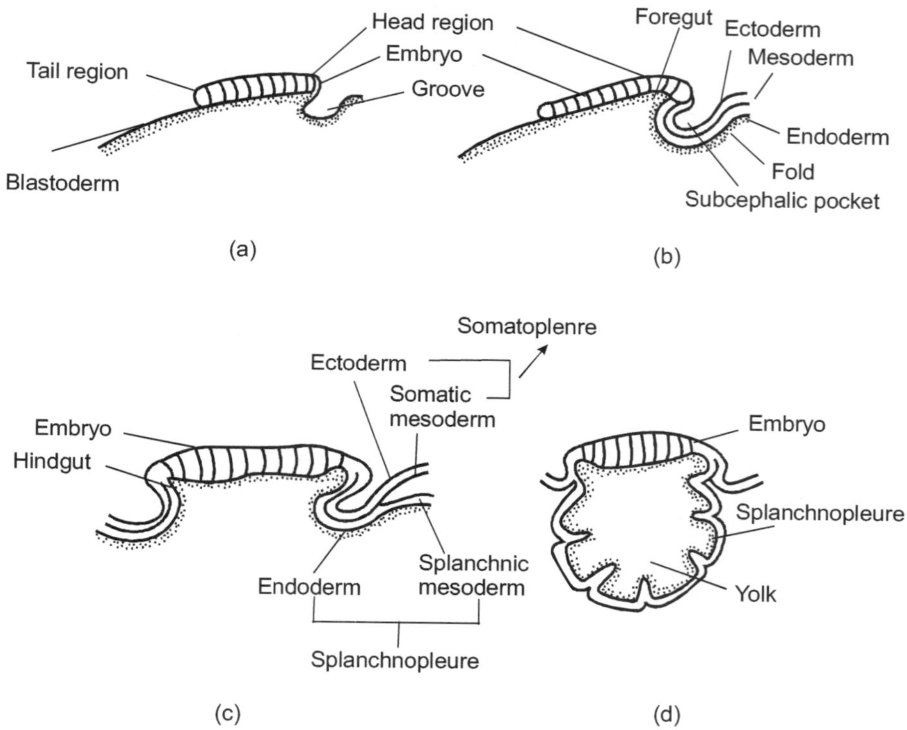

Figure 15.2 Development of yolk sac in chick. a) Formation of groove in the head region of the embryo b) Formation of subcephalic pocket and foregut c) Formation of hindgut and spliting of mesoderm and d) Formation of yolk sac.

Serosa and Amnion

When the yolk sac is extending over the yolk, the somatopleure around the embryo simultaneously gives rise to the serosa and amnion.

The amnion first appears in front of the gut of the embryo as a ridge of the somatopleure at about 30 hours of incubation. This fold grows over the head like a cap at about 32 hours of incubation. This is called **head fold**. A similar fold is also formed in the tail region and is called **tail fold** which extends forwards. Similar folds arise from the two sides of the embryo during the 4th day of incubation (Figure15.3a). All these folds meet at a point and form the structure called **seroamniotic junction** near the tail region. Thus a complete dome-like structure is developed. This structure consists of four membranes arising from the somatopleure. Out of these four membranes, the outer two layers form the serosa (with outer ectoderm and inner mesoderm) and the inner two layers form the amnion (with outer mesoderm and inner ectoderm). In between the amnion and the embryo, there is a cavity called **amniotic cavity** filled with **amniotic fluid** which prevents desiccation of the embryo. An extension of the coelom is found between the serosa and amnion and is called as the **extra-embryonic coelom** (Figure 15.3b and 15.3c).

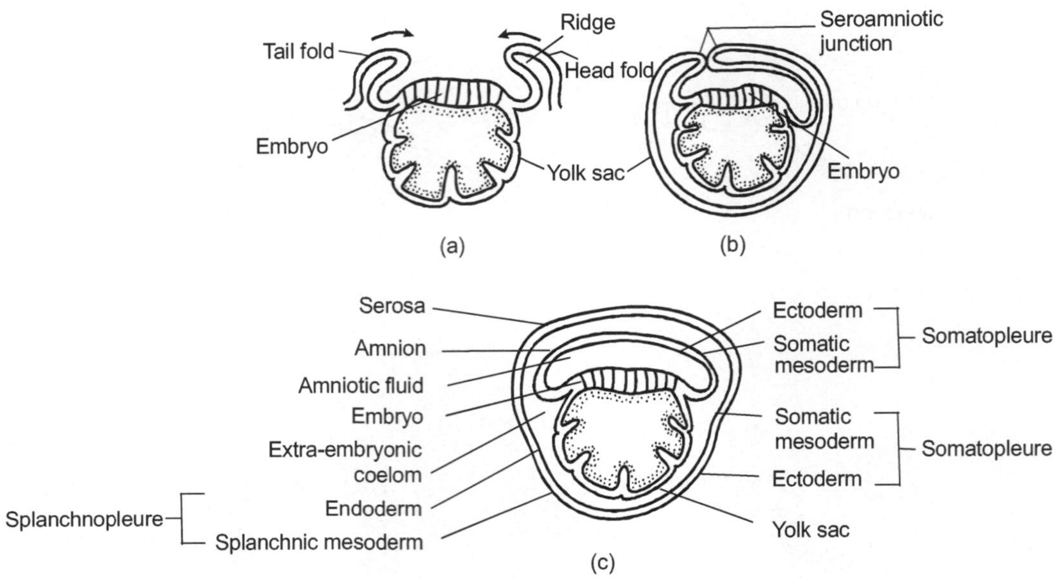

Figure 15.3 Development of amnion and serosa in chick. a) Formation of head and tail folds b) Formation of seroamniotic junction and c) Fully formed ammion and serosa.

Allantois

The allantois makes its appearance at about 72 hours of incubation as an outgrowth of the hindgut. It is formed off by the splanchnopleure with an inner endoderm and the outer mesoderm. It grows rapidly into the extra-embryonic coelom, becomes fairly a big bag on the 4th day of incubation and expands very quickly throughout the extra-embryonic space (Figure 15.4).

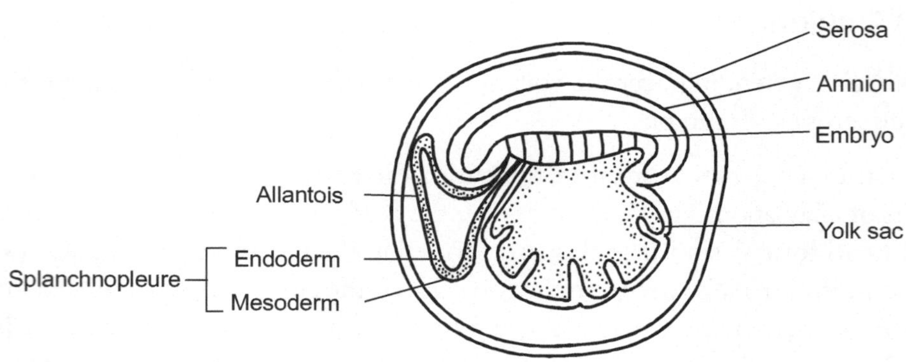

Figure 15.4 Development of allantois in chick.

The stalks of the allantois and the yolk sac together constitute **the umbilical cord** in mammals. The main function of the allantois is respiratory and it also helps in embryonic excretion. The excretory product of the embryo is uric acid which is deposited in the allantois and the water is reabsorbed by the blood vessels.

The egg yolk is completely exhausted towards the end of incubation so that the yolk sac becomes smaller in size. A couple of days before hatching, the yolk sac is absorbed and becomes part of the ventral wall of the gut. During hatching, the other membranes are left inside the egg and by this time they have dried up.

MAMMALIAN FOETAL MEMBRANES

In mammals, the foetal membranes are very similar to that of chick (Figure 15.5). Though the mammalian egg is secondarily yolkless, the foetal membranes are not lost but they have acquired new functions. In mammals, the amnion, chorion, yolk sac and allantois develop exactly in the same way as that of chick. But one major difference is that it is the tail fold of the amnion that develops first followed by the formation of head fold. The chorion and allantios form a complex structure with the uterine wall forming the **placenta**.

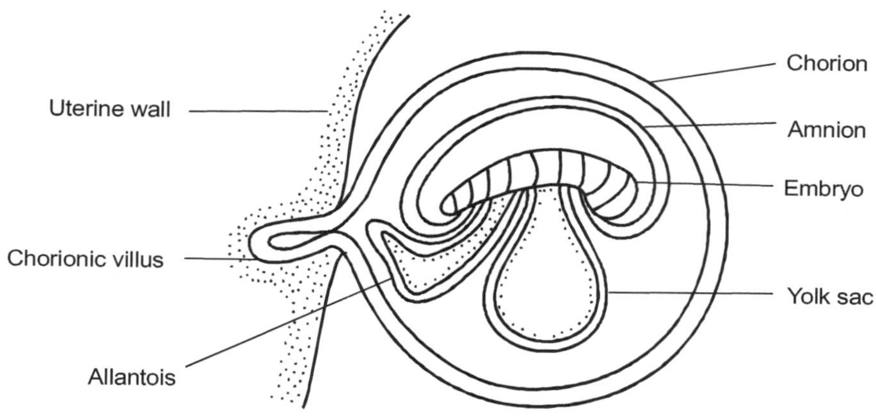

Figure 15.5 Foetal membranes in pig.

REVIEW QUESTIONS

1. What are foetal or extra-embryonic membranes? Explain their structure and functions with examples.
2. Describe the development of yolk sac/amnion and serosa/allantois in chick.
3. Write a brief account on the role played by the foetal membranes.
4. Write notes on
   i. Yolk sac
   ii. Amnion
   iii. Allantois
   iv. Head and tail folds
   v. Sero-amniotic junction

16

IMPLANTATION AND PLACENTATION IN MAMMALS (EUTHERIAN MAMMALS)

IMPLANTATION

Embryonic development in all viviparous animals occurs within the uterus of the mother in order to get physiological requirements such as food, oxygen, etc. Therefore, the embryo becomes attached to the wall of the uterus for further development. In mammals, the fertilized egg after blastulation (blastocyst) moves to the uterus and gets attached to the uterine wall. This process is called **implantation** which is shown to be under the control of ovarian hormones namely progesterone and estrogen. These hormones influence the preparation of the uterine wall to receive the fertilized egg.

The process of implantation varies in different mammals and can be categorized into three types namely **superficial implantation, interstitial implantation** and **eccentric implantation** as shown in Figure 16.1.

Superficial implantation In this type, the blastocyst attaches to the surface of the uterine epithelium so that it is found in the uterine cavity (Figure 16.1.a) as in carnivores, insectivores, ungulates and monkeys.

Interstitial implantation Here the blastocyst deeply penetrates into the uterine wall and further development of the embryo proceeds within the uterine wall (Figure 16.1.b) as in man, apes, bats, guinea pigs, etc.

Eccentric implantation when the blastocyst is found to lie in the uterine sac which loses contact with the main uterine wall, as in squirrels and rats, it is called eccentric type (Figure16.1.c).

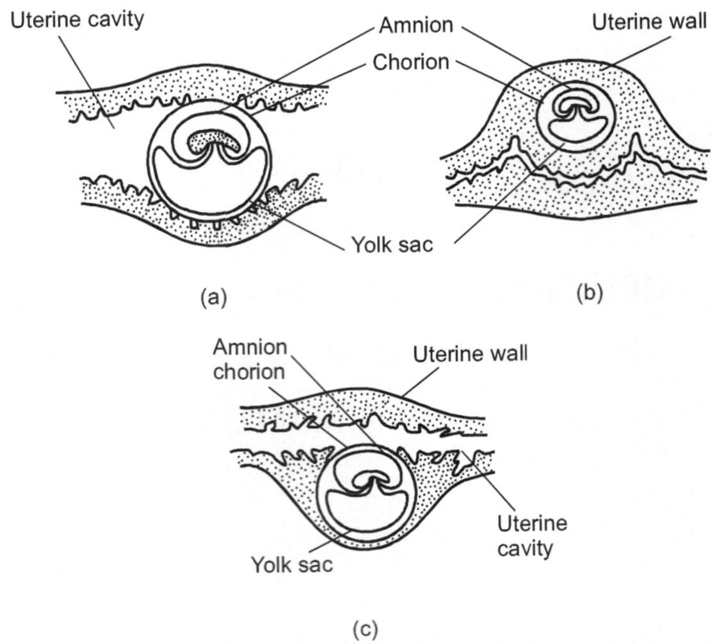

Figure 16.1 Categorization of implantation. a) Superficial implantation b) Interstitial implantation and c) Eccentric implantation.

PLACENTATION

Placenta is a complex structure consisting of both maternal and foetal tissues namely uterine wall, chorion and allantois. In other words, it is the structure formed by the foetal membranes and the uterine mucosa for physiological interchange between the mother and embryo. After the entry into the uterus, the embryo utilizes the organic substances secreted by the glands of the uterine wall during the initial stages until the connection between the foetal and maternal tissues is made through the placenta. Later, the developing embryo depends solely on the substances provided by the mother. Placentation in mammals can be studied under the following headings.

Mode of Formation

The mammalian placenta is formed by the extra-embryonic membranes (chorion, allantois or yolk sac) and the endometrium of the uterus with a large blood sinus called intervillous space in between them. The chorionic blood supply is either due to the vitelline circulation of the yolk sac or the allantoic circulation of allantois. Accordingly, the placenta of mammals can be divided into the following types

i. *Chorio-vitelline placenta or yolk sac placenta* Here, the blastocyst or cystoblastula is fitted into a shallow depression of the uterine wall and it develops a large yolk sac and a small allantois. The yolk sac is in contact with the chorion and is directed towards the uterine wall in the depression. The contact is made still more efficient by additional wrinkling of that part of the chorion (Figure16.2).

The food and oxygen are absorbed from the mother through this way and carried out by means of the yolk circulation (vitelline circulation) into the embryo. Eg: Some marsupials.

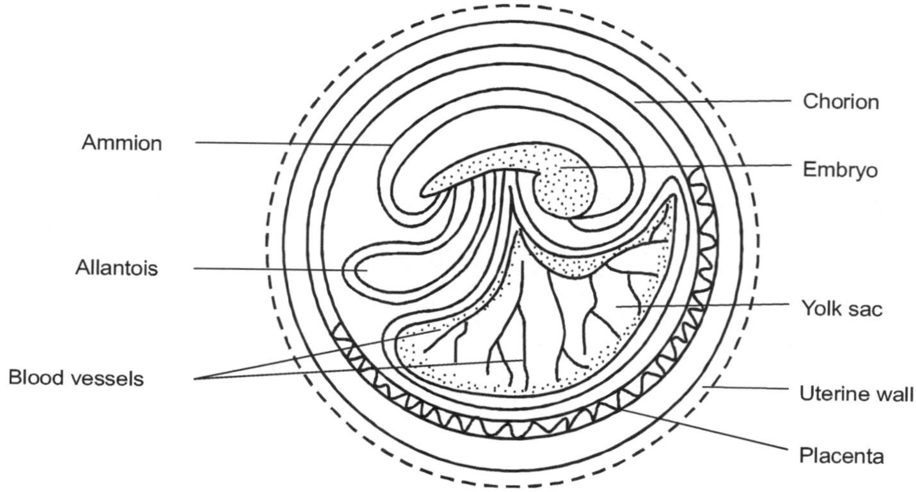

Figure 16.2 Structure of yolk sac placenta.

ii. *Allantoic placenta* In almost all **eutherian mammals**, the allantois plays a general role in absorbing food and oxygen from the mother's blood and also in storing the nitrogenous waste materials. The allantois persists in adults as the urinary bladder. This function is brought about by the allantois by its application with the uterine wall where the chorion and uterine wall come in contact (Figure 16.3). This kind of placenta is called the allantoic placenta.

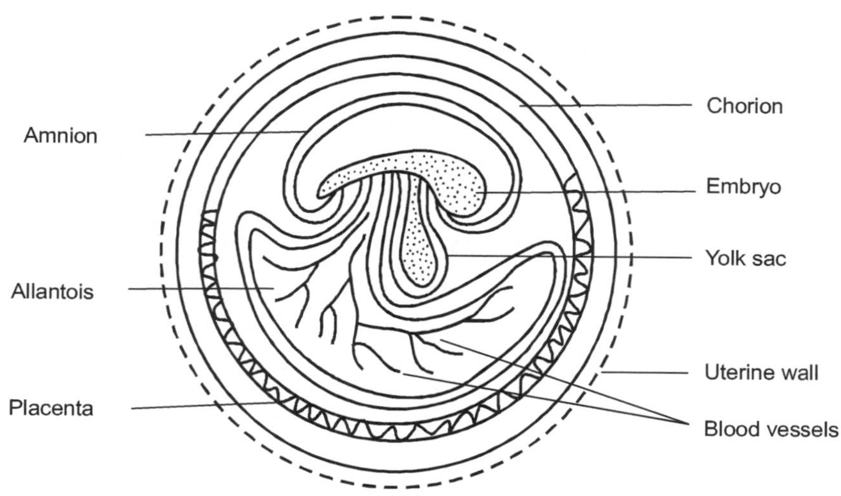

Figure 16.3 Structure of allantoic placenta.

iii. *Chorio-allantoic placenta* Here the allantois is reduced or vestigeal and never grows out to meet the chorion. But the blood vessels of the allantois grow and vascularize the chorion where the placental attachment is developed (Figure 16.4). Therefore, this type of placenta is referred to as chorio-allantoic placenta.

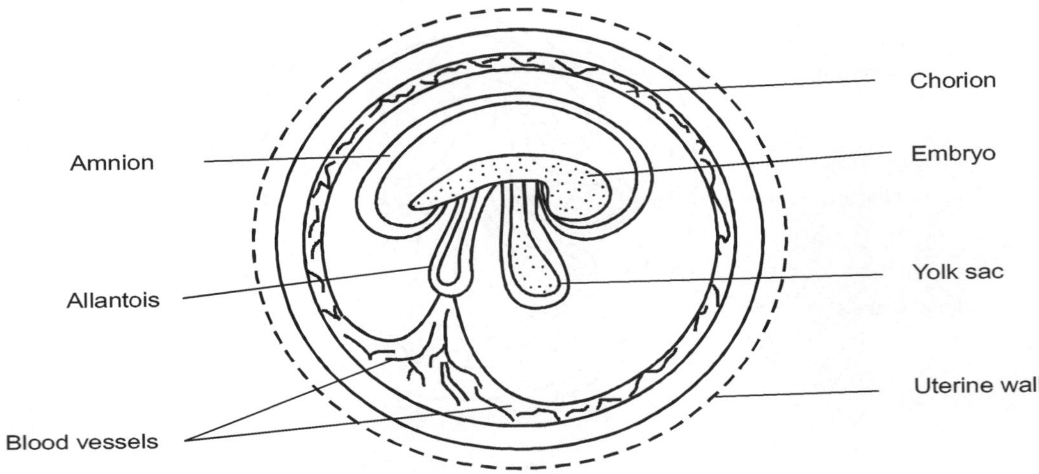

Figure 16.4 Structure of chorio-allantoic placenta

The chorion develops into finger-like outgrowths called **chorionic villi** which penetrate into the uterine wall. Through these villi, interchange takes place between the developing foetus and mother, e.g. some **marsupials** and all **eutherians** including **man**.

Shape of the Placenta

The surface contact between the maternal and foetal tissues is increased by the development of chorionic villi which may be simple or branched and containing the chorionic epithelium, connective tissue and blood vessels. These villi fit into the wall of the uterus in depressions called **crypts**. Based on the distribution of villi which determine the shape of the placenta, the placenta are classified into the following types:

i. *Diffuse placenta* If the placenta contains villi which are scattered all over the chorion, it is called diffuse placenta (Figure 16.5a), e.g. **pig**.

ii. *Cotyledonary placenta* As in **sheep** and **cattle**, the villi may become localized and restricted into patches called cotyledons and the rest of the chorion is smooth (Figure16.5 b). The placenta of this type is called as cotyledonary placenta.

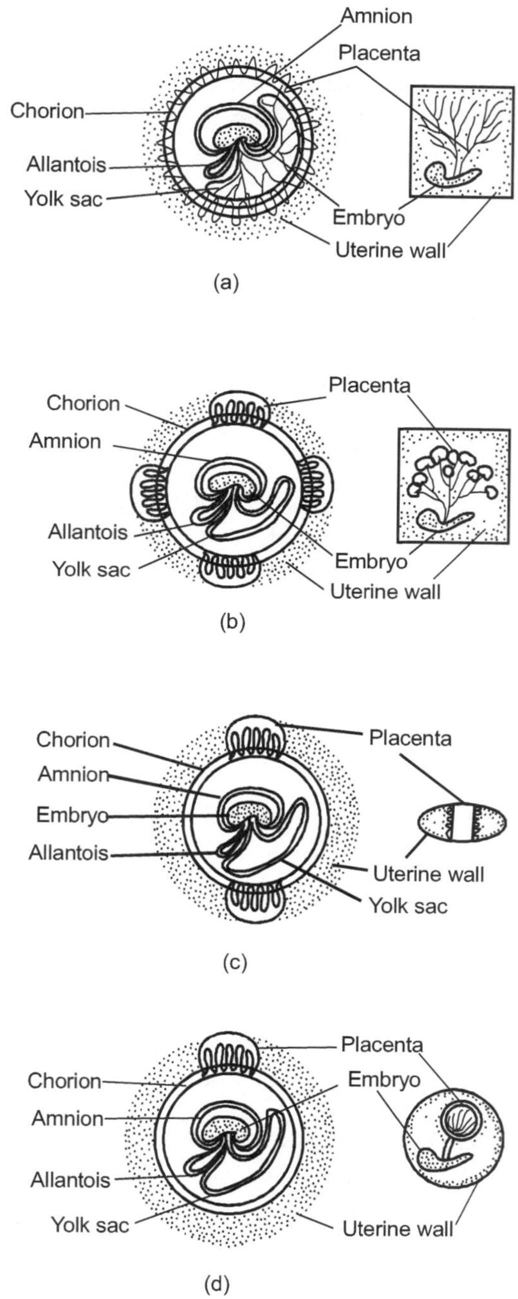

Figure 16.5 Types of placenta based on the shape. a) Diffuse placenta b) Cotyledonary placenta c) Zonary placenta and d) Discoidal placenta.

iii. ***Zonary placenta*** In some animals like carnivorous mammals (**dog**), the villi are developed as a belt or a zone (Figure 16.5 c). This is zonary placenta.

iv. ***Discoidal placenta*** In **man** and other **primates**, the villi develop on one side only, that is, the side away from the uterine cavity (Figure 16.5d). Hence the placenta is disc-like and so is called discoidal placenta. A discoidal placenta also occurs in **rodents**. In **monkeys**, there are two discs and so it is referred to as **bi-discoidal placenta**.

Structure

The placental efficiency is increased by reducing the layers between the foetal and maternal blood. The tissues separating these two blood are **chorionic epithelium, connective tissue** and **endothelium** which constitute the **foetal tissues** and the **uterine epithelium, connective tissue** and **endothelium** of the uterus which constitute the **maternal tissues**. Based on the intimacy of these two tissues, the placenta are classified into the following types:

i. ***Epitheliochorial placenta*** If all the layers are present in the placenta, then the chorionic epithelium is in contact with the uterine epithelium. In other words, the diffusion barrier is fairly extensive as in Figure 16.6a. This condition is called as epitheliochorial placenta which includes diffuse and non–deciduate types of placenta, e.g. **pig** and **horse.**

ii. ***Syndesmochorial placenta*** Here, the chorionic villi start invading the mother's tissues. That is, the uterine epithelium is eaten up so that the villi are in contact with the connective tissue of the uterus (Figure16.6 b). This is syndesmochorial placenta which includes cotyledonary and deciduate types of placenta, e.g. **Sheep** and **cattle.**

iii. ***Endotheliochorial placenta*** In this type of placenta, there is a further reduction of uterine layer (the connective tissue of the uterus) so that the villi comes in close contact with the endothelium of the maternal tissue (Figure16.6 c). This includes zonary and deciduate types of placenta, e.g., **carnivorous animals** like **dog, cat,** etc.

iv. ***Haemochorial placenta*** The destruction of the tissue of the uterine wall may involve even the endothelium of the uterine tissue. As a result, the chorionic villi dip in pools of the maternal blood and the diffusion distance is minimum (Figure 16.6 d). This is haemochorial placenta which includes discoidal and deciduate types of placenta, e.g., **mammals** like **rodents, rats, primates** and **man.**

v. ***Haemendotheliochorial placenta*** In some mammals, the embryonic blood is separated from the maternal blood only by the endothelial wall of the foetal capillaries. This condition is known as haemendotheliochorial placenta (Figure 16.6 e), e.g., **rats** and **rabbits.**

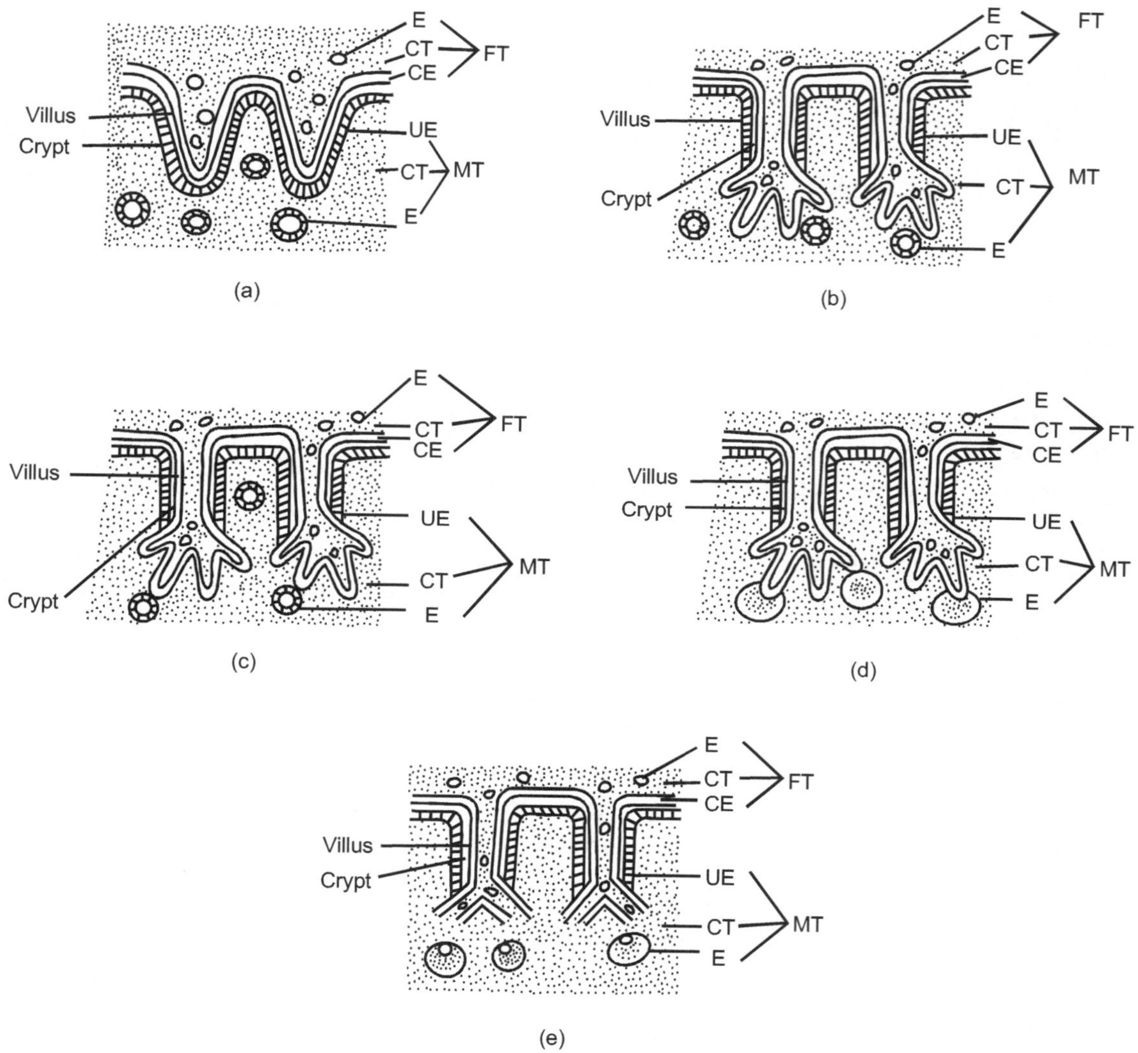

Figure 16.6 Types of placenta based on structure (CE—Chorionic epithelium, CT—Connective tissue, E—Endothelium, FT—Foetal tissue, MT—Maternaltissue, UE—Uterine epithelium)

IV. Parturition

In the case of epitheliochorial type of placenta, the villi can be easily pulled out and there is no break in the uterine wall. As a result, there is no bleeding and loss of maternal tissues at the time of birth. Hence, this type of placenta is otherwise called as **nondeciduate placenta**. In other types of placenta, the intimacy between the foetal and maternal tissues is greater. Therefore, part of uterine wall is also torn away at the event of shedding of the placenta and an open wound is left on the wall of the uterus with the resultant loss of blood and maternal tissues. The wound is healed due to clotting and contractions of the uterine wall which at the same time helps in birth or parturition. This type of placenta is called **deciduate placenta**.

PHYSIOLOGY OF PLACENTA

1. Placenta plays a key role in foetal nutrition, respiration and excretion. It provides the nutritive substances and required oxygen to the foetus and helps in the elimination of carbon dioxide and nitrogenous waste materials from the foetus.
2. It acts as a temporary endocrine gland in all mammals except a few and secretes a number of protein hormones like chorionic gonadotropins as well as steroid hormones like estrogen and progestrone.
3. It mediates the metabolic changes between the mother and foetus. The oxygen consumed by the placenta is utilized by the foetus for energy metabolism. The placenta acts as a store for fat, glycogen and iron. Water, gases and simple solutes diffuse through the placenta at varying rates. Substances such as sugars, amino acids and water-soluble vitamins are actively transported.
4. Placenta is a complex structure that exists as a barrier between the foetal and maternal bloods. It is a protective barrier for the foetus against disease- producing agents which circulate in the maternal blood. The antibodies from the blood of mother enter the foetus via the placenta and develop positive immunity in the foetus against many diseases like diphtheria, measles, smallpox, etc. The placenta is impermeable to bacteria and macromolecules during the first half of the pregnancy, thus preventing any ill effects in the foetus. But later, it becomes more permeable and so harmful organisms and substances can easily cross the placenta. Thus, the transfer of Rh antibodies, pathogenic viruses, bacteria and drugs through the placenta from the maternal blood to the foetus would bring adverse effects in the developing embryo in the form of many diseases.

REVIEW QUESTIONS

1. What is implantation ? Classify it with examples.
2. Write an essay on placentation in mammals.
3. On what basis are placenta classified ?
4. With suitable diagrams, explain yolk sac placenta, allantoic placenta and chorio-allantoic placenta.
5. Describe different types of placenta based on their shape.
6. The placental efficiency is increased with reduction in foetal and maternal tissues. How ?
7. Write a brief account on the following:
   i. Parturition and placenta
   ii. Physiology of placenta

17

TERATOLOGY

The word teratology literally means the study of **monstrosities** and it is, in general, used to denote the study of any abnormality that arises during the course of development. In the broadest sense, the term refers to the abnormalities of the internal organs or to the formation of congenital defects or to the developmental malformations. **Teratogenesis** (Teros–monster) is the interference with the normal development of either embryo or foetus with abnormalities in newborns. It may cause morbidity and mortality in neonates. The toxic substances which induce abnormal development in foetuses are called **teratogens** or **teratogenic agents** and the induction of malformations by the toxicants is termed as **teratogenicity**. The teratogenic agents include natural toxins like nicotine, solvents like benzene, carbon tetrachloride, di-methyl sulfoxide, propylene, xylene, glycol, etc., insecticides, herbicides, fungicides, azo dyes like Trypon blue, Evan blue, etc., antibiotics like penicillin, streptomycin, tetracycline, etc., and drugs and chemicals such as caffeine, carbutamide, chloropromazine, hydroxy urea, nitrosamines, quinine, alkaloids, etc.

STAGE SENSITIVITY OF FOETUS IN TERATOGENESIS

The tremendous multiplication and differentiation of embryonic cells make the gestating embryo more susceptible to teratogens. The sensitivity of the embryo to the teratogenic agents include the following stages.

Pre-differentiation stage At this stage, the embryo is not susceptible to teratogens because the teratogenic agents may either cause death of the embryo by killing all or most of the cells or they may have no apparent effect on the embryo. Thus this period is the resistant stage which includes 5 to 9 days of gestation of the embryo.

Embryonic stage During this stage, the embryonic cells undergo intensive differentiation, mobilization and organization with the occurrence of most of the organogenesis. Therefore, the embryo becomes more susceptible to the teratogenic agents at 10th to 14th days of gestation in rodents and at 14th week of gestation in humans. However, all organs of the embryo are not susceptible in the same period of pregnancy. Table 17.1 illustrates the percentage of susceptibility in the organs of rat embryo during 10th day of teratogenic treatment.

Table 17.1 Susceptibility of embryonic organs to the teratogens in rat embryo at 10th day treatment

Embryonic Organs	% defects
Brain	35
Eyes	33
Heart	24
Skeletal structures	18
Urinogenital system	6
Palate defects	0

Foetal Stage This is the stage of growth and functional maturation of the embryo so that the teratogens do not cause morphological defects but may cause functional abnormalities.

TWINNING AND DOUBLE MONSTERS IN MAN

In humans, two or more embryos may develop inside the uterus instead of a single embryo. "**Similar**" or "**identical**", or "**duplicate**" or **monovular twinning** is due to the division of a single fertilized egg at a very early stage of development into two independently growing cell masses which form complete individuals. On the other hand "**fraternal twins**" or "**diovular twins**" arise due to the ovulation of two ova at a time fertilized by two spermatozoa. The same principles can be applied to **multiple births** also. For example, **quadruplets** (4 embryos) may arise from four separate ova (fraternal) or they may be monovular. They may also be of mixed origin, two being fraternal twins and the other two being identical. In multiple births (development of more number of embryos), the offsprings may be monovular or fraternal or a combination of the two. It is reported that approximately three-fourths of twins are fraternal and only one-fourth monovular.

A rare incident during the development of identical twins is the appearance of "**double monsters**" in which the twins are joined or fused together at certain regions of the body. The degree of fusion varies from a slender connection of superficial tissues that join the two independent individuals to fusions involving the skeleton and viscera. Such type of twins are called as "**Siamese twins**". In some, the fusion may involve most of the organs of the trunk so that only the head or only the posterior part of the body appears as double. These double monsters are of two major types namely **equal conjoined twins** and **unequal conjoined twins**.

Equal Conjoined Twins

These include **symmetrical double monsters** which may be grouped into three general types based on the nature of the fusion of the part of the body namely **upper union**, **middle union** and **lower union**. The upper unions involve fusion at the head–neck level, middle unions between the neck and the umbilicus and posterior unions from caudal to the umbilicus. These kinds of fusions may be back-to-back, face-to-face or side-to-side. The head-to-head fusion is called as **craniopagus**; chest to chest union is **thoracopagus**; rump to rump union is **pygopagus** (Figure 17.1). Side-to-side fusions are prevalent

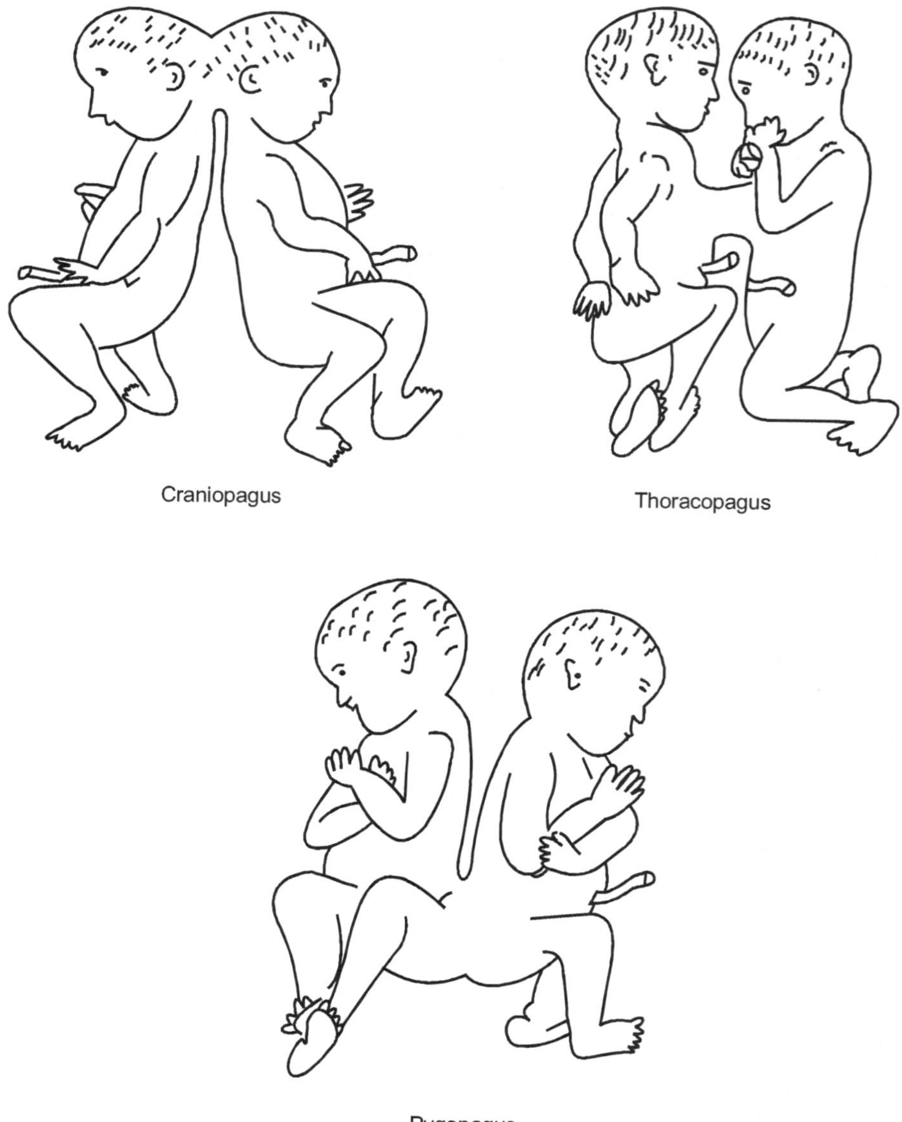

Figure 17.1 Types of conjoined twins in man

at the head or the rump end and never at the thoracic levels. Lateral fusions seem to be quite extensive involving thorax frequently. Based on the part that remains double, these twins are named as **duplicitas anterior** or **duplicitas posterior**. The fusions involving both thorax and head is called as **cephalothoracopagus** (Figure 17.2). However, the more intimately joined double monsters like cephalothoracopagus fail to survive whereas less extensively joined twins live occasionally.

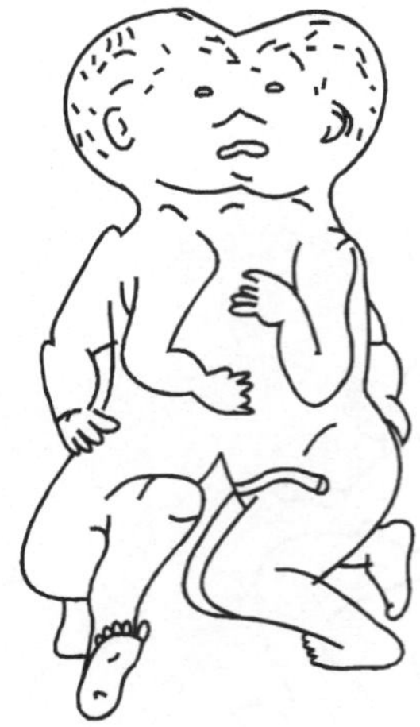

Figure 17.2 Conjoined twins in man with more extensive fusion

Unequal Conjoined Twins

The nature of union of unequal conjoined twins is the same like those of symmetrical double monsters. But the only major difference is that the growth is inhibited or the normal differentiation fails to occur in one of the twins resulting in unequal pairs. In such unequal twins, the smaller individual of a conjoined pair is called as "**parasitic twin**" and the normal one is known as "**autosite**". If a parasitic twin is attached to the jaws of "autosite", then it is referred to as **epignathus parasiticus**. It is **thoracopagus parasiticus** when the parasitic twin is attached to the thorax of autosite. In **pygopagus parasiticus**, the parasitic twin is attached to the rump of autosite (Figure 17.3).

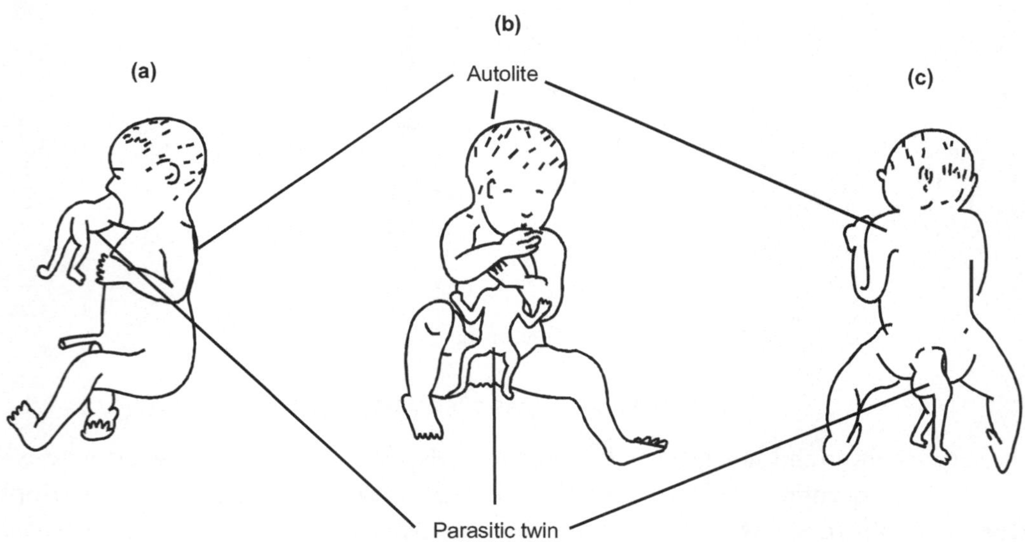

Figure 17.3 Some unequal conjoined twins in man. a) Epignathus parasiticus b) Thoracopagus parasiticus c) Pygopagus parasiticus

EMBRYOMATA AND TERATOMATA

Embryomata is one kind of mixed tumour containing clearly differentiated organs or parts of organs representing all primary germ layers. There is no definite distinction between a parasitic twin and an embryoma. Intermediate conditions such as "**included foetuses**" (*foetus in fetu*) may arise when one member of a pair of conjoined twins lags behind the other during very early development and becomes encased in the body of the normal twin. These foetuses usually have greatly distorted body organization. **Teratoma** refers to any kind of mixed tumours with tissues or fragmentary parts of organs derived from more than one germ layer but without normal architectural arrangement. For example, **dermatoid cyst** is one of the teratomatous masses containing structures like skin, hair, sebaceous glands, nails and teeth along with cartilage or bone. The above structures notably represent only ectoderm and mesoderm but not the endodermal derivative. The dermatoid cysts commonly occur in the gonads especially in the ovary and also in the embryos with ectodermal fusions.

MALFORMATIONS IN THE EXTERNAL STRUCTURES OF THE BODY

Anomalies are also evident in specific organs and the abnormalities may involve external body form, body proportions or appendages. No doubt that they are developmental malformations that can be studied under the following heads:

Malformations in Legs and Arms

Many malformations occur involving a leg or both the legs and the arms. The two posterior appendage buds, instead of growing independently, may fuse with each other to form a single tapering mass so that the body is fish-like in its caudal half (Figure17.4a). As this anomaly is suggestive of the mermaid (siren) with the upper body of a beautiful woman and the tail of the fish, it is called as **Sirenomelus**. A very rare anomaly is a condition called **amelia** in which both paris of appendages fail to develop completely (Figure17.4b).

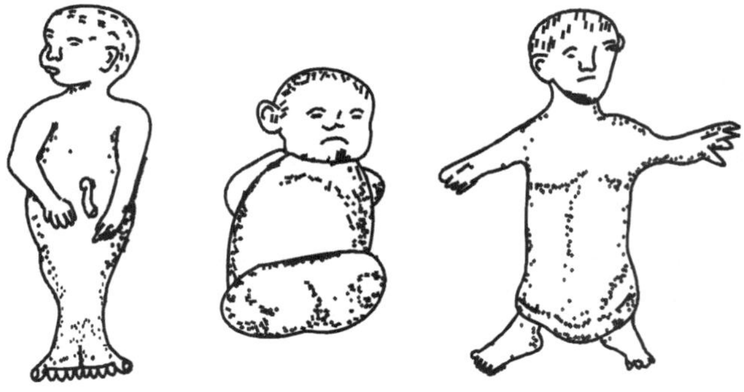

(a) (b) (c)

Figure 17.4 Anomalies in legs and arms of man a) Sirenomelus b) Amelia and c) Phocomelia.

The normally appearing hands and feet may be attached directly to the trunk due to the failure of the limbs to elongate (Figure 17.4c).These malformed appendages resemble the flippers of seal and so this condition is known as **phocomelia.** Most of the developmental defects which are not so extreme may affect the arms or the legs alone or even a single arm or leg with all other appendages normal.

Malformations in Hands and Feet

A rare but most striking malformation is division of distal extremity of hands and feet with the resultant duplication of digits. If it involves the hands, then the condition is known as **dichirus** (Figure17.5a) and the same malformation in the foot is called **diplopodia** (Figure 17.5b). The duplication of a single digit is known as **polydactyly** (Figure 17.5c). The developing digits may fail to separate from each other, resulting in **syndactyly** (Figure17.5d). Another malformation is the failure of development of one or more digits and is known as **oligodactyly** (Figure 17.5e).

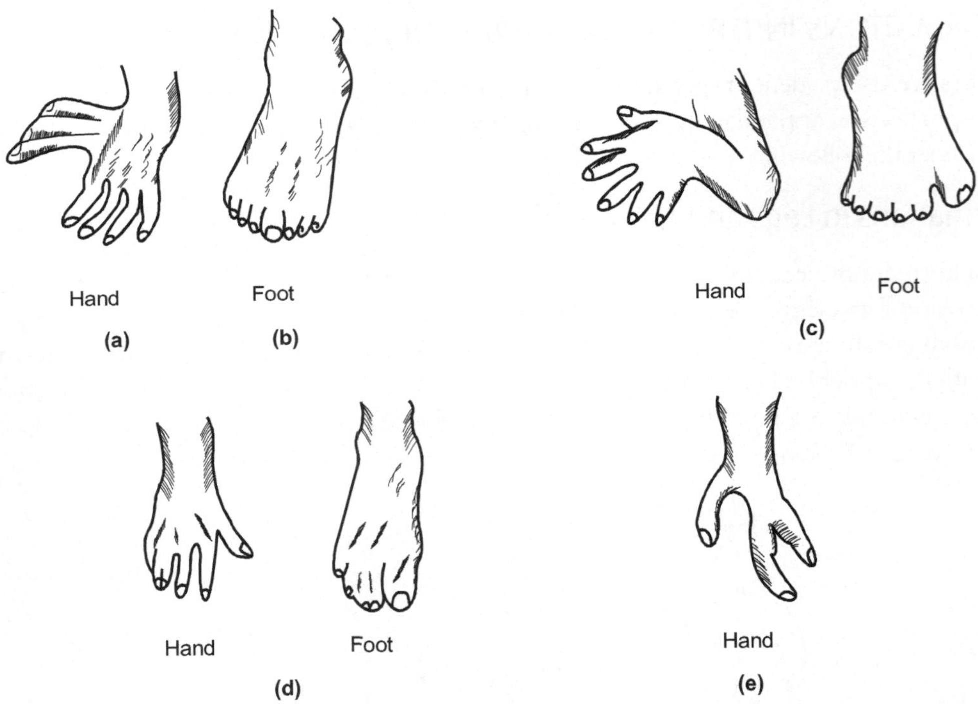

Figure 17.5 Types of defects in hands and feet of man. (a) Dichirus (b) Diplopodia (c) Polydactyly (d) Syndactyly and (e) Oligodactyly.

Persistence of Tail

During the development of human embryo, there is a well developed tail at the second month of gestation. At the third month, it disappears due to regressive changes. Sometimes, the tail, instead of undergoing regression, actually continues to grow in relation to the rest of the body (Figure17.6). However, the tail can be easily removed surgically.

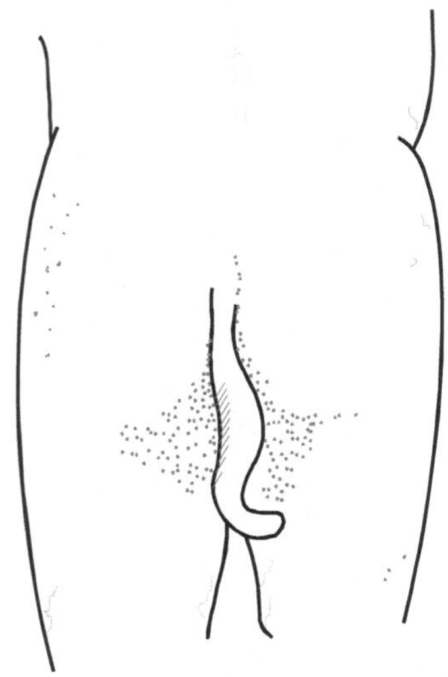

Figure 17.6 Persistence of a well developed tail in man.

Gigantism and Dwarfism

These two abnormalities seem to be due to the endocrine disturbance especially the growth-promoting hormone of the anterior lobe of the pituitary during the growth period. The excessive production of growth hormone results in **gigantism**. If this begins early and continues throughout the growth period, then the disturbance will result in an individual having nearly nine feet height. If this hormone is not produced until the normal growth period, then the individual attains less height but the hands, feet and jaws undergo marked overgrowth so that a characteristic appearance results. This condition is known as **acromegaly**. A deficiency in the production of growth hormone is the cause for **dwarfism** which results in slender individuals with fairly normal proportions. These individuals are sterile due to lack of sexual development. This is referred to as **pituitary dwarfism**. Dwarfism may also be due to congenital deficiency of the thyroid gland and resulting individuals are called **cretins**. They possess heavy bodily proportions with protruded lip and thick and puffy skin due to overdevelopment of the dermal connective tissue. An extreme type of dwarf is known as "**midget**" which results in individuals with the height of two feet, although they possess fairly normal proportions. However, the underlying causes for this type is not known. Another type of dwarfism is known as **chondrodystrophy** or **achondroplasia** in which the trunk of the individual is of perfectly normal size but the bones are extremely short. Thus this is connected with the development of bones.

CAUSATIVE FACTORS IN TERATOGENESIS

Though the discussion of causative factors for the malformations is only tentative, it can be concluded that these anomalies are due to the interplay of **heredity** and **environment**. Some malformations like syndactyly, achondroplasia, cleft lip and palate, etc. are shown to be inherited with regularity, suggesting gene defects by means of mutation. There may be lack of adequate regulation of functioning of growing tissues like excess production of growth hormone from pituitary or deficiency of thyroid hormone. The disturbance in the regulation of the activity of one organ may produce structural abnormalities in other organs, as the development is a progressively constructive process. In general, these disturbances are of **intrinsic type** because they operate from within the embryo itself. However, experimental evidences indicate that the abnormalities may also be produced by modifying the environment. The **physical factors** that are involved in the production of anomalies include pressure, mechanical damage, temperature, radiation, etc. In fish embryos, a change in the amount of various **chemicals** in sea water is found to produce malformations of different types. Similar effects are shown to occur in a variety of individuals due to **insufficient supply of oxygen**. Skeletal defects are seen in rat embryos due to **defective diets** fed to the mothers. It is noticed that different disturbances produce the same malformations at the same phase of development whereas different defects are produced by the same disturbing factor applied at different phases of development. Moreover, the effect of all disturbing agents seems to be slowing down or stopping of growth. Any effective treatment whether it is drop in temperature or lowering of oxygen supply or alterations of salts in the sea water would exert the retarding action on any developmental processes. In the causation of malformations, **diseases** also play a possible role. The disease of the uterus or placenta can disturb the normal environment causing chemical disturbances in mammalian embryos.

REVIEW QUESTIONS

1. Define the terms:
   i. Monstrosities
   ii. Teratogenesis
   iii. Teratogenicity
   iv. Twinning
   v. Embryomata
   vi. Teratoma
   vii. Teratogens
2. Write a brief essay on teratology and its causative factors.
3. Explain the stage sensitivity of the embryo to the teratogens.
4. Give an account of "double monsters".
5. Describe various malformations met within the external structures of the body.
6. Write brief notes on the following:
   i. Double monsters
   ii. Equal conjoined twins
   iii. Unequal conjoined twins

iv. Embryoma
v. Teratoma
vi. Teratogenic agents

18

PRENATAL DIAGNOSIS OF ABNORMALITIES

Prenatal detection is highly useful for the diagnosis of a number of foetal abnormalities in humans and for the prevention of further damage in the develoment of the embryo. Various techniques have been evolved to detect the defects during foetal life or the intra-uterine life of the human embryo. As a result, the effects of genetic disorders and other abnormalities could be prevented in human populations.

AMNIOCENTESIS

It is the most commonly used method to analyse the amniotic fluid collected from the uterus. This technique is otherwise called as "**Amniotic Fluid Test**" (AFT) used in prenatal diagnosis of chromosomal abnormalities and foetal infections. The word "amniocentesis" literally means "puncture of the amnion". It is a specialized test carried out during pregnancy, in which a little amount of amniotic fluid sample is removed from the amnion or amniotic sac around the developing foetus for analysis.

Fuchs and **Riis** (1956) were the first workers to use amniotic fluid in the diagnosis of genetic diseases. They determined the foetal sex from the cells of amniotic fluid based on the presence or absence of Barr body. In 1956, **John Edward** discussed the antenatal detection of hereditary diseases for the first time. **Steele** and **Breg** (1966) have shown that the cells in the amniotic fluid are suitable for karyotyping. The enzyme assays using cultured foetal cells from the amniotic fluid have been demonstrated by **Nadler** (1968) who presented the first diagnosis of **Trisomi 21** (a chromosomal abnormality). In 1972, **Milunsky** and **Littlefield** have discussed the diagnosis of inborn errors of metabolism. Presence of excess quantity of alpha-fetoproteins (AFP) has been reported in 1972 by **Brock** and **Sutcliffe**. Early amniocentesis has been described by **Benacerraf** and his coworkers in 1988. In 2007, the American College of Obstetricians and Gynaecologists (ACOG) has recommended that all the pregnant women irrespective of age should have the screening for foetal abnormalities.

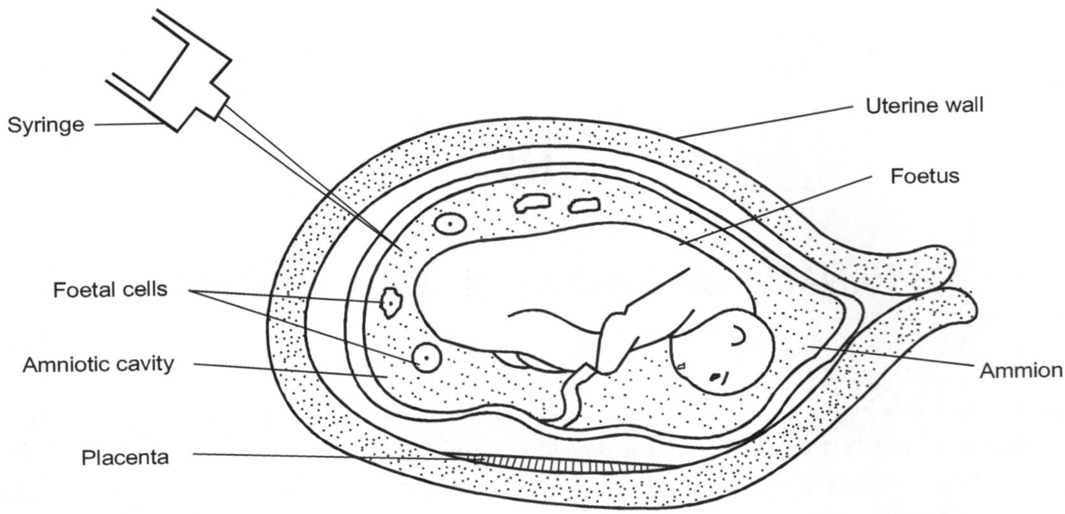

Figure 18.1 Diagram to illustrate the procedure of amniocentesis

This technique involves the removal of about 20 ml of the amniotic fluid from the amniotic sac without damaging the foetus. Here a needle (smaller than 2.7 mm) is usually inserted through the mother's lower abdominal wall, then through the wall of the uterus and finally into the amniotic sac (Figure 18.1). The amniotic fluid is withdrawn with the help of **ultrasonic guidance**. Amniocentesis is possible at any stage of pregnancy but is usually performed during the 15th week of pregnancy. Early amniocentesis before the 12th week of gestation is advisable to have minimum risks and complications. This method is 99.4% accurate and may be unsuccessful occasionally due to technical problems.

The amniotic fluid contains live foetal skin cells that are normally shed during growth as well as other substances such as alpha- fetoproteins (AFP) which provide information about the baby's health before birth. The amniotic fluid is centrifuged so that the foetal cells are separated in the form of sediment. The supernatant is used for the determination of proteins associated with genetic disorders. The cells are grown in culture medium, fixed, stained and used for karyotypic as well as biochemical analyses.

Detection of Disorders from the Supernatant

i. Presence of a high level of alpha-fetoproteins in the amniotic fluid indicates a neural tube defect either in the brain (**anencephalia**) or in the spinal cord (**Spina bifida**) of the foetus or the defects of abdominal wall or pregnancy complications.
ii. A high alpha-feto protein level with or without the activity of acetylcholine esterase shows an increased risk of **neural tube defects** (anencephaly or spina bifida) or abnormalities in organs such as esophagus and abdominal wall.
iii. Estimations of estriol and β-human chorionic gonadotropin (β-hcg) in the amniotic fluid show the risk of **Down's syndrome** and other chromosomal abnormalities.
iv. An increased 17-ketosteroids in the amniotic fluid indicate **adrenogenital syndrome.**

v. Absence or low level of activity of enzymes in the amniotic fluid would reveal specific **metabolic disorders.**

Detection of Disorders from the Amniotic Cells

i. The amniotic cells are useful to identify the foetal **ABO blood groups** and **Rh incompatibility.**

ii. The **foetal sex** is identified through the determination of sex chromatin (Barr body) in the foetal cells.

iii. In cultured amniotic cells, biochemical tests would reveal certain **enzyme defects** such as glucose 6 – phosphate dehydrogenase, galactose phosphate, uridyl transferase, glucosidase, cystathionase, Valine transaminase, etc.

iv. Presence of metachromatic granules identified by the histochemical analysis of amniotic cells reveals certain disorders like **Gaucher's Disease, mucopolysaccharidosis, fibrocystic disease** of pancreas, etc.

v. When Tritium (H^3)-labelled substrate is administered to the amniotic cells, the cells do not undergo labelling in the case of **uricaciduria** in the foetus.

vi. The analysis of DNA in cultured foetal cells by recent molecular techniques helps to detect **thalassemias** and **hybridomas.**

vii. A number of chromosomal abnormalities like **Turner's syndrome, Klinefelter's syndrome, Down's syndrome** (Trisomy-21), **Edward's syndrome** (Trisomy-18), etc. can be detected.

viii. Recently, it has been found that the amniotic fluid contains multipotent mesenchymal, haemopoietic, neural, epithelial and endothelial stem cells which could be engineered to be useful for patients suffering from congenital diseases or malformations of organs.

AMNIOCENTESIS AND ULTRASOUND

At present, amniocentesis and associated techniques are greatly aided by ultrasound. As early as 1967, **Vidoson, Hofmann** and **Hollander** have reported the importance of placental localization using ultrasound before amniocentesis. In 1972, **Jens Bang** and **Allen Northeved** have employed ultrasonic guidance in amniocentesis. Ultrasound- guided pure foetal blood **'Cardocentesis'** has been pioneered by **Daffos** (1983). In recent times, ultrasound is invariably used at the time of amniocentesis to detect birth defects that are not detected by amniocentesis such as cleft palate, cleft lip, club foot or heart defects.

FETOSCOPY AND FOETAL TISSUE SAMPLING

Fetoscopy is a procedure to obtain blood and skin samples from the foetus for prenatal diagnosis. The first attempt of fetoscopy was made by **Westin** (1954) using a hysteroscope (10 mm diameter) introduced through the cervix. A transabdominal approach has been tried by **Mandelbaum** (1967). In 1972, **Valenti** obtained foetal skin samples with the help of a 5 mm needlescope called **'endoamnioscope'** and made the first aspiration of foetal blood and diagnosis of haemoglobinopathy in the foetus. The term fetoscopy was introduced by **Scrimgeous** (1973). The successful diagnosis of diseases by fetoscopy include **sickle cell anaemia** (**Hobbins** and **Mahoney**, 1977), **haemophilia** (**Firshein**, 1979), **chronic granulomatous disease** (**Newburger**, 1979), **galactosaemia** (**Fensom**, 1979) and **Tay–Sach's disease** (**Perry**, 1979). **Rodeck** (1982) reported **foetal liver biopsy** and detected **orinithine carbanyl transferase deficiency**. In the late 1980s, fetoscopy was used mainly for tissue or organ sampling and the foetal blood sampling is always done via ultrasonic guidance needle procedure. In 1990, **Cullen** and coworkers described a new transabdominal thin gauge embryo fetoscopy procedure called "**embryoscopy**".

The technique (fetoscopy) involves the introduction of a fibre optic needlescope in a cannula having 2.7 mm diameter into the uterus. The instrument has a lens which helps to view the foetus and a needle is connected to a syringe for drawing the blood. The placenta is located by the ultrasound and about 10–50 microlitre blood is drawn from the placental vein which is traced by the lens (Figure 18.2).

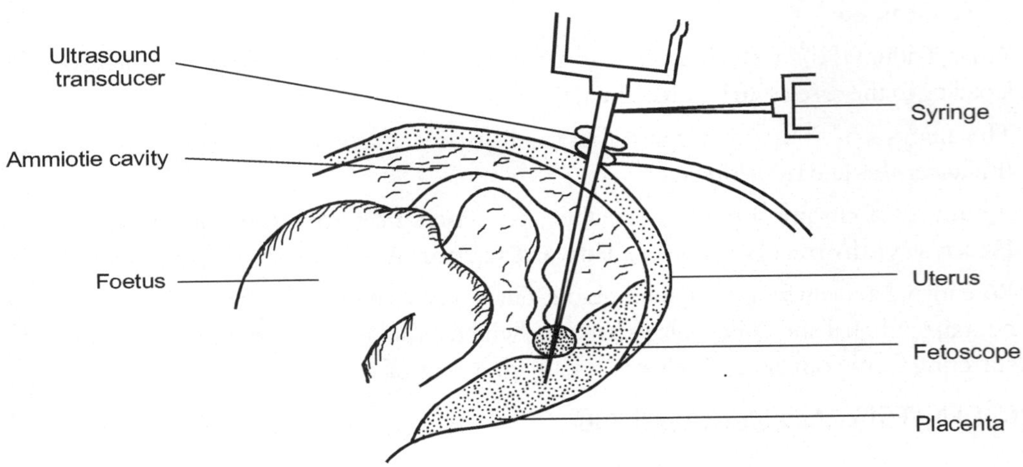

Figure 18.2 Diagram showing the insertion of fetoscope into the uterus.

CHORIONIC VILLUS SAMPLING (CVS)

This technique involves the removal of a small amount of placental sample from the uterus. It is a kind of prenatal diagnosis to detect genetic disorders in the foetus and can be carried out earlier than amniocentesis. It is considered to be 98% accurate in the diagnosis of chromosomal defects like **Down's syndrome** and other genetic diseases such as **cystic fibrosis**. The concept of antenatal genetic diagnosis using chorionic villus sampling method was first introduced by **Mohr** (1968). He performed transcervical biopsy of chorion under direct endoscopic view. In 1975, the foetal sex was diagnosed in China through chorionic villi biopsy. Foetal sexing and enzyme assays on chorion biopsies were reported by **Kazy** (1980). **Niazi** and coworkers (1981) for the first time, used ultrasound during chorionic sampling. In 1983, **Ward** made transcervical chorionic sampling under ultrasonic guidance.

This type of sampling can be performed between the 8th and 12th week of pregnancy and the results can be obtained earlier than amniocentesis. There are two ways of performing CVS, the choice of which depends on the position of the placenta in the uterus. One is **transcervical CVS** which involves obtaining of the sample through cervix by inserting a catheter (a small tube) or a needle into the vagina with the aid of ultrasound. The other method is **transabdominal CVS** in which the sample is obtained by inserting a needle through the abdomen into the placenta under ultrasound guide.

REVIEW QUESTIONS

1. What is amniocentesis? Describe the method with a note on its uses.
2. In what ways does amniocentesis help to detect prenatal disorders?
3. Describe the uses of ultrasound and fetoscopy in prenatal diagnosis of diseases.
4. Write an essay on chorionic villus sampling.
5. Write notes on the following:
   i. Amniotic fluid test
   ii. $\propto$-feto protein
   iii. Fetoscopy
   iv. CVS (Chorionic Villus Sampling)

19

METAMORPHOSIS

The embryological development of animals can be classified into two main types based on the presence or absence of metamorphosis, namely **direct development** and **indirect development**. In direct development, the fertilized egg directly develops into the adult without larval stages whereas in indirect development, the zygote develops into a larva which is entirely different from the adult and the larva metamorphoses into the adult after a brief independent existence. Thus metamorphosis can be defined as a process by which an adult individual develops from a larva through a number of successive changes. This phenomenon is found only in those animals which include a larval stage in their embryonic development and is prevalent in some invertebrate groups especially in arthropods and insects and many vertebrates like ascidians, cyclostomes and amphibians.

METAMORPHOSIS IN INSECTS

Insects are terrestrial animals in which growth is inhibited by the presence of an outer chitinous covering, the **cuticle**. As a result, the cuticle of insects is to be shed periodically through the process called **moulting** in order for the cells of the body to undergo growth and differentiation. The period between two moults is called **stadium** and the form acquired at a particular stadium is **instar**. Thus insect metamorphosis involves changes in form and structure starting from the first instar to the adult and varies in different insect groups. As a rule, the development in insects can be studied under the following types:

Ametabolous Development (Absence of Metamorphosis)

In this type, the life history involves no larval stages or metamorphosis and the eggs directly develop into young ones which are exactly similar to their adults except the size and non – development of gonads and external genitalia. Examples are **Apterygote insects** like silver fish.

Hemimetabolous Development (Incomplete Metamorphosis)

Here also the eggs give rise to the young ones resembling the adults and these young ones undergo simple metamorphosis through gradual growth by the development of wings, gonads and genitalia. The young ones are called as **nymphs**. This type of development is seen in **exopterygote insects** and includes the following two types.

i. ***Gradual metamorphosis*** In some insects like **cockroaches, grasshoppers, crickets**, etc., the nymphs resemble the adults in structure and habit and metamorphose into winged adults by gradual development of wings, gonads and genitalia.

ii. ***Heterometamorphosis*** The nymphs of some insects (**dragonflies, damsel flies** and **mayflies**) differ from the adults in structure and habit as they are aquatic and herbivorous. They undergo massive alterations in development to acquire adult structures with aerial mode of life. These nymphs are also called as **naiads**.

Holometabolous Development (Complete metamorphosis)

In all **endopterygote insects**, the fertilized eggs give rise to voraciously feeding larvae which are entirely different in structure and habit from the adults. These larvae undergo several moults and develop into physiologically inactive pupal stages. Then the pupae are transformed into adults by histolysis and histogenesis as in insects like **bees, butterflies, moths, flies, beetles**, etc.

Hormonal Control of Insect Metamorphosis

The first evidence to show the hormonal control of metamorphosis in insects was given by **Kopec** (1927) through his ligature experiments in caterpillars. When a ligature was made behind the head in a caterpillar of a particular instar after seven days of last larval moult, the larva exhibited normal moulting. If the ligature was made within four days of last larval moult, there was no moulting and the larva remained as larva. From this, he concluded that some factors in the head are responsible for moulting and this head factor requires seven days to diffuse into the haemolymph. This was again proved by **Wigglesworth** (1940) by his decapitation experiments in **Rhodnius larva**. It is shown that the brain of insects contains large neurosecretory cells which secrete the **brain hormone (BH).** These cells have been identified by their staining properties as well as by the implantation experiments in **Rhodnius (Wigglesworth).** The work of **Fukuda** (1944) on **silkworm larvae** demonstrated that the **thoracic hormone** from the thoracic gland induces larval moulting, pupation and imaginal development. It was also shown that the hormone from the brain is necessary for the activation of the thoracic gland. The parabiosis experiments of **Wigglesworth** have proved that the **juvenile hormone** from the corpus allatum of insect brain maintains the development of larval characters.

Thus moulting and metamorphosis in insects are under the control of hormones secreted by the brain, corpora allata and prothoracic glands and the entire process is depicted in Figure 19.1. The hormone secreted from the neurosecretory cells of the brain is called brain hormone (BH) or **prothoracotrophic hormone** which activates the thoracic glands to secrete the **moulting hormone** (MH) or **ecdysone**. However, the thoracic glands require a continuous supply of the brain hormone until definite period (**critical period**). The ecdysone initiates the changes in the epidermis leading to the growth and deposition of the new cuticle and casting off the old cuticle. The corpora allata are the sources of the **juvenile hormone** (JH) or **neotenin** that maintains the development of larval characters. This hormone acts directly on the epidermal cells ensuring the retention of larval features. Another important effect of JH is the maintenance of the thoracic gland. At high concentration of JH, the epidermal cells secrete the larval cuticle (**larval moult**). A pupal cuticle is secreted in the presence of low quantity of JH (**pupal moult**) and an adult or imaginal cuticle (**imaginal moult**) in the complete absence of JH. In other words, the response of JH depends on its quantitative titre. That is, hormonal differences exist in the blood of insects and are responsible for the morphological changes. It is also evident that an insect can develop imaginal characters (can undergo metamorphosis) at any stage, if the required hormones circulate in the blood.

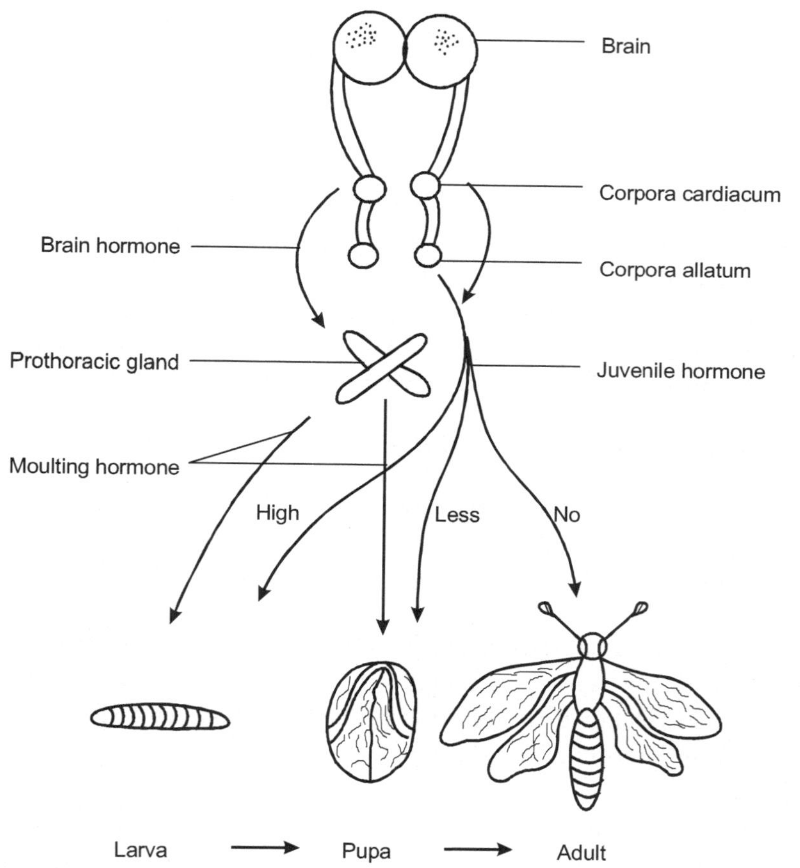

Figure 19.1 Hormonal control of moulting and metamorphosis in insects

METAMORPHOSIS IN AMPHIBIANS

In anurans like **frog**, metamorphosis involves morphological, physiological and biochemical changes with a transitional life from an aquatic, herbivorous and tailed tadpole stage to a terrestrial, carnivorous and tail-less adult. These changes can be studied in the following account.

Morphological Changes

These include a number of **regressive changes** such as reabsorption and disappearance of tail with fin folds and disappearance of external gills, horny teeth, ventral sucker, lateral line sense organs, etc.

Progressive changes include development of limbs, middle ear and tympanic membrane, protruding eyes, hyoid apparatus, and long sticky tongue as well as changes in circulatory and respiratory systems.

Physiological Changes

During metamorphosis, feeding is stopped by the animals so that only the **reserve food materials** are utilized with resultant reduction in the body weight. The **phagocytic activity** is shown to be prevalent in the amoeboid macrophages for the autolysis of gills and tail with the aid of lysosomal enzymes. **Glycogenesis** is found to occur at high level due to the initiation of endocrine function of pancreas which induces the functioning of the liver.

Biochemical Changes

The biochemical changes that occur during metamorphosis form the basis for all other alterations to cope up with the transition from aquatic to terrestrial life. A major biochemical change during metamorphosis is the change-over from ammonotelism to **ureotelism** which is mainly due to differential functioning of the liver. The quantity of **thyroxine hormone** increases as the liver enzymes are more pronounced. Increased **serum proteins, altered haemoglobin function** and **secretion of new digestive** and **respiratory enzymes**, etc. are other changes that occur during metamorphosis.

Mechanism of Amphibian Metamorphosis

In amphibians, the process of metamorphosis depends on the species, specific time, size and environmental conditions especially temperature. Above all, amphibian metamorphosis is influenced by the **thyroid hormone** which is found to increase as the metamorphosis proceeds and reaches the climax. The thyroid hormone is an iodine-containing derivative of **tyrosin**. The activity of thyroid gland is activated by a hormone called **thyrotropin** or **thyroid stimulating hormone** (TSH) produced by the anterior lobe of the pituitary. The level of activity of pituitary–thyroid axis (PT) is under the control of the feedback effect of thyroid hormone and the regulatory TSH activity is by the way of **Thyrotropin Releasing Factor** (TRF) produced from the hypothalamus. It is experimentally proved that the pituitary gland of tadpoles controls thyroid activity which, in turn, is the immediate agent for metamorphic changes. It is also demonstrated that the feeding of thyroid gland preparations induce metamorphosis in young tadpoles. Another hormone namely **prolactin** from the anterior lobe of pituitary is known to stimulate body growth with an antithyroid activity in tadpoles.

Though the early tadpoles possess all the elements necessary for metamorphosis (hypothalamus, pituitary, thyroid and tissues), there is no immediate transformation of adults. This is because of the production of low concentration of thyroxine in early tadpoles. The premetamorphic period may be regarded as one in which the activity of **pituitary–thyroid axis** is maintained at an extremely low level. The level of this steady state is so low that the amount of thyroid hormone produced is not sufficient for metamorphosis. This is indicative of the fact that the low activity level of PT axis is an essential factor in maintaining the characteristic high growth rate of the premetamorphic period. It is also shown that there is an antagonism between thyroid hormone and prolactin and that prolactin stimulates growth in normal tadpoles. The neuroendocrine relationship responsible for the high growth rate and the low metamorphic tendency in premetamorphic tadpoles can be summarized as follows.

The hypothalamus is only minimally active in producing TRF or prolactin inhibiting factor. As a result, it partially retards the production of prolactin and does not appreciably stimulate TSH production. Therefore the PT axis is kept at a very low level. The high amount of prolactin and a low quantity of thyroid homone favour a high growth rate without appreciable metamorphic change during this period.

It is found that a structure called **median eminence**, a vascular region between the hyphothalamus and pituitary, is poorly developed in the premetamorphic tadpole. This capillary network derives blood from hypothalamic arteries and feeds the capillary system of the anterior pituitary. In the premetamorphic animal, this system would carry only a minimum hypothalamic substance. When the animal enters metamorphic climax, the median eminence system becomes well-developed and the amount of the hypothalamic material increases to reach a level for a high level of PT axis. This median eminence part of the hypothalamic mechanism is, in turn, controlled by the thyroid hormone. The median eminence region is insensitive to thyroid feedback in the premetamorphic stage and the feedback begins about a week before the commencement of metamorphosis and reaches the maximum through prometamorphosis climax.

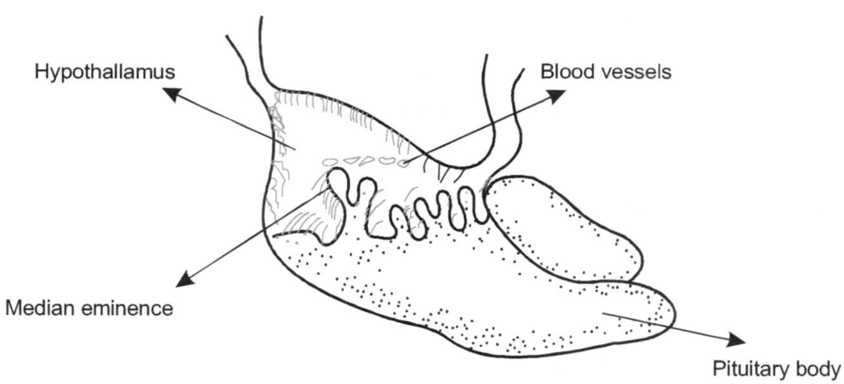

Figure 19.2 Structure of median eminence

NEOTENY OR PAEDOGENESIS

In general, precocious reproduction in larval stages is called **paedogenesis**. It is the ability of individuals to reproduce before attaining adulthood and is otherwise referred to as **neoteny** and such individuals are called as **neotenic** or **paedomorphic forms**. The nature of neoteny in which the young ones become sexually active with incomplete adult characters is called **Prothetely**. The presence of a number of infantile characters in individuals with capacity of reproduction is known as **Metathetely**. In short, in neotenous forms, metamorphosis is stopped at the larval stage and at the same time, reproductive capacity is achieved. Among amphibians, paedogenesis is not seen in anurans whereas it is widespread in **urodeles** or **caudates** to different degrees. For example, the **axolotl larva** of **Ambystoma** remains as permanent larva without undergoing metamorphosis. This condition is not only seen in Ambystomidae but also in Plethodontidae and Sirenidae urodeles in which metamorphosis can be induced. In some Ambystomidae and Salamandridae, the individuals are occasionally neotenous due to ecological conditions.

Thyroid Gland and Neoteny

It is well-known that the thyroid extract induces metamorphosis in amphibians whereas the removal of thyroid gland in larval forms prevents metamorphosis. Amphibians have no ability to respond to thyroxine during their early development but they acquire the capacity at a specific period of development. Therefore, the failure of metamorphosis in neotenous forms could be either due to the deficient thyroid function or due to the loss of sensitivity of tissues to respond to thyroid. As an example, the axolotl larvae do not possess reactivity to thyroxin, so they do not metamorphose. Another species ***Necturus*** never has reactivity, so it never metamorphoses. The failure of metamorphosis in *Necturus* is the result of failure of tissue response because the thyroid of *Necturus* accelerates metamorphosis in *Rana*. In amphibians, the production and liberation of thyroid hormone are under the control of pituitary gland which in turn depends on the hypothalamus. There is also a feedback mechanism between thyroid and hypothalamus. In short, it may be said that the proper functioning of the thyroid is dependent on sufficient amount of iodine that is provided through food. Hence, insufficient iodine in the food taken by the larva would affect metamorphosis.

REVIEW QUESTIONS

1. Define the following terms:
   i. Metamorphosis
   ii. Moulting
   iii. Instar
   iv. Neoteny or paedogenesis
   v. Prothetely
   vi. Metathetely
2. Explain the various kinds of metamorphosis met within various insects.
3. Write an essay on hormonal control of insect metamorphosis.
4. Enumerate the different types of changes that occur during amphibian metamorphosis.
5. In what ways do hormones control metamorphosis in amphibians?
6. Give an account of neoteny or paedogenesis.

20

REGENERATION

Regeneration is the ability of an organism to repair, renew or replace the damage in its body at varying degrees. This may include the replacement of the loss of an organ or major part of the body or the whole organism or it may be simply a wound healing. Regeneration may either be **reparative regeneration** or **physiological regeneration**. Reparative regeneration involves cell migration, morphogenetic movements, tissue interactions, growth, differentiation and so on. If reparative regeneration accomplishes addition of parts to the remaining part of the organ, it is referred to as **Epimorphic regeneration** or **Epimorphosis** as seen in the regeneration of the amphibian limb, lost tail of the lizard, replacement of the damaged cells or wound healing. In animals like hydra, planaria and earthworms, the adult is capable of producing new individuals from body pieces, involving reorganization of the remaining part of the body. This type of regeneration is called **morphallactic regeneration** or **morphallaxis**. In rare cases, even a portion of an amputated organ could develop into an entirely different organ. For example, the removal of eye in **Palinurus** (a crustacean) results in the formation of an antenna-like structure instead of developing into the eye. This type of regeneration is called as **heteromorphic regeneration** or **heteromorphosis**. The phenomenon of periodical replacement of a number of variety of cells that possess specific lifespan (blood cells, glandular cells, skin cells, intestinal cells, etc.) is known as **physiological regeneration**. In the case of earthworm or planaria, a lateral cut near the head regenerates, giving rise to the additional heads. This process of development of a number of parts or organs in the body is called **super regeneration**.

REGENERATION IN VARIOUS GROUPS OF ANIMALS

Though prevalent throughout the animal kingdom, the ability of regeneration is found to differ in various groups of animals. Table 20.1 shows the occurrence and nature of regeneration in various animal groups. A high degree of regeneration is noticed among coelenterates. In Hydra, each part of the cut in the body develops into a complete individual where the posterior end regenerates the mouth and tentacles and the anterior end, the foot and basal disc. A small portion of the body of Hydra is capable of regenerating the whole animals through morphallaxis. In general, highest regenerative power is evident in **polyps**, and the **medusae** exhibit very low capacity of regeneration among the coelenterates. The **planarians** are another group that shows a remarkable power of regeneration. When the body of planarians is cut across or lengthwise, each part of the body regenerates the lost parts so that any missed

Table 20.1 Nature of regeneration in different animal groups

Animal groups	Nature of regenerative capacity
Invertebrates	
Protozoans	Reconstitution of cellular parts
Sponges	Whole organisms from archeocytes
Coelenterates	Polyps with high regenerative power
Platyhelminthes (Planarian)	Whole organism
Nemertines	Whole organism
Annelids (polychaetes and oligochaetes)	Whole organism
Mollusca (Gastropoda)	Eye stalks, parts of head and foot
Arthropoda	Renewal of lost parts
Echionoderms	Arms and parts of the disc
Vertebrates	
Fishes	Restricted to fins
Amphibia (Newts and Salamanders) Anurans (Tadpoles)	Limbs, tails, external gills, upper and lower jaws, lens and retina, limbs and tails only
Reptiles (Lizards)	Tails
Birds	Part of the beaks
Mammals	Mostly wound healing

part of the body either head, tail or middle part can be replaced through epimorphosis and morphallaxis. In **nemertines**, small pieces of body can regenerate into a complete worm, thus showing high degree of regenerative capacity. Among the annelids, **Hirudinearians** are incapable of regeneration whereas **polychaetes** and **oligochaetes** exhibit a good degree of regeneration. But regeneration is somewhat restricted in majority of annelids. For example, only a limited number of segments are formed from the anterior cut end of the body whereas equal number of segments are replaced from the posterior cut end as that of lost segments through epimorphosis. Thus the process of regeneration is very much limited and restricted in annelids. The regenerative power is evident only in the eye stalks and parts of the head and foot among **gastropods** and in the arms of **cephalopods**. The renewal of lost appendages is widespread in arthropods. **Crustaceans** are capable of regeneration of limbs at any stage of development including adults. The **larval insects** exhibit limb regeneration, and the regenerated limb is always smaller in size. **Autotomy** or **self-mutilation** is prevalent in **crabs** and **spiders** which escape from their enemies by breaking off the legs at the expense of the loss of the limbs. Echinoderms like **starfishes**, **brittle stars** and **sea lilies** are capable of regenerating the arms and parts of the disc. The internal organs such as respiratory tree and the alimentary canal regenerate after they are ejected out through the anus in **holothurians**.

Among vertebrate animals, regenerative power is very much restricted in **fishes**, the fins of which can be regenerated on cut or damage. On the other hand, **newts** and **salamanders** (urodele amphibians) and their larvae have enormous power to regenerate not only the limbs but also the upper and lower jaws, external gills and tails. Even a new eye can develop in these animals from a small part of the eye which is left with lens and retina. In **frogs** and **toads** (anuran amphibians) only the tadpoles are able to regenerate the limbs and tails. In **lizards**, the power of regeneration is restricted to the tails only and this is followed by autotomy. **Birds** show a poor capacity of regeneration which is evident in the renewal of parts of the beaks. In the case of **mammals**, the regenerative capacity is represented by **tissue regeneration** in which the defects in various tissues are rectified as in the case of wound healing. A few examples include covering of wounds in skin by new epidermis and connective tissue, the restoration of defects of the bones, rectification of the defects of injured muscles by the proliferation of cells at the remaining part of the muscle, replacement of lesions by tendons with connective tissue and so on. In some internal organs such as liver of vertebrates, the loss of parts is compensated by extensive proliferation from the remaining part.

MECHANISM OF REGENERATION

Regeneration is an immediate event followed by an injury and it involves a number of histological alterations along with morphogenetic and histogenetic processes. The phenomenon of regeneration is given in Figure 20.1 and can be studied under the following headings.

Wound Healing or Preblastema Phase

Immediately after an injury, the cells from the interior body accumulate at the surface of the wound. In addition, the dead cells that are damaged due to destruction or squashing, also accumulate as debris at the wound surface. If blood vessels are involved in the injury, the blood which is oozing out from the damaged vessels, coagulate at the wound site. Now, the epithelial cells of the skin grow over the surface of the wound forming a covering.

Blastema Formation

During this process, a large number of undifferentiated cells are formed under the epithelial covering from the adjoining tissues of the wound surface through **dedifferentiation** and **redifferentiation**. These cells with the epidermal layer constitute the **blastema** or **regeneration bud**. When the wound is covered by the epidermal cells, the bone and cartilage cells disintegrate with the dissolution of connective tissue and muscle cells. At this stage, the cells of all the tissues resemble the embryonic cells and accumulate as a mass of undifferentiated blastema cells. This process is called **dedifferentiation**. When the blastema attains a specific size, the process of dedifferentiation stops and the blastema begins to grow further. The rate of growth is the highest immediately after the formation of blastema and the growth seems to decrease later. Now, various kinds of cells at the blastema become seggregated to their respective specific types, differentiate and develop into the required part. All these events constitute **redifferentiation**.

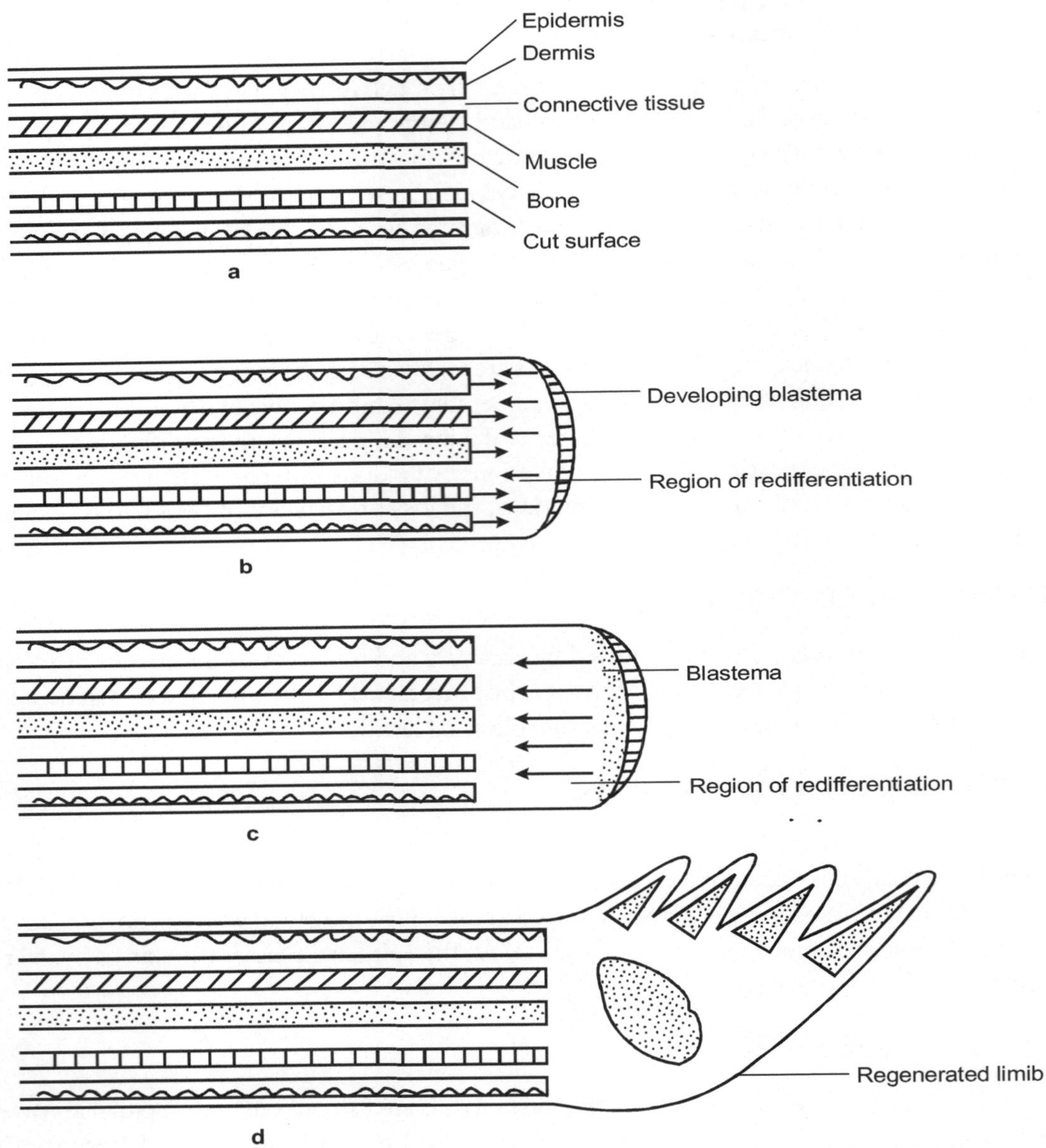

Figure 20.1 Digrammatic representation to explain the mechanism of regeneration. (a) A position of cut limts, (b) Process of redifferentiation, (c) Formation of blastema and redifferentiation, and (d) Completion of regeneration

There are **two major theories** with regard to the origin of the blastema cells. According to one theory, the cells of the blastema are derived from the tissues immediately adjoining the wound surface and all the other cells are set free from the dedifferentiating tissues.

The second theory postulates that the blastema cells migrate from different parts of the body to the site of regeneration via the blood or by amoeboid movement and possess capacity for development. However, these theories have not been universally accepted as the blastema cells are derived from both sources in different animal groups.

HISTOLOGY OF REGENERATION

The process of regeneration in all animals is characterized by the accumulation of cells at the site of injury. The nature of blastema and the characteristics of its cells are not clearly understood. In **planarians**, there are a group of undifferentiated cells called **neoblasts** which remain in their embryonic state and appear to be **omnipotent cells**.

During regeneration, the neoblasts actively divide and migrate towards the zones of injury to form the blastema. In **hydroid coelenterates**, the interstitial cells located in the epithelium appear to be the embryonic totipotent cells which migrate to form the blastema. In the case of **amphibians**, the blastema is formed by the process of dedifferentiation in which the cells become more homogeneous with progressive loss of specialization.

Later the dedifferentiation ceases and the established blastema enters into the growth phase followed by differentiation into various tissues of the organ (redifferentiation). In general, the blastema cells do not lose their morphological nature and specific potency and thus a cartilage cell gives rise to cartilage tissue alone and the dedifferentiated muscle cell gives rise to muscles only.

PHYSIOLOGICAL ASPECTS OF REGENERATION

1. During the initial stages of regeneration where there is considerable dedifferentiation, the activity level of proteolytic enzymes is found to increase suddenly.
2. Free amino acids and proteins along with their products undergo changes both qualitatively and quantitatively.
3. An abrupt fall in respiratory quotient (RQ) during regeneration is indicative of presence of incomplete oxidation in the tissues. During the early stages of regeneration, the rate of oxygen consumption decreases with increased accumulation of lactic acid.
4. The metabolic alterations like changes in the accumulation of free amino acids, lactic acid, etc. result in lowering of the pH in the blastema cells and the differentiating tissues.
5. During the later period of regeneration, the cells exhibit an increase of oxidation, normal pH, higher level of RQ and decreased quantity of lactic acid.
6. The blastema cells possess large amount of RNA which promotes enhanced growth and its quantity diminishes at the stage of differentiation of the regenerating part.

FACTORS THAT INFLUENCE REGENERATION

i. In general, the process of regeneration is temperature-dependent and its ability is increased with the increase of temperature up to a certain limit. As a rule, regeneration is inhibited at very high or very low temperatures.

ii. It seems that regeneration mainly involves the utilization of reserve food material and so food plays no influencing role in the process. However, experiments have shown that the provision of adequate food accelerates regeneration in animals.

iii. The nervous system and the neurosecretory hormones are found to have a major influence on regeneration.

iv. While increased oxygen content and electric field stimulate the process of regeneration, X-rays, mustard gas, etc. inhibit the process.

POLARITY IN REGENERATION

If the whole organism is taken into account, it shows differential polarity as in the case of an egg. In Hydra, it is observed that the bits of tentacular end develop only tentacles and the aboral end, the basal disc. However, this polarity can be altered, simply by exposing the two ends to differential amount of oxygen (Figure 20.2).

Now, the basal end in high concentration of oxygen develops tentacles whereas the tentacular end forms a base. The same results have also been obtained through ligature experiments in Hydra. When the body of Hydra is ligatured at the centre (Figure 20.3), both basal end as well as tentacular end developed tentacles, thus resulting in two individuals from one mass of tissue. These clearly indicate that the organization within a tissue is quite labile.

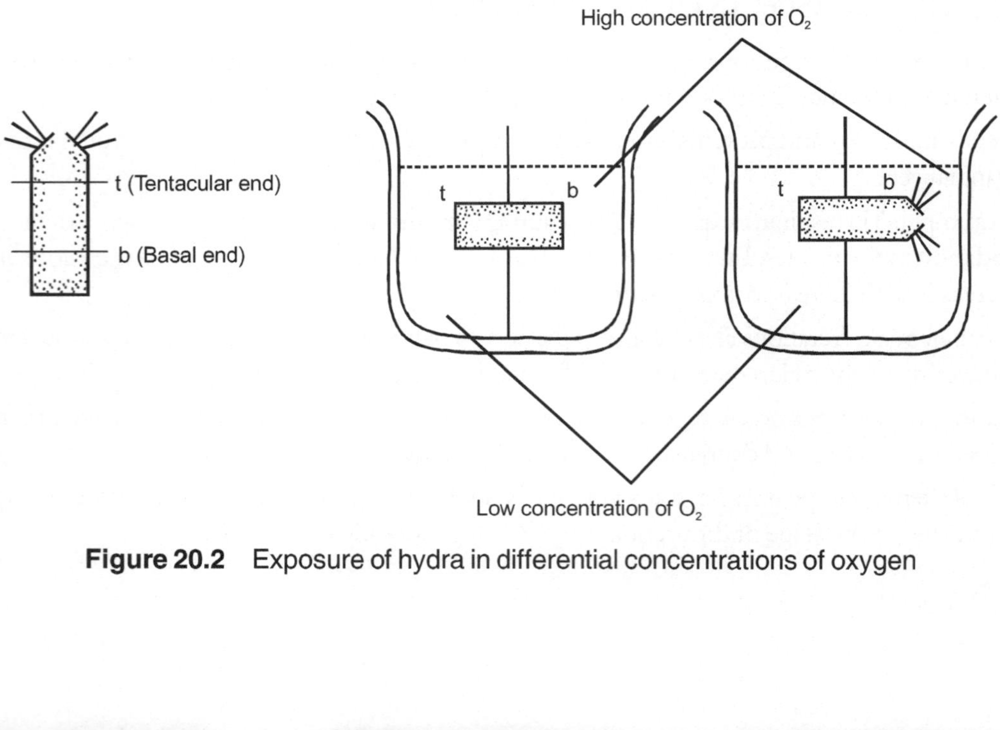

Figure 20.2 Exposure of hydra in differential concentrations of oxygen

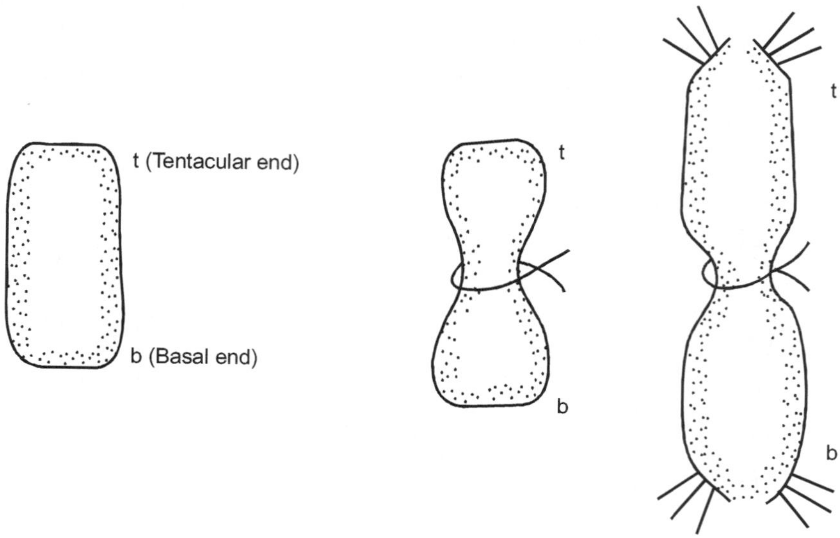

Figure 20.3 Development of tentacles in ligatured hydra.

INDUCTION IN REGENERATION

Regeneration in animals exhibits a phenomenon of induction or cell interaction. When the growth region of ***Hydra pirardi*** is grafted to the posterior region of ***Hydra fusca*** in which the base has been cut, then *H. fusca* develops tentacles in the basal region (Figure 20.4).

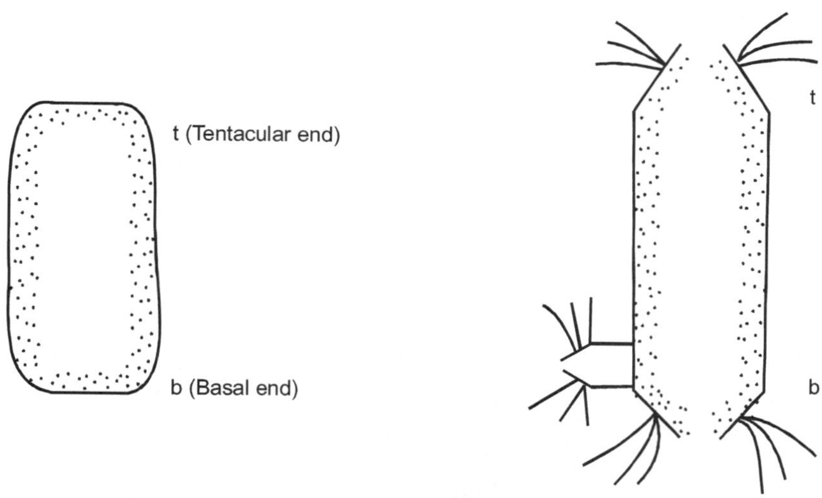

Figure 20.4 Grafting of hypostome to the posterior region in Hydra

This could be due to the diffusion of growth stimulating factor from the tissue of transplanted hydra. Here the stimulating factor overcomes the influence of the inhibitory factor at the base to stimulate the formation of new hypostome. Thus regeneration in hydra is controlled by **hypostomal factor** that stimulates head formation. In **planarians,** the **brain** has an inducing action on the regeneration of eyes, the head on the pharyngeal region, the prepharyngeal region on the pharynx and the genital glands on the copulatory organs. The mechanism of inhibition intervenes parallel to the inductive processes, thus preventing repetitive regeneration of an organ. Figure 20.5. shows the pattern of induction and inhibition exerted on anterior and posterior regions of Planaria.

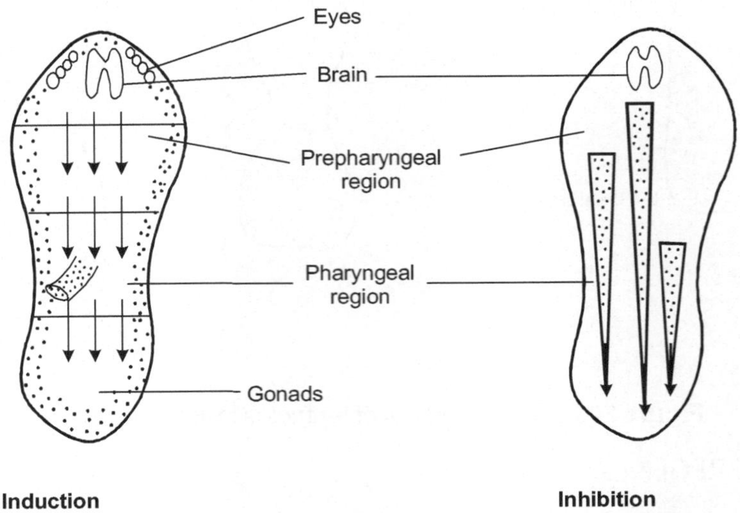

Figure 20.5 Diagrams to show the phenomenon of induction and inhibition of regeneration in Planaria

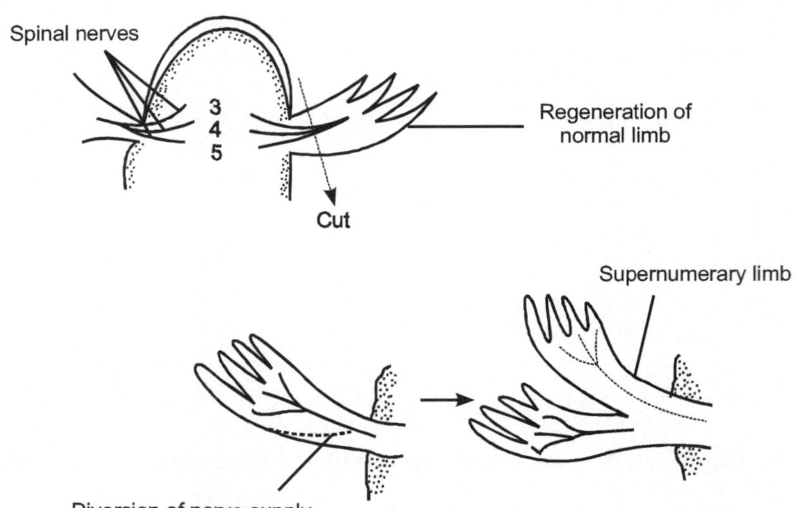

Figure 20.6 Regeneration induced by nerves in salamander

The role of various tissues in the limb regeneration of amphibians is poorly understood. But evidences are available to indicate the special role of adult tissues of the limb in the regeneration. The epithelium that covers the wound is found to be necessary for blastema formation and possibly it accounts for a kind of inductive reaction with the underlying tissues aiding in differentiation. The appropriate differentiation seems to be due to the mesodermal cells of the same morphogenetic field. When the blastema cells are replaced by the mesenchymal cells derived from the tail region, tail-like characteristics appear in the limb. The relationship of the nervous system to regeneration is another aspect. In **Salamander**, if the amputation of the limb is made with the spinal nerves, there is regeneration of a normal limb. But, if the limb is amputated after cutting the spinal nerves at the base of the brachial nerve, no regeneration occurs. The diversion of the nerve supply in the limb is found to regenerate supernumerary limbs. However, if the appropriate region of the neural tube is removed, then the limb exhibits regeneration but without nerve (Figure 20.6). These studies show that the nerve induces the surrounding cells, thus making them to depend on nerves in regeneration.

REGENERATION FIELD

In addition to various factors that are discussed so far for the occurrence of regeneration, the position of the wound in some way determines its nature. For example, if a cut is made in Salamander through a limb or a tail, then a limb or tail will regenerate respectively. When a part of the shoulder girdle is removed, the whole arm with the shoulder girdle is renewed. On the other hand, if the entire shoulder girdle with its muscles are completely removed, there is no renewal of arm. This clearly shows that regeneration requires the presence of a remnant of the original organ. With regard to regeneration, the shoulder girdle and the arm constitute one unit which is referred to as **regeneration field** or **regeneration territory**. When the territory of any specific organ is removed, then the wound simply heals in the region of cut without the formation of blastema and regeneration. In the case of Palinurus, heteromorphosis is due to the removal of the whole territory (ganglion and eye). In the presence of a part of the territory (ganglion), the complete system comprising the ganglion and eye is renewed.

Experiments in planarians and newts have proved that the regeneration cells are more plastic and retain a wide range of possibilities for differentiation in lower animals. In other words, the regeneration territories are not strictly restricted in these animals and the competence for the formation of a tail or a head gradually decreases from the anterior or posterior end of the body. In short, it may be mentioned that the regenerating cells possess the capacity of renewal within very definite limits and these limits are more narrow in higher animals than in lower forms. There is no doubt that the regeneration cells resemble the eggs or early cleavage cells in acquiring capacity for development. But a major difference is that the early embryonic cells are capable of undergoing development in complete isolation whereas the regeneration cells require the presence of a remainder of the body part to initiate and complete the development.

REVIEW QUESTIONS

1. Define the following terms:
   i. Ephimorphosis
   ii. Morphallaxis
   iii. Heteromorphosis
   iv. Autotomy
2. Give a survey on regeneration in the animal kingdom.
3. Explain the mechanism of regeneration in animals.
4. Give a brief account of various aspects of regeneration.
5. How does the regeneration territory influence regeneration?
6. Write a note on the role of nervous system in regeneration.
7. Write a brief account of the following:
   i. Reparative regeneration
   ii. Ephimorphic regeneration
   iii. Morphallactic regeneration
   iv. Heteromorphic regeneration
   v. Super regeneration
   vi. Wound healing
   vii. Blastema

21

REPRODUCTIVE AND DEVELOPMENTAL PATTERNS IN INVERTEBRATES

Based on the development, the invertebrate animals are divisible into two major groups namely **annelid superphylum** and **Echinoderm superphylum**. The annelid superphylum includes the phyla like Platyhelminthes, Annelida, Arthropoda, Mollusca and a few minor phyla. The individuals of these phyla have a **trochophore type of larva, mosaic development, spiral cleavage** and **schizocoelic coelom**. The Echinoderm superphylum includes the phyla namely Echinodermata and Chordata which possess a **pluteus type of larva, regulative development, radial cleavage** and **enterocoelic coelom**. The schizocoelic coelom found in vertebrates is secondary in nature. The annelid superphylum is otherwise known as **Protostomia** in which the blastopore becomes subdivided into two openings, one developing into mouth and the other into anus. The echinoderm superphylum is referred to as **Deuterostomia** in which only the anal opening is connected with the blastopore during development and the mouth develops later as an independent perforation of the body wall. The two types of larvae namely the trochophore larvae and the pluteus larvae found in these two groups strikingly resemble each other and the tornaria larvae of Prochordata is only a modified pluteus type of larva.

Asexual reproduction of one kind or another is prevalent in a number of invertebrate groups. Protozoans divide mitotically for many generations by **binary fission** or **multiple fission**. The reproduction in some protozoans like paramecia approach **sexual reproduction** via conjugation. Though sexual reproduction is prominent in all multicellular phyla including sponges, a number of more primitive groups reproduce asexually or by regeneration. In sponges, some exhibit regeneration and many reproduce by **budding**. All fresh water and some marine species reproduce via special asexual bodies called **gemmules**. In different invertebrates like coelenterates, helminth worms and few annelids and tunicates, agametic reproduction by **budding** and **fragmentation** is common. Some coelenterates like Hydra produce lateral **buds** whereas some others like flatworms and oligochaetes may multiply through a series of **transverse divisions**. In some groups of invertebrates, **parthenogenesis** is the only method of reproduction as seen in some helminth worms, rotifers, certain wasps and saw flies. In many cases, there is cyclical **alternation of generation** in which the asexual generation alternates with the sexual one. In many insects, the unfertilized eggs develop into haploid males whereas the fertilized eggs develop into females. **Gynogenesis** is a phenomenon in which a sperm activates an egg without the contribution of genetic materials so that the resulting embryo would possess only maternal chromosomes. The reverse condition of gynogenesis is known as **androgenesis.** Genetically speaking, the processes namely gynogenesis, androgenesis and regeneration are the same, since the offspring in each case possesses chromosomes from only one parent. In nature, gynogenesis is seen in a few non-segmented worms and insects. **Hermaphroditism** is another phenomenon found in all the major groups of invertebrates and vertebrates. It may either be a **protogynous type** or **protandrous** type in which the gonad produces only one type of gametes as seen in many invertebrates. In protogynous type, the ovarian tissue begins its function first so that the individuals produce eggs. In later life, if the population is reduced, the ovary is suppressed and the gonad begins to produce sperms. The reverse condition forms the protandrous type.

EARLY DEVELOPMENT IN SPONGES

Fresh water sponges reproduce asexually by producing **gemmules**. During gemmule formation, a new individual develops from groups of cells which become completely cut off from the mother so that the development is entirely independent of the maternal body even from the beginning of the development.

The **archeocytes** (undifferentiated amoeboid cells) dispersed among the differentiated cells of the sponge body accumulate as the rudiment of gemmule and the other cells arrange themselves in the form of columnar epithelium, thus forming the **shell** on the surface. The epithelial layer or the shell is strengthened by the deposition of **spicules** (amphidiscs) secreted by scleroblasts. The developing gemmule has a temporary opening called **micropyle** (Figure 21.1).

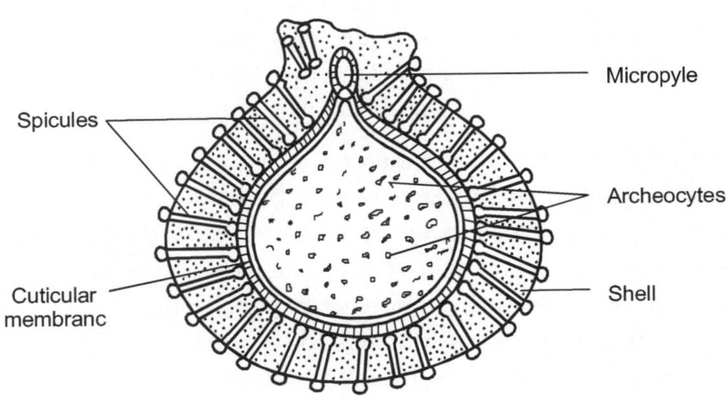

Figure 21.1 Structure of a gemmule.

The archeocytes are found to accumulate reserve food in the form of glycoproteins supplied by the trophocytes. Thus the interior of the developing gemmule contains only the archeocytes filled with glycoproteins in the form of discoidal platelets. Now some of the archeocytes become activated and divide repeatedly to form a number of smaller cells resembling blastomeres. As the division progresses, the size of the cells decreases with depletion of glycoprotein and the nuclei of the cells concentrate rich chromatin. These active small cells are called as **histioblasts** from which all the tissues and cell types of the new sponge develop. The fully developed gemmules are capable of survival even after the mother sponge dies due to unfavourable conditions. On destruction of the parental body, the gemmules are set free and produce new individuals during favourable conditions. When the gemmule germinates, its inner contents come out through the micropyle and form an irregular mass around the empty shell of the gemmule. Thus the histioblasts and the remaining archeocytes with remnant glycoprotein are brought to the outside of the shell where the formation of histioblasts from the archeocytes continue. The hostioblasts now become arranged into an irregular meshwork in which cavities appear. Some of the histioblasts differentiate into choanocytes surrounding these cavities. The epidermal cells, scleroblasts, pore canals, etc. develop from other histioblasts. The mass of cells thus soon becomes a small sponge.

In the formation of gemmule, the renewal of morphogenetic processes depends on the persistence of undifferentiated cells which are capable of developing into a variety of cells types. These undifferentiated cells are **totipotent** and so they are equivalent to the egg cell. Here the initial development is already multicellular and so cleavage is not necessary. However, the formation of gemmule somewhat resembles cleavage in the respect that the archeocytes accumulate reserve food materials as in the oocytes of ovary. Again, gastrulation is also not necessary because the cells are arranged in more than one layer during the formation of gemmule. Then the main aspects of gemmule development seem to be organogenesis, differentiation and growth. It can be mentioned that the formation of a new individual from gemmule is most complicated, approaching that of the development of the egg. However, the germination of gemmule occurs only after the death and decomposition of the parental body. In the absence of the parent body to influence the polarity of the offspring, the polarity of the new individual has to be acquired by itself. Moreover, the homogeneous contents of the gemmule do not possess any morphological organization so that the structure of a new sponge has to be established by the interaction of independent cells. Anyhow, the organization of the sponge body is mainly determined by the hereditary constitution of the species-specific cells.

In general, **sexual reproduction** in sponges involves **internal fertilization**. From the fertilized egg, a tiny ciliated larva develops and is liberated to the surrounding sea water. This larva freely swims in water for some time, becomes attached to the substratum and metamorphoses into adult. The occurrence of a free-swimming larval stage during development helps for the dispersal of the species. In the development of sponges, two major types of larvae namely **Parenchymula larva** and **Amphiblastula larva** are met with.

The **parenchymula larva** occurs in some simple forms of calcarea like **Olynthus**. The fertilized egg develops into a hollow **coeloblastula** with a large central cavity surrounded by a single layer of elongated, narrow and flagellated cells. At the posterior end, it has few rounded and non-flagellated archeocytes. Then some of the flagellated cells lose their flagella and become amoeboid cells which enter the central cavity along with archeocytes and fill the cavity.

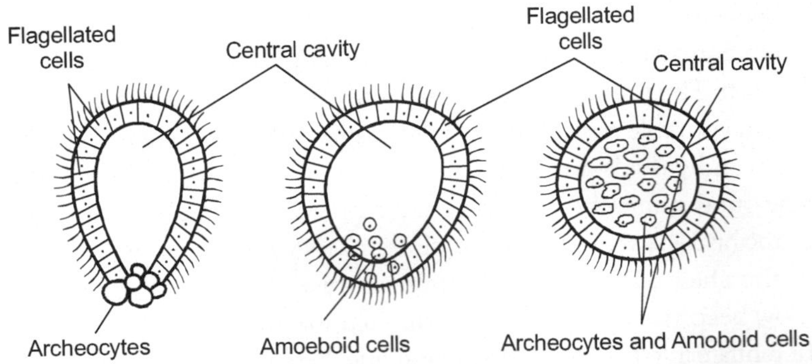

Figure 21.2 Formation of parenchymula larva in a sponge

This stage is called **parenchymula larva** which comes out of the parent body as a free-swimming larva (Figure 21.2). This larva actively swims in water for some time and then becomes attached to the substratum. It undergoes gastrulation by **invagination** so that the outer flagellated cells becomes inpushed. This invaginated layer becomes modified into choanocytes and the inner amoeboid cells migrate to the surface forming the **ectoderm** and **mesenchyme**. A central cavity, the spongocoel appears along with the osculum. With the development of spicules and other structures, the parenchymula larva develops into the adult sponge.

The **amphiblastula larva** occurs in most of the calcarea. The fertilized egg undergoes cleavage resulting in a 16-celled embryo with 2 tiers of 8 cells each. The cells in the upper tier are smaller blastomeres (**micromeres**) and the cells in the lower tier are larger blastomeres (**macromeres**). Soon, a cavity called blastocoel appears in between the cells of the two tiers. The smaller cells now multiply rapidly and each cell develops a flagellum facing the blastocoel. But the larger cells remain undivided, become rounded and granular. With the development of a large opening (mouth) in the middle of the larger cells, the embryo is now called as **stomoblastula**. It undergoes a phenomenon called **inversion** by which it turns inside out through the mouth.

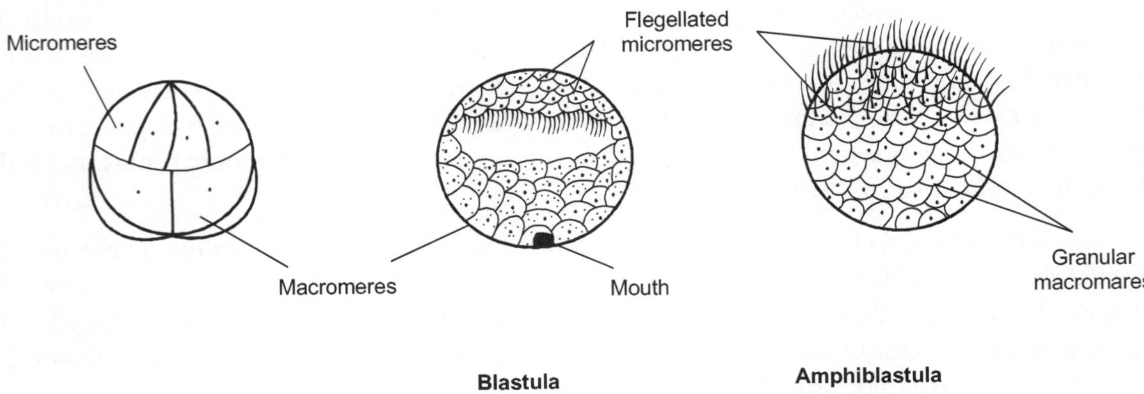

Figure 21.3 Formation of amphiblastula larva in a sponge

As a result, the flagellar ends of micromeres are brought to the outside and the mouth disappears. Now the embryo is called as **amphiblastula larva** which is more or less oval in shape with small, narrow and flagellated micromeres in one half and large, rounded, granulated and unflagellated macromeres in another half (Figure 21.3). When fully formed, it escapes from the parent body, leads a free-swimming life for few hours and undergoes gastrulation by **invagination**. Hence the flagellated micromeres become inpushed resulting in a typical double-walled **gastrula** with a blastopore. The non-flagellated granular cells are arranged as the outer layer and flagellated cells as the inner layer. Soon it attaches to the substratum and undergoes metamorphosis. The ectoderm and mesenchyme are developed from the macromeres and the choanocytic layer from the micromeres. Now the larva elongates into a cylinder with the development of osculum at the free end and the dermal ostia in the body wall. At this stage, the young sponge is called as **olynthus stage** which closely resembles a simple ascon type. With the formation of radial canals, shifting of flagellated cells into the radial canals, thickening of the body wall and appearance of spicules and canal system, the adult stage (**syconoid**) is developed.

It is noteworthy that the sponge development exhibits a peculiar feature in the form of **inversion of germ layers** which is not found in all other metazoans. In sponges, the choanocytes arise from the larval outer layer which becomes internal during metamorphosis and the inner mass of cells of the embryo becomes the dermal epithelium. But in other metazoans, the gastral layer develops from the non-flagellated layers of the larva and the dermal layer from the flagellated layer of cells. Therefore, sponges occupy a unique position in the animal kingdom as an isolated branch of Metazoa namely Parazoa.

EARLY DEVELOPMENT IN COELENTERATES

In coelenterates like **Obelia**, **Aurelia**, etc., the fertilized egg undergoes cleavage and a ball of cells enclosing a cavity called **blastocoel** is produced. In Obelia, the cavity of the blastula is filled up with cells budded off from the outer layer and this inner mass of cells represent the endoderm. The outer layer, the ectoderm, becomes ciliated. But in some coelenterates like Aurelia, the blastula undergoes invagination resulting in a two-layered embryo with a central cavity. The outer ectodermal layer develops cilia and the inner layer forms the endoderm enclosing the **archenteron** which opens to the outside by a **blastopore**. At this stage, the embryo is set free from the egg as a free-swimming, mouthless and ciliated larva called **planula larva** (Figure 21.4).

It elongates, swims for sometime in water, loses the cilia and settles down to the substratum. In Obelia, the larva develops an inner cavity. Mouth and tentacles appear at its free end. In Aurelia, the larva settles down after the closure of the blastopore and develops mouth and tentacles at the free end. The planula larva develops into the adult colony in Obelia whereas in Aurelia, it transforms into another type of larva called **scyphistoma** which by strobilization gives rise to another larva known as **Ephyra larva.** These larvae in turn develop into adults.

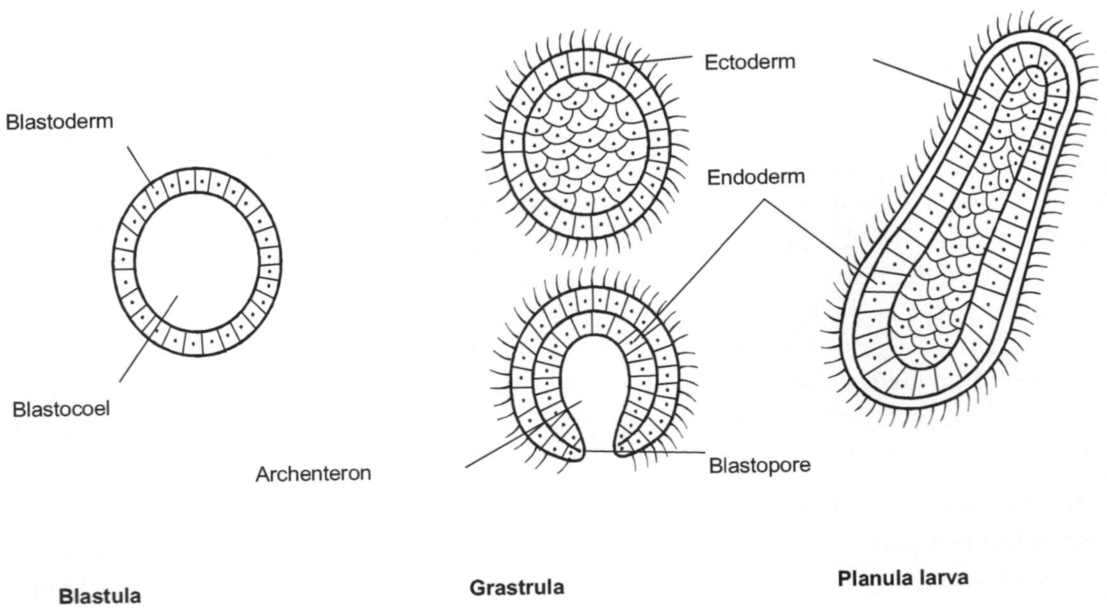

Figure 21.4 Formation of planula larva in a coelenterate animal

Ctenophore coelenterates are hermaphrodites and reproduce sexually by producing ova and sperms. The gonads are endodermal in origin and the fertilization is external. The egg is **telolecithal** as against other coelenterates and so the yolk is not uniformly distributed in the egg, i.e., the yolk is accumulated more towards the vegetal pole and the nucleus is at the animal pole. The fertilized egg undergoes cleavage and the first two cleavages are meridional resulting in four cells. The third cleavage is vertical in two places so that 8 cells are formed. Among these 8 cells, the middle 4 cells are large and the outer cells are small. This type of cleavage is called **bimodial cleavage** which is characteristic of ctenophores. The long axis of the 8-celled embryo forms the tentacles in the adult and thus bilateral symmetry is formed even in this early stage. Due to the **telolecithal** nature of the egg, the resulting cells are **unequal, total** and **determinate**. The animal pole divides more rapidly resulting in smaller micromeres and the vegetal pole produces larger macromeres. Later, a solid ball of cells are formed without a cavity inside, thus developing into a **solid blastula**. This blastula undergoes gastrulation by which the micromeres by further division grow over the macromeres, forming the outer layer. Thus a central mass of larger macromeres become surrounded by a single layer of micromeres with a blastopore which disappears later. The micromeres form the ectoderm and the macromeres develop into the endoderm. This process of formation of gastrula by the growing of the micromeres over the macromeres forming the inner layer is called **epiboly**. Now the ectoderm at the lower pole invaginates and forms the mouth and stomodaeum (Figure 21.5). By further development, the embryo is transformed into a free-swimming larva called **cydippid larva** which gradually develops into the adult.

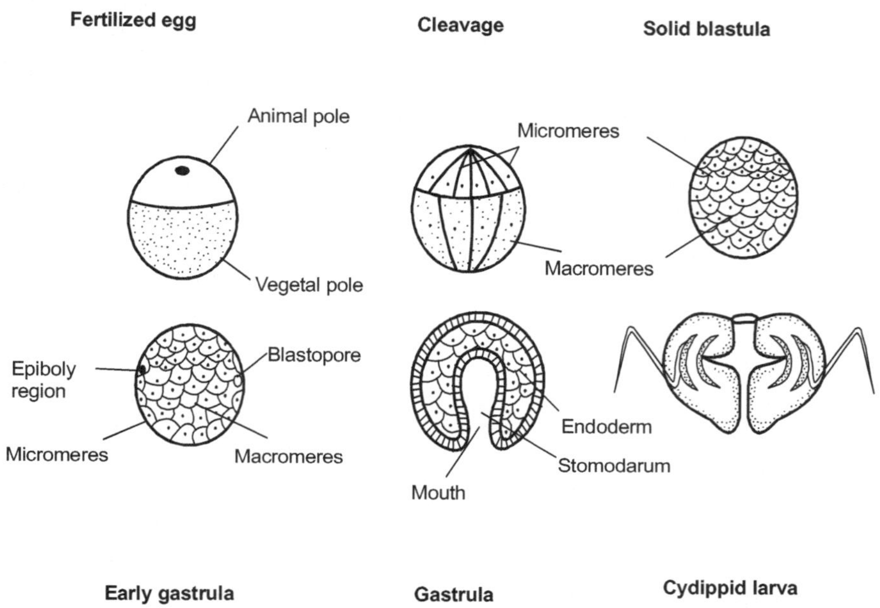

Figure 21.5 Early development of a ctenophore.

The planula larva in coelenterates represents the gastrula stage of higher animals. The free-swimming larvae in the life history of coelenterate representatives is helpful for the disbursal of the species.

EARLY DEVELOPMENT OF FRESH WATER MUSSEL

In fresh water mussel, fertilization occurs in the outer gill lamina which acts as a brood pouch for further development of zygote. Immediately after fertilization, the zygote undergoes cleavage which is **complete** and **unequal** so that a hollow ball of cells are produced. This **blastula** has a fluid-filled cavity called **blastocoel** and consists of two types of cells namely micromeres on the animal pole and macromeres on the vegetal pole. The **micromeres** are small, clear, yolkless and rapidly multiplying cells whereas the **macromeres** are large yolk-filled and slowly dividing cells. Now the blastula undergoes **invagination** so that the macromeres become impushed into the micromeres resulting in a **gastrula** enclosing a small archenteron. A few larger cells bud off into the blastocoel and they differentiate into the mesoderm. Simultaneously, a deep invagination occurs on the postero-dorsal side of the embryo, forming the characteristic molluscan organ namely the shell gland. Initially, the shell gland secretes a single embryonic shell which is replaced later by a bivalved shell (Figure 21.6). Long cilia arise from the posterior end of the embryo and the mesoderm cells form the adductor muscle.

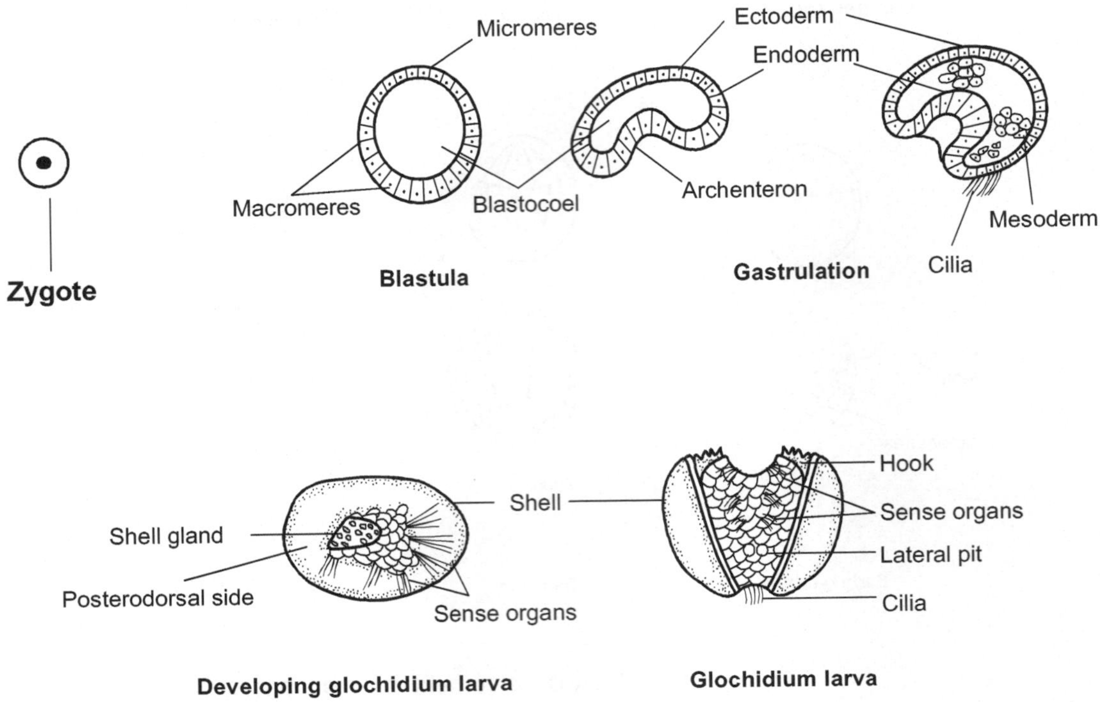

Figure 21.6 Early development of fresh water mussel.

The mouth of the gastrula soon closes and a new definite mouth is formed by the invagination of the ectoderm. Gradually, the embryo develops into a larva called **glochidium larva** which metamorphoses into the adult animal.

EARLY DEVELOPMENT OF STARFISH

In starfish, fertilization is external occurring in the sea water. Here, the egg is small, spherical and homolecithal and the cleavage is **total, equal, holoblastic** and of **indeterminate type.** As a result of cleavage, a typical, spherical, single-layered, hollow and ciliated **coeloblastula** with a blastocoel is formed . The ciliated blastula swims freely in water and undergoes gastrulation by **invagination.** As a result, the outer layer becomes impushed resulting in an elongated, two-layered gastrula. It has an outer ectoderm and an endoderm enclosing the archenteron which opens to the outside by a wide opening, the blastopore. During invagination, the tip of the archenteron gives rise to the mesenchyme cells into the blastocoel. The growing archenteron differentiates into two parts. The upper part develops two lateral pouches which give rise to the right and left coelomic sacs. The narrower lower part becomes the stomach and intestine with the blastopore becoming the anus (Figure 21.7).

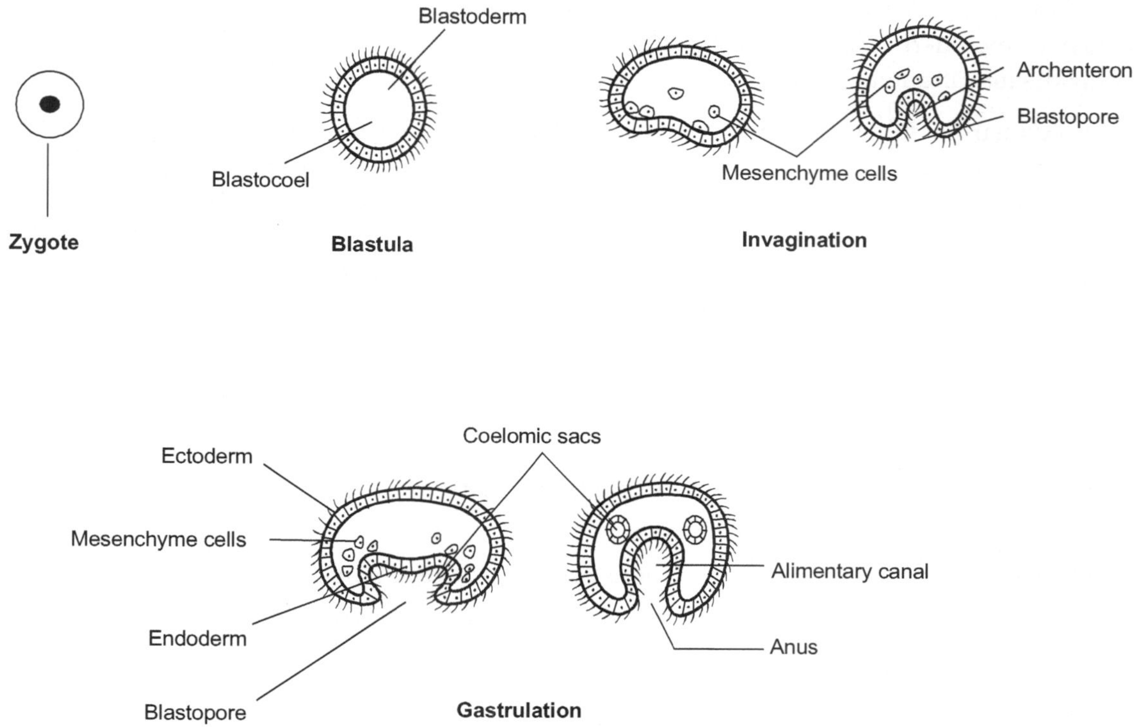

Figure 21.7 Early development of starfish egg with the formation of coelom and mesoderm.

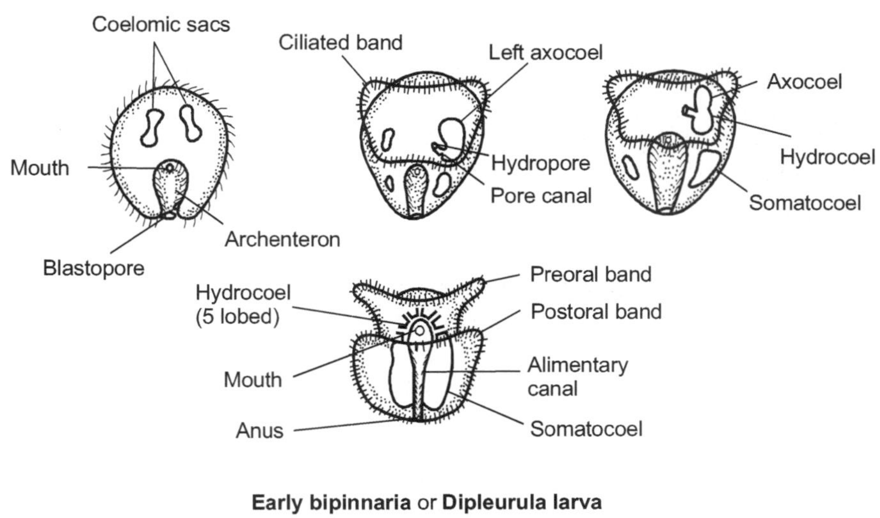

Figure 21.8 Development of coelom and water vascular system in starfish.

Of the two coelomic sacs, the left one grows more rapidly than the right and gives rise to the coelom. Its mesodermal lining develops into the water vascular system. The fully grown left coelomic sac divides into an anterior portion called **axocoel** and a posterior portion, the **somatocoel**.

Now a narrow tubular outgrowth develops from the anterior portion of axocoel to the dorsal surface where it opens by the hydropore. This is the **pore canal** through which water passes into the coelom and it becomes the stone canal of the adult. Soon the left axocoel gives rise to another hollow outgrowth called **hydrocoel** which is the beginning of the water vascular ssytem (Figure 21.8). The hydrocoel develops into the ring canal and radial canals of the adult. The right coelomic sac is represented only by a small vesicle.

This embryo is free swimming and is called **early bipinnaria larva** which soon develops into bipinnaria larva. This free-swimming larva metamorphoses into the adult through the **Brachiolaria stage**.

REVIEW QUESTIONS

1. Explain the various developmental patterns met within invertebrates.
2. What is a gemmule? How do fresh water sponges reproduce through gammules?
3. Write an essay on sexual reproduction and development in sponges.
4. Give an account of early development of coelenterates.
5. Brief the early development of fresh water mussel and starfish.
6. Write notes on the following :
   i. Gemmule
   ii. Histioblasts
   iii. Parenchymula
   iv. Amphiblastula
   v. Planula larva
   vi. Glochidium

22

INVERTEBRATE LARVAE AND THEIR SIGNIFICANCE

The major phyla of invertebrates are classified into two major divisions namely **annelid superphylum** or **Protostomia** and **echinoderm superplylum** or **Deuterostomia** on the basis of their development. During development, the individuals of annelid superphylum possess **trochophore type of larvae** whereas the echinoderm superphylum exhibit **pluteus type of larvae**. Trochophore larva occurs in the development of animals belonging to various diversified groups such as Polycladida, Turbellaria, Nemertinea, Bryozoa, Annelida and Mollusca and resembles very closely certain adult rotifers. In these groups, the early stages of development especially the trochophore stages are almost similar in many respects. According to the **Trochophore theory** (**Hatschek**, 1878), the trochophore is the larva of an ancestral form namely the trochozoan which could be the common ancestor for most of the bilateral phyla. The widely accepted version of Trochophore theory is known as the **Ctenophore–Trochophore theory** which reiterates that the trochophore larva might have evolved from a Ctenophore-like ancestor through the Trochozoan. Thus this theory bridges the gap between the radiates and bilateral animals. However, the trochophore larva somewhat resembles the larvae of other Protostomous phyla namely Muller's larva of Polycladida and Pilidium larva of nemertines. These three distinct larval types clearly represent the modified **Ctenophore** ancestral group from which Polycladida, Nemertinea and Annelida arose.

TROCHOPHORE LARVA OF ANNELIDA

In polychaetes, the fertilized egg develops into a trochophore larva which is typically a minute, unsegmented, ciliated and pear-shaped, pelagic larva with a broader and a narrower end (Figure 22.1). The middle of the apical region has an epidermal thickening called apical plate which has a tuft of sensory **apical cilia**. The mouth is ventral in position lying in the middle of the body. It opens into a short ectodermal stomodaeum which opens into an endodermal stomach or midgut and then into the ectodermal proctodaeum or hindgut. The hindgut opens to the outside through the anus which is placed at the posterior end of the body. The entire alimentary canal is ciliated. The larva has no coelom, but a large space representing the blastocoel is present between the ectoderm and endoderm. It has a pair of protonephridia. A statocyst is also present with a tuft of cilia near the anus.

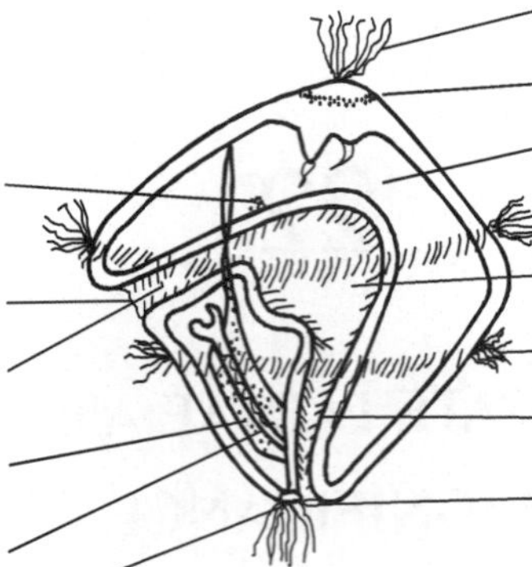

Figure 22.1 Structure of trochophore larva

Typically, the trochophore larva has a pre-oral circlet of cilia or **prototroch** in front of the mouth and a post-oral circlet or **metatroch** just behind the mouth. These ciliary bands are in the form of girdles surrounding the body. They help in swimming and also in food capturing. However, the arrangement of cilia in the larva varies in different polychaetes. Therefore, the trochophore larvae are classified into 4 types based on the ciliary distribution. In **atrochal type**, the body is uniformly ciliated without the differentiation of pre-oral and post-oral bands. **Mesotrochal type** of trochophore has a single band of cilia at the middle of the body where there is no prototroch and metatroch. In **telotrochal** type, the larva has a telotroch around the anus in addition to prototroch and mesotroch. When the Trochophore possesses several circlets of cilia between the mouth and anus, it is **polytrochal type**.

Trochophore larva after a free-swimming existence in sea water, undergoes metamorphosis. The pre-oral end becomes differentiated into the prostomium of the adult. The post-oral region elongates and becomes constricted into segments which soon develop parapodia. The internal mesoderm band divides into somites each of which now develops a coelom and the original blastocoel is eliminated. Then the ciliary bands disappear and the larva grows in size and length with the addition of new segments in front of the caudal segment. This young worm now sinks to the bottom and becomes a burrowing adult.

CRUSTACEAN LARVA

In most crustaceans, the development includes a little or more metamorphosis. In the case of large eggs with much yolk, the development is direct without a larval stage whereas in small eggs with little amount of yolk, the development is indirect with one or more larval forms. The following account gives a description of various types of larvae seen among the crustaceans.

Nauplius Larva

It is the most common larva seen in crustaceans. All crustaceans start their development with a free-swimming nauplius larva. Typically it has an oval unsegmented body with an anterior broader end and a posterior narrow end (Figure 22.2). Anteriorly, it has a simple median eye and 3 pairs of appendages—antennullary feet, antennary feet and mandibular feet—with a pair of telson at the posterior end. The larva actively swims in water with the help of appendages. Mouth develops anteriorly and anus posteriorly but the larva cannot feed. It undergoes a series of moults and develops into several types of larvae such as metanauplius, protozoea, zoea and mysis which metamorphoses into the adult in **Penaeus** (Prawn).

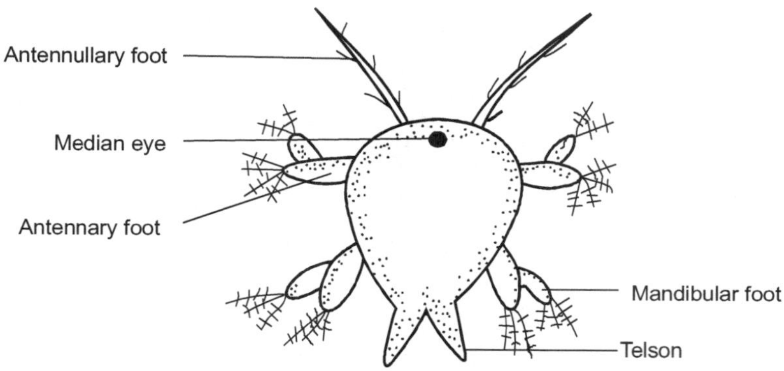

Figure 22.2 Nauplius larva.

Metanauplius Larva

It is very similar to the nauplius structurally but it exhibits some segmentation of the body. It develops 4 pairs of additional rudimentary appendages which become the I maxillae, II maxillae, I maxillipedes and II maxillipedes of adult respectively. The frontal organ begins to appear and the mandibles acquire mastigatory function so that the larva begins to feed. Some decapods like **Lucifer** begin their development as metanauplius.

Protozoea Larva

In **Penaeus**, the metanauplius larva develops into a protozoea larva with the formation of a carapace covering the dorsal surface of the body anteriorly. (Figure 22.3). The seven pairs of appendages of metanauplius become well-developed and begin to function. The larva has paired lateral eyes and six appendages. However, the abdomen is unsegmented. In older protozoea, III maxillipedes also appear along with the demarcation of five anterior abdominal segments.

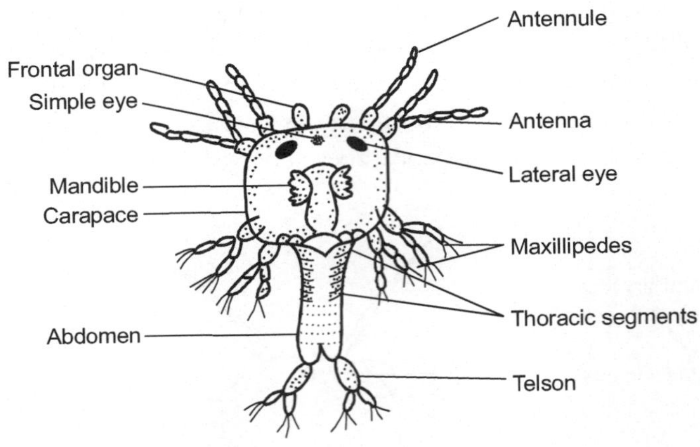

Figure 22.3 Protozoea larva.

Zoea Larva

This is the second important larva in crustaceans and its structure is depicted in Figure 22.4. In this larva, the head has fused with the thorax to form a distinct caphalothorax. The carapace is produced into a rostral spine and the lateral compound eyes becomes stalked and movable. The maxillipedes are well-developed and six pairs of walking legs appear. The segmentation of abdomen begins at this stage. The fully developed older zoea is called **metazoea** in which six pairs of abdominal appendages begin to develop. In crustaceans like crabs, the development begins with a zoea larva.

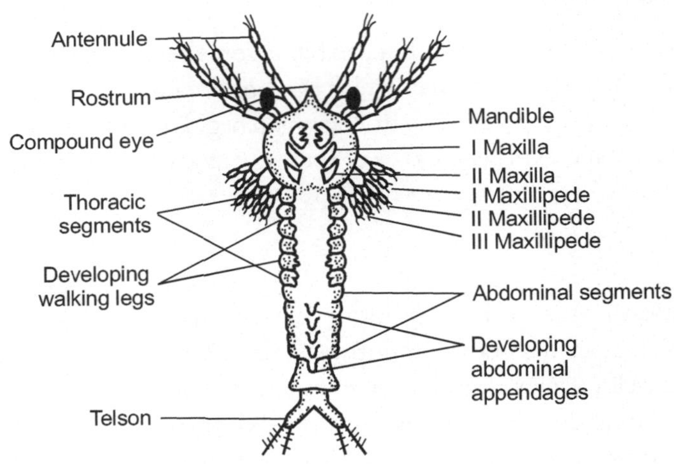

Figure 22.4 Zoea larva.

Mysis or Schizopod Larva

In **Penaeus**, the zoea larva moults into a mysis larva because this stage structurally resembles an adult **Mysis** as shown in Figure 22.5. In this larva the cephalothorax becomes covered by carapace dorsally.

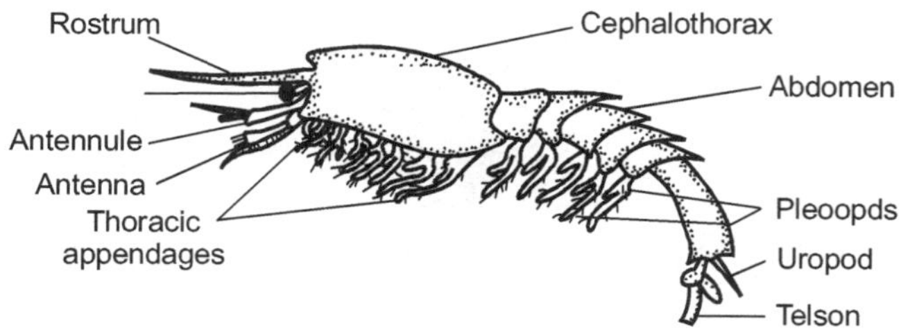

Figure 22.5 Mysis larva.

All the cephalothoracic appendages have developed and the thoracic appendages are used in locomotion. The abdomen elongates and pleopods begin to develop with uropod. This larva metamorphoses into an adult in the life history of prawn. But in the life history of **lobster,** the development begins with mysis stage.

Phyllosoma Larva

In the rock lobster (**Palinurus**), the newly hatched larva is called as **phyllosoma** or **glass crab** which is nothing but a modified mysis stage (Figure 22.6). It is larger in size with a leaf-like, delicate and flattened body with a glassy transparency and so the name glass crab. The larval body is divisible into head, thorax and abdomen. The head has paired antennules, stalked compound eyes, antennae, I maxillipeds and II maxillipeds. The thoracic appendages are extremely elongated and biramous.

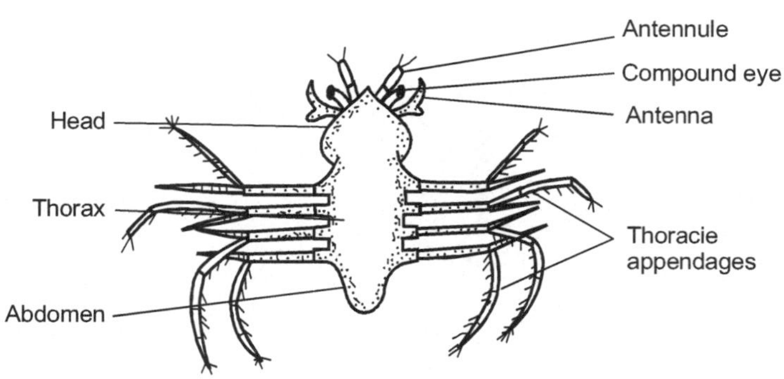

Figure 22.6 Phyllosoma larva

Alima Larva

It is the larva of **squilla** and is a modified zoea larva (Figure 22.7). Its body is slender and transparent. The cephalothorax is dorsally covered by a broad carapace with a dorsal spine and stalked compound eyes. The II maxillipedes are long and prehensile and the II maxillae are raptorial in function. The abdominal appendages are present and the telson is provided with spines.

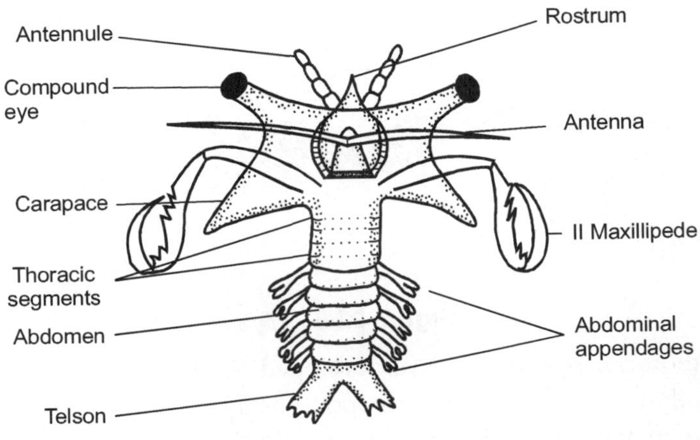

Figure 22.7 Alima larva

Megalopa Larva

It is the larva of **crab** in which the zoea larva develops into the megalopa stage. It has a broad and crab like cephalothorax which is dorsally covered by a carapace (Figure 22.8). The carapace is anteriorly produced into a median spine. The eyes are large and stalked. The abdomen is well-developed with biramous pleopods. The larva lives on surface water but later sinks to the bottom and metamorphoses into the adult in which the abdomen begins to reduce and comes to lie just below the cephalothorax.

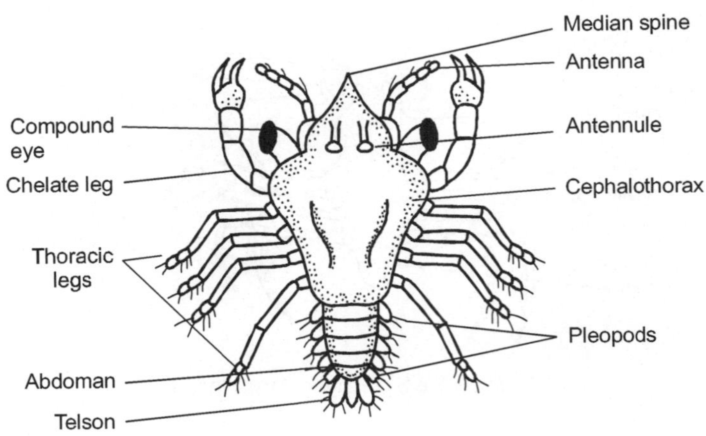

Figure 22.8 Megalopa larva

Cypris Larva

In **Lepas**, the nauplius larva develops into a stage called cypris larva in which the body is differentiated into head, thorax and abdomen and is enclosed by a bivalved shell attached by adductor muscles. The head bears compound eyes and a peduncle which continues as the antennule, ending in a disc. The larva has six pairs of thoracic appendages and four abdominal segments (Figure 22.9).

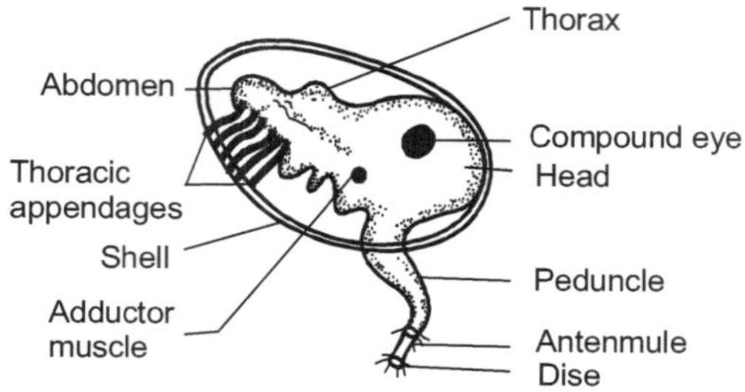

Figure 22.9 Cypris larva

Kentrogen Stage

In **Sacculina**, the cypris larva is transformed into a larva called kentrogen stage in which the shells are lost and the body is covered by new cuticle. The body structures are entirely modified into an undifferentiated mass (Figure 22.10). It develops a tubular structure known as dart through which the cell mass is passed into the body cavity of the crab, the host.

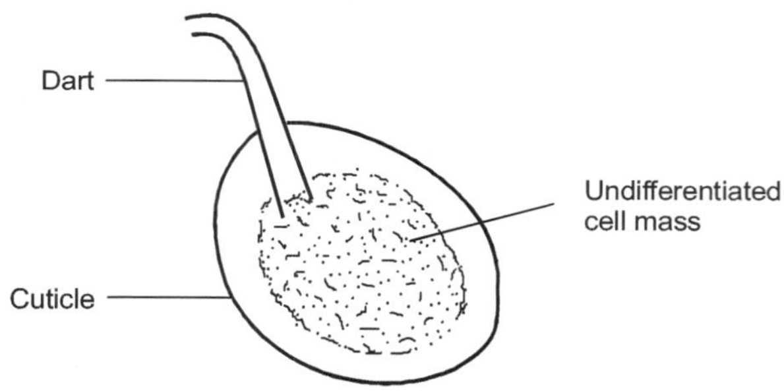

Figure 22.10 Kentrogen larva.

Significance of Crustacean Larvae

According to **Haeckel's biogenetic law**, every organism in its development (ontogeny) repeats to some extent its ancestral characters (phylogeny). Therefore, it can be said that all crustaceans might have evolved from a nauplius-like ancestor because all crustaceans start their development as nauplius larva. In addition, the study of larval stages in crustaceans is useful in the identification of certain groups of crustaceans. For example, **Sacculina**, a parasitic crustacean on crabs, can be identified as a crustacean only on studying the characteristics of its larval stages.

ECHINODERM LARVAE

In most echinoderms, the development includes a free-living, pelagic, transparent and bilaterally symmetrical larval stage. From the fertilized egg, an embryo with its uniformly ciliated body develops and freely swims in water with the help of cilia. Within a short period, the uniformly arranged cilia become concentrated into longitudinal bands. In some echinoderms like **starfishes**, there are two longitudinal bands of cilia and the others have only one ciliated band.

Bipinnaria Larva

It is the larva of **starfish** and is bilaterally symmetrical. The postoral region of the body is broad while the pre-oral region is elongated (Figure 22.11).

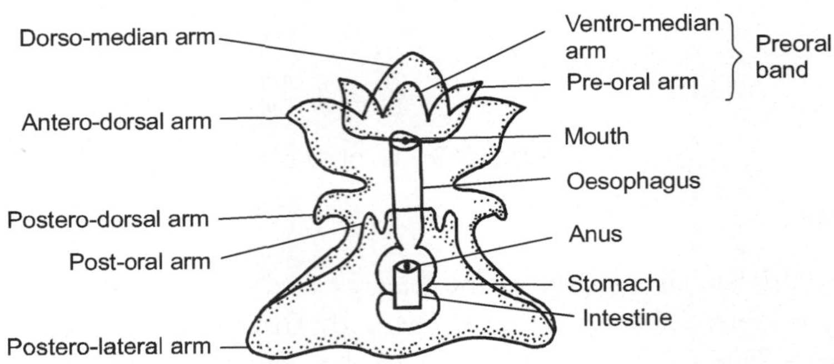

Figure 22.11 Bipinnaria larva of starfish

The body is encircled by **pre-oral** and **post-oral ciliated bands** which are thrown into definite arms and are used for locomotion and food capture. The preoral band is thrown into an unpaired ventro-median arm and a pair of pre-oral arms. The post-oral band is thrown into a dorso-median arm and paired antero-dorsal, postero-dorsal, post-oral and postero-lateral arms. It has a simple alimentary canal which is bent so that both the mouth and anus open on the same side.

This bipinnaria larva freely swims in water for six or seven weeks, settles to the sea bottom, temporarily fixes itself by the pre-oral lobe and undergoes metamorphosis. At this stage, the larva is called as **brachiolaria larva**. It resembles the bipinnaria larva in structure except that there are three additional arms called brachiolar arms at the anterior part of the larva. Each arm is provided with a sucker at its tip for attachment. The bilaterally symmetrical brachiolaria larva gradually metamorphoses into a radially symmetrical adult. During metamorphosis, the larva rotates through 90° clockwise with the loss of larval arms and ciliated bands. The larval mouth and anus close and a new mouth appears on the oral side while a new anus is formed on the aboral side. By the development of skeletal elements, radial canals, tube feet and other internal structures, the larva becomes a young starfish.

Ophiopluteus Larva

It is the larva of **brittle star** and has a single ciliated band (pre-oral band only) encircling the body (Figure 22.12). This ciliated band is thrown into long, paried, pre-oral, postero-dorsal, postero-lateral and post-oral arms supported by calcareous rods. The postero-lateral arms are always long and directed forward so that the larva has the appearance of a 'V'. It metamorphoses into the adult and there is no attachment stage.

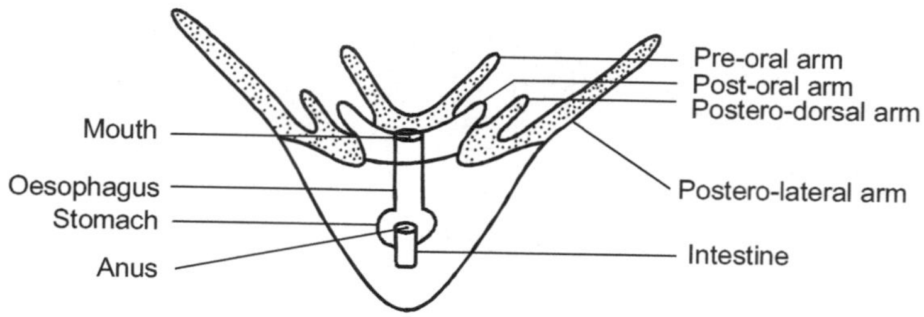

Figure 22.12 Ophiopluteus larva of Brittlestar.

Echinopluteus Larva

This larva occurs in the life history of **sea urchin** and resembles the ophiopluteus larva in having a single ciliary band supported by calcareous rods (Figure 22.13). In this larva, the postero-lateral arms are usually absent and if present, they are much reduced and directed backwards. The paired antero-lateral arms which are wanting in the ophiopluteus larva are seen. In addition, the larva has two ciliated structures called epaulettes which are meant for locomotion. It also metamorphoses directly into adult without an attachment stage.

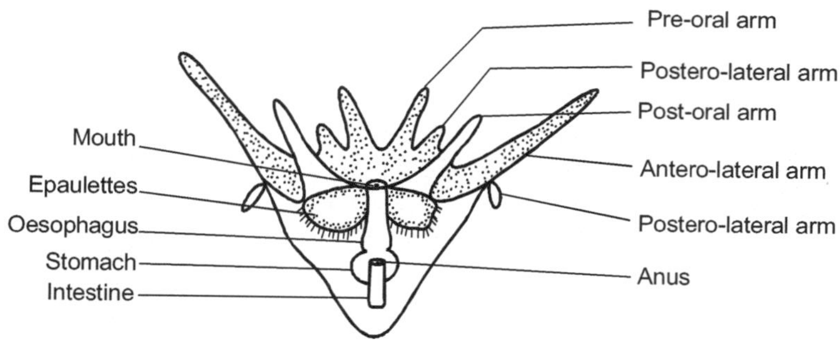

Figure 22.13 Echinopluteus larva of sea urchin.

Auricularia Larva

The development of **sea cucumber** exhibits auricularia larva which closely resembles the bipinnaria larva but the arms are not so much elongated (Figure 22.14). Moreover, it has only a single ciliary band which is thrown into paired processes without being supported by calcareous rods. The paired processes include pre-orals, antero- dorsals, postero-dorsals and postero-laterals.

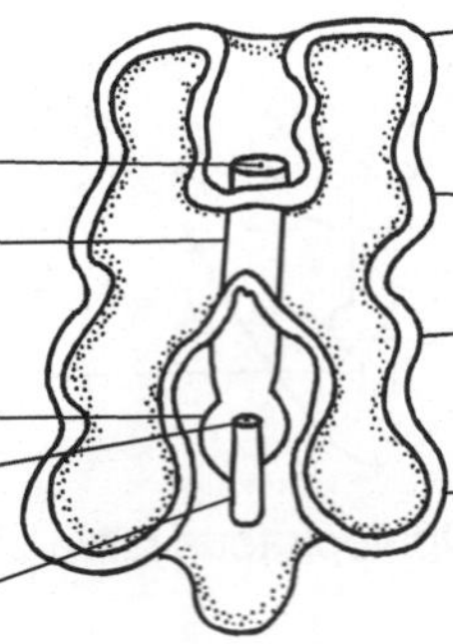

Figure 22.14 Auricularia larva of sea cucumber

Doliolaria or Antedon larva

In **sea lily** (Antedon), the development has a doliolaria larva which possesses a tuft of cilia called apical tuft of cilia at the pre-oral end. The body of the larva is encircled by five ciliated bands which are used for locomotion. Above the first ciliary band, there is an adhesive pit midventrally near the apical tuft. The vestibule is located in between the first and third ciliated bands (Figure 22.15).

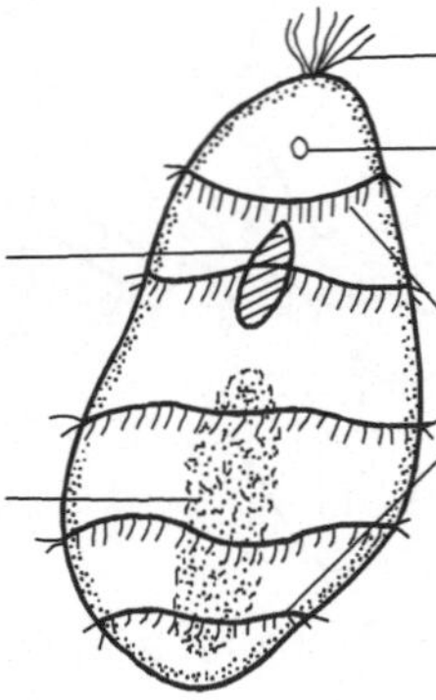

Figure 22.15 Doliolaria larva of sea lily.

The larva freely swims in water for sometime, attaches to the substratum and rotates through 90° clockwise. It develops a stalk and this stage is called **pentacrinoid larva** or **cystidean larva** which metamorphoses into adult.

Significance of Echinoderm Larvae

The larval forms of echinoderms are useful to derive some ideas with regard to the phylogeny of echinoderms. A close study of echinoderm larvae exhibit so many fundamental resemblances like free-living and pelagic habitat, ciliary bands thrown into arms, simple alimentary canal, bilateral symmetry and so on. These common characteristic features suggest that all the echinoderms might have originated from a common ancestor. Echinoderms are believed to be evolved from a free-living, coelomate and bilateral ancestor. So, the bilateral condition may be recapitulated in these echinoderm larvae. The radial symmetry of echinoderms is clearly indicative of the attached life of early echinoderms. Thus the existing echinoderms might have evolved from these early attached forms, the ancestors of which were bilaterally symmetrical and free-swimming forms. It is to be noted that the fossils of the earlier echinoderms are all attached forms.

In addition, the echinoderm larvae are also useful to trace the origin of chordates. According to **Garstang's auricularia theory**, a ciliated auricularia-like larva might have been converted into a fish- like creature through progressive stages with muscular locomotion. According to Garstang, the fish-like form arose by the development of muscles along the sides of the elongated body of the larva in which the ciliated bands were being pushed upwards and eventually rolled up with their underlying sheets of nerve plexus to form the neural tube. The adoral ciliated band might then be transformed into the endostyle. Thus the larval tunicate organization may be directly derived from an echinoderm-like auricularia larva. Then fish-like forms might have evolved by **neoteny** or **paedogenesis**. It is an accepted view that the early free-swimming adult chordates arose from some tunicate larva-like metamorphosing form by **paedomorphosis**.

REVIEW QUESTIONS

1. Describe the trochophore larva of annelids.
2. Give an account of crustacean larvae.
3. Write an essay on echinoderm larvae.
4. Enumerate the significance of the study of invertebrate larvae.
5. Write notes on the following:
   i. Trochophore theory
   ii. Nauplius
   iii. Bipinnaria
   iv. Auricularia
   v. Auricularia theory

Appendix I

SELECTED BASIC EMBRYOLOGICAL METHODS

1. Examination of Fresh Sperms of Frog from a Squash Preparation

Aim To examine fresh sperms from a squash preparation of frog's testis.

Materials Mature male frog, Petri dish, dropper, dissection instruments, compound microscope, glass slides, cover glasses and 10% Holtfreter's solution.

Method A sexually matured male frog is pithed and the testes are dissected out to a Petri dish containing 10% Holtfreter's solution. The testes are macerated thoroughly until a milky white suspension is obtained. The sperm suspension is kept aside for about 15 minutes allowing the sperms to become motile. A drop of this sperm suspension is placed on a glass slide and is covered by a cover glass. The slide is examined under the microscope. The characteristic movement of the live sperms is noted and sketched.

Alternately, the testes after removal to the Petri dish are cut into small pieces. Two pieces are placed on a clean glass slide with a drop of solution and covered with a cover glass which is gently pressed to make a squash. The slide is examined under the microscope and thousands of actively swimming sperms are seen.

2. Observation of Fresh Eggs, Fertilization and Early Cleavage in Frog

Aim To observe fresh eggs, fertilization and early cleavage by using frog in the laboratory.

Materials Sexually matured male and female frogs, Petri dishes, dissection instruments, compound microscope, 10% Holtfreter's solution, etc.

Method A healthy sexually matured male frog is dissected and the testes are removed into a Petri dish containing 10 ml of 10% Holtfreter's solution. The testes are crushed with the help of a clean glass rod so that the solution would contain active spermatozoa. This sperm suspension is taken in several Petri dishes. By dissecting a healthy sexually matured female frog or by induced ovulation, the eggs are directly stripped into the sperm suspension taken in the Petri dishes. Now the eggs are fertilized within 5 minutes.

At this stage, the fresh eggs and fertilized eggs are observed. The fertilized eggs could be easily identified. After fertilization, the eggs rotate so that the animal hemisphere (black colour) comes uppermost within an hour. Moreover, the jelly coat of the fertilized eggs gradually absorbs water and swells so that the jelly coat is allowed to swell to its maximum. Now the eggs are separated and transferred carefully into fresh Petri dishes containing 500 ml Holtfreter's solutiuon with 25 eggs in each Petri dish. The early cleavage of the egg is examined under the microscope. The fresh eggs, fertilized eggs and early cleavage stages are sketched.

3. Induced Ovulation in Frog

Aim To study induced ovulation in frog by injecting pituitary extract (pituitrin).

Materials Mature male and female frogs, dissection instruments, aquarium jars with lids, hypodermic syringe and needle, mortar and pestle, Petri dishes, chloroform and 10% Holtfreter's solution.

Method: The required male frogs are anaesthetized by using chloroform. In each frog, the pituitary gland is carefully dissected out into a Petri dish. For this, the upper jaw is cut just behind the tympanum and the brain is exposed from the ventral side to trace the optic chiasma. The pituitary body is located just posterior to the optic chiasma as a pinkish, kidney-shaped structure. The gland is removed with the help of sharp forceps into the petridish containing 10% Holtfreter's solution. In this way five pituitary glands are dissected out and ground with Holtfreter's solution contained in a mortar and pestle. The preparation is injected with the help of syringe and needle into the body cavity of a large, healthy and sexually matured female frog without injuring the internal organs. At the place of injection, the skin is pinched while drawing the needle to prevent the loss of the injected fluid. This injected frog is now placed in a wire-covered aquarium jar containing little quantity of water. Small insects are provided as feed to the frog.

After a period of time (24 hours to 48 hours), a few eggs are released by the frog instantaneously. If not so, the frog is taken and its abdomen is gently squeezed by holding the animal in both the hands in a lateral position. If any egg passes out of the cloaca, it confirms the occurrence of ovulation. If not, the frog is again kept in the jar for one more day to observe ovulation. The amount of pituitary extract injected and the time taken for ovulation are recorded.

4. Temporary Mountings of Chick Embryos of Different Stages

Aim To prepare and examine temporary mountings of chick embryos of different stages after proper staining.

Materials Fertilized eggs of chick, egg incubator, dissection instruments, Petri dishes, cavity slides, cover glasses, dropper, filter paper, thermometer, dissection microscope, 1% saline solution, 70% alcohol, glycerol, and alcoholic eosin (70%).

Method The incubator is set at 38°C or 100.4°F with 50% humidity by placing a large pan of water in the lowest shelf of the incubator. The fertilized eggs are kept in the incubator after marking the date and time on them. After the stipulated period of time, the egg is removed from the incubator and the shell is removed in pieces with the help of forceps by breaking the shell at the broader end of the egg by means of a scalpel. The embryo with the yolk is now allowed to float in 1% saline solution contained in a Petri dish. The blastoderm is cut along the margin and is separated from the yolk. Then the embryo with the blastoderm is carefully transferred to a watch glass and the saline is removed from the embryo with the help of filter paper. Now the embryo is treated with 70% alcohol for few minutes and then the alcohol is removed. The embryo is stained by adding 70% alcoholic eosine. After proper staining, the embryo with the blastoderm is transferred to a cavity slide, added with glycerine and mounted by placing the coverglass.

The mounted embryo is examined under a dissection microscope. In this way, temporary mountings of chick embryo of different stages (18, 24, 36, 48, 72, 96 and 120 hours) are prepared, examined and sketched.

5. Vital Staining of Chick Embryo of Various Stages

Aim To observe the development of various organs through preparing temporary mountings of chick embryos of various stages (18, 24, 36, 48, 72, 96 and 120 hours) after vital staining.

Materials Fertilized eggs of chick, egg incubator, dissection instruments, Petri dishes, cavity slides, cover glasses, dropper, filter paper, thermometer, dissection microscope, 1% saline solution, 70% alcohol, glycerol, and 1% neutral red (vital stain)

Method The temporary mounting of chick embryos of different stages are made as in the previous experiment but the embryos are stained with neutral red solution. The mounted embryos are examined under dissection microscope and sketched.

6. Study of Different Stages in the Development of Frog

Aim To identify and record various stages in the development of frog by rearing tadpoles of very early stages in the laboratory.

Materials Aquarium tanks, aquatic plants, pieces of wood or cork, raw meat, dissection microscope, metric ruler, 1/10 mm graph paper and early-stage tadpoles.

Method : Tadpoles of very early stages are collected from a pond and are kept in an aquarium tank containing water and some aquatic plants. When the tadpoles become free-swimming with the development of legs, a few pieces of raw meat are provided to them as they require animal food. When the young frogs develop from the tadpoles, small pieces of wood or cork are made to float on the water as the substratum.

During rearing of tadpoles, the characteristics of initial stages of development as well as the gradual changes undergone during development and metamorphosis are observed. The tadpoles are measured at various stages and sketched. The measurements can easily be made by transforming the tadpoles to the Petri dish placed on a piece of 1/10 mm graph paper.

7. Effect of Thyroxine on the Development of Frog tadpoles

Aim To examine the effect of thyroxine on the development of tadpoles of frog.

Materials Aquarium tanks, aquatic plants, dissection microscope, metric ruler, 1/10 mm graph paper, dried thyroid extract, rice flour and early-stage tadpoles.

Method Fully developed tadpoles of frog are collected from a pond and reared in the laboratory in the aquarium tanks containing water and aquatic plants. Two separate aquaria are set up containing a few tadpoles in which the hind legs are just beginning to appear. To one of the groups of animals, a pinch of thyroid extract and a little flour are provided. The other group is the control group which is provided with rice flour only during rearing. The water in the aquaria, feed flour and thyroid extract in each aquarium is changed daily. In addition, a little quantity of finely crumbled boiled egg yolk is also supplied to the tadpoles as dietary supplement once a week.

The tadpoles are observed for one or two weeks. The total body length and relative size of the tail as well as the length of the hind limbs are recorded by using the graph paper. The body length is measured from snout to anus and the total length from the snout to the tip of the tail. Moreover, changes in the shape of the body, development of legs and general behaviour of tadpoles are also recorded. By comparing the data of the control and thyroid-treated tadpoles, the effect of thyroxine on tadpoles is assessed.

8. Observation of Regeneration of Tail in Frog Tadpoles

Aim To study the phenomenon of regeneration in the tail of frog tadpoles.

Materials Tadpoles, aquarium tank, aquatic plants, boiled green lattice, Petri dishes, 1/10 mm graph paper, dissection instruments and sodium sulphadiazine powder.

Method Frog tadpoles are collected from a pond and reared in the laboratory. A few tadpoles of same stage of development are selected and the fore limbs, hindlimbs or tail are severed without damaging the tissues. They are left in the aquarium tank, the water of which is sprinkled with a small amount of sodium suphadiazine powder in order to avoid infection of wound in the tadpoles. The tadpoles are fed with boiled green lattice and are observed periodically for the regeneration of parts severed. The size and shape of the blastema are noted and sketched. The length of the tail is also measured by placing the tadpoles on a piece of graph paper fixed in a Petri dish.

Appendix II

SELECTED EMBRYOLOGICAL SPOTTERS

The following spotters either in the prepared slides or as specimens have to be identified and described. The descriptions and diagrams are given only to those spotters which are not found in the text. For others, the diagrams and descriptions shown in the text are to be followed.

Amphioxus

1. Unfertilized egg
2. Fertilized egg—4-celled stage and 8-celled stage
3. T.S. of blastula and gastrula
4. T.S. of embryo showing the development of neural tube and coelom
5. T.S. of embryo showing the development of myotomes
6. Amphioxus larva

Frog

1. Sperm
2. Unfertilized egg
3. Fertilized egg with grey crescent
4. Fertilized egg—4-celled and 8-celled stages
5. T.S. of blastula
6. T.S. of early gastrula
7. T.S. of late gastrula
8. T.S. of gastrula—yolk plug stage
9. T.S. of gastrula showing neurulation
10. T.S. of embryo through optic cup
11. T.S. of embryo through heart tubes

Chick

1. *Egg*

2. *Blastoderm WM—Primitive streak (16 h)* At the beginning, the blastodermal cells invaginate in the space between the epiblast and the hypoblast. Then the cells move downwards towards the middle line of the under surface of the blastoderm (convergence) and then undergo involution in an antero-lateral direction as a separate sheet of mesoderm. This causes the formation of primitive groove and primitive ridges in the primitive streak. Then the pre-chordal and chordal cells roll inward so that they forming the Hensen's node. The centre of the node forms a funnel-shaped depression, the primitive pit. Now the notochordal cells converge on the node and develop into a dense mass of tissue called head process under the epiblast. Thus the primitive streak is formed by the various morphogenetic movements namely convergence, involution and divergence.

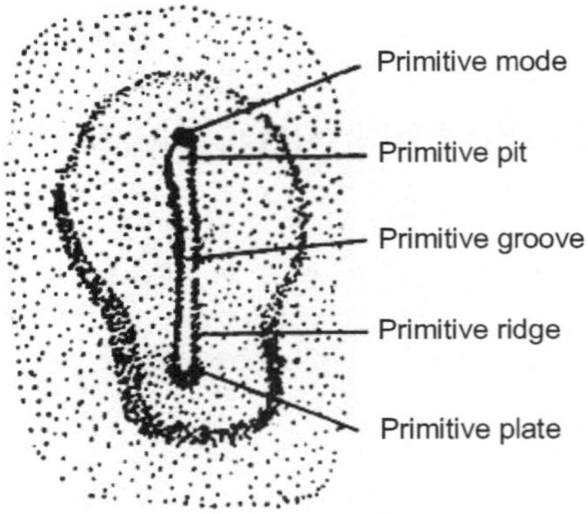

Figure A1 Chick: Blastoderm WM—Primitive streak (16 h)

3. *Chick embryo WM –24 h* In this stage, 4 pairs of somites have developed. The head process rises above the blastoderm so that the subcephalic pocket or space is formed between the head and blastoderm. The neural plate begins to fold and is more prominent at the cephalic end forming the neural groove. This groove runs all along the length of primitive streak. The notochord lies at the bottom of the neural groove. Simultaneously, the primitive foregut is differentiated. The mesoderm differentiates into dorsal mesoderm (somites), intermediate mesoderm (with nephrotome) and lateral mesoderm (with somatic and splanchnic layers). The pericardial coelom develops ventral to the foregut. Blood islands are formed in the region of area opaca.

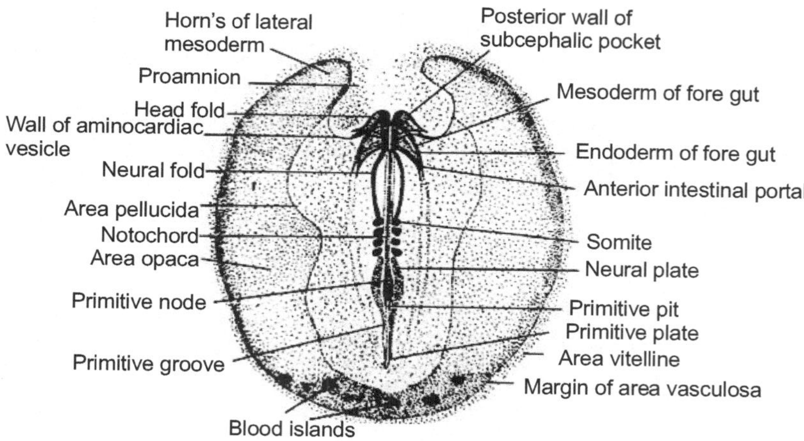

Figure A2 Chick embryo WM—24 h

4. *Chick embryo WM–32 h* The embryo at 32 h of incubation resembles that of 24 h stage but exhibits certain advancements. The vascular area becomes well-developed. The subcephalic pocket is well-distinguished at the region of optic vesicle. The foregut increases in size with the appearance of midgut and hindgut. The neural folds have fused to form the neural tube which opens to the outside anteriorly by the neuropore. The neural tube begins to differentiate into prosencephalon, mesencephalon and rhombencephalon. The primitive streak exists at the caudal region. The embryo at this stage possesses nearly 12 pairs of somites. The somatopleure and the splanchnopleure are well-formed. The heart is in the form of a straight double tube which is present ventral to the gut. The omphalomesenteric veins and ventral aorta are seen. The enlarged coelom forms the pericardial cavity in the region of heart.

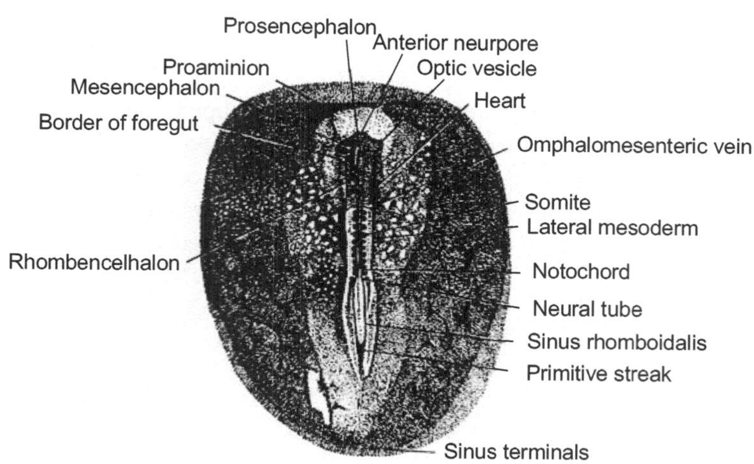

Figure A3 Chick embryo WM—32 h

5. *Chick embryo WM –48 hrs* Here, the embryo acquires a number of changes especially bending of the body, with 25 pairs of somites. The differentiated brain exhibits cranial and cervical flexures so that the fore- and hindbrains lie parallel. The extra-embryonic vascular system has been developed. The head is more prominent but the proamrion is very much reduced with the disappearance of the primitive streak.

The neuropore closes and the brain differentiates further into five regions. The epiphysis begins to develop. The optic cup, lens placode and auditory placode appear. The pharynx develops pharyngeal pouches with branchial arches. The 'S' shaped tubular heart differentiates into sinus venosus, atrium, ventricle and bulbous arteriosus. Three pairs of aortic arches develop and connect the ventral aorta to the dorsal aorta. New somites are formed with the differentiation of sclerotome, myotome and dermatome. The yolk sac, chorion and amnion are formed on either side of the head.

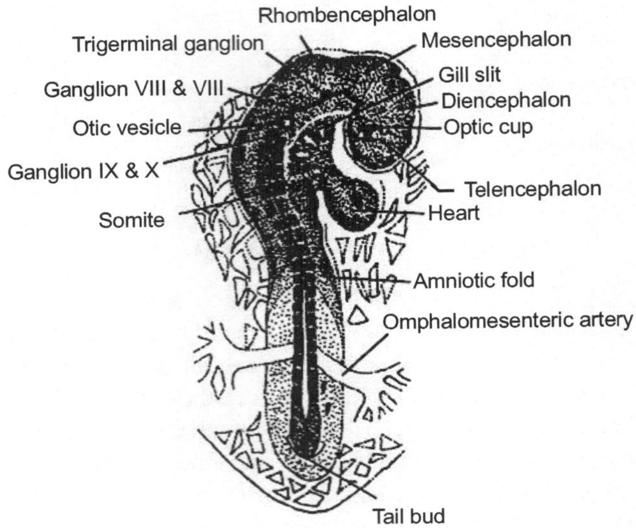

Figure A4 Chick embryo WM—48 hrs

6. *Chick embryo WM—72 h* On day 3, the embryo has 35 pairs of somites with extended vascularization over the yolk. The body exhibits two major flexures namely lumbar and caudal flexures along with well-pronounced cervical flexure. The limb buds begin to develop. The ventricles of the brain are well-developed. Auditory vesicles make their appearance and the eyes have developed completely. The digestive system becomes demarcated into various regions. The laryngo-tracheal groove produces two lung buds which become surrounded by the pleural cavity. Partition of the heart tube occurs, differentiating into chambers by the septa. Vitelline circulation is well marked off. The mesonephric ducts become elongated and extra-embryonic membranes (amnion, yolk sac, chorion and allantois) appear in this stage.

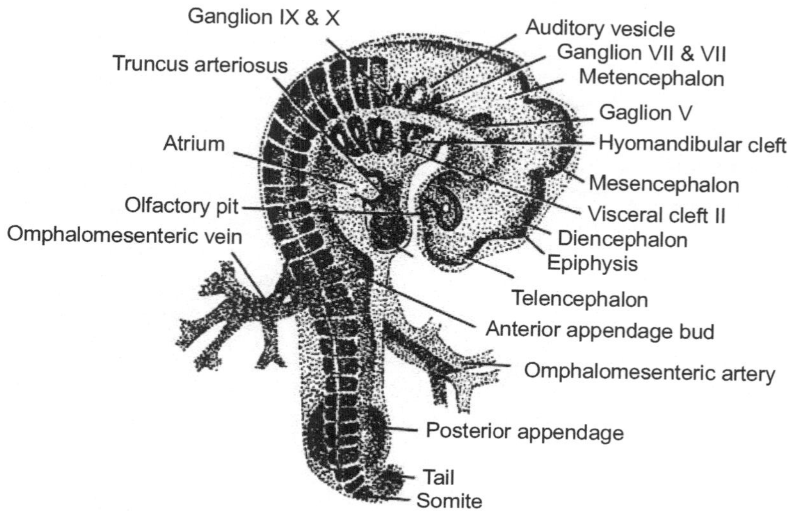

Figure A5 Chick embryo WM—72 h

7. *Chick embryo WM—96 h* Here, the embryo has 41 pairs of somites and the body is demarcated into head, trunk and tail with completion of torsion and flexures. As the embryo is 'C' shaped, the head and tail are nearer to each other. The limb buds become paddle-like and the somites continue to differentiate with dermatome, myotome and sclerotome. The nervous system is well-developed with nerves and ganglia. The digestive and respiratory organs are well-pronounced. The aortic arches, arteries and veins are distinctly developed. The metanephros and gonads make their appearance. The extra-embryonic membranes have become fully developed.

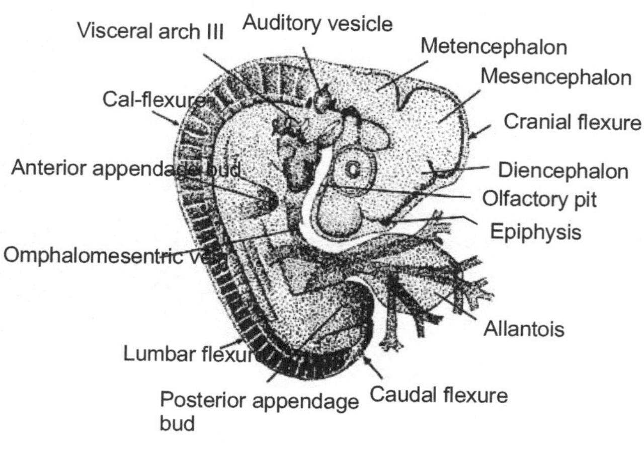

Figure A6 Chick embryo WM—96 h

8. *Sections of chick embryo* For the description of sections of chick embryos of various developmental stages, the text of the book and the notes given in the whole mounts are to be referred.

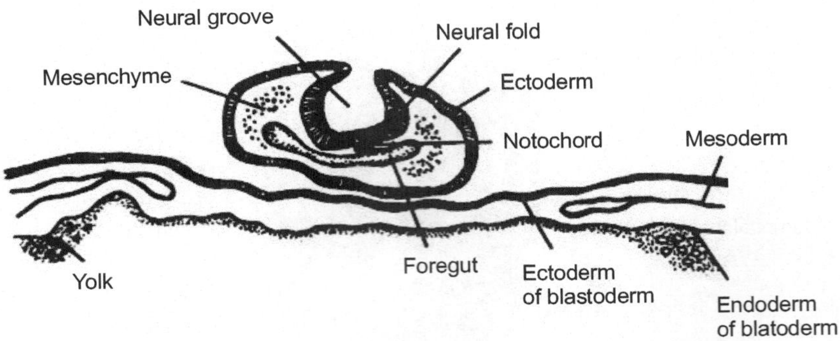

(a) C.S. through neural tube

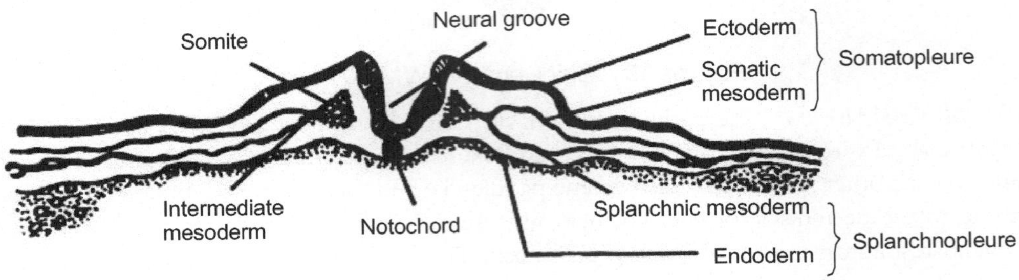

b) C.S. through somites

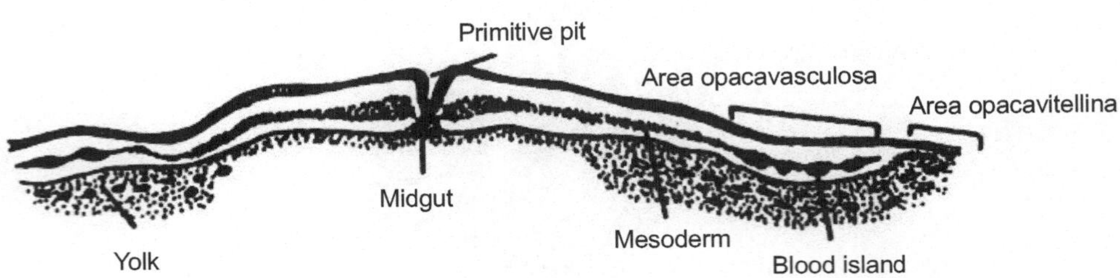

c) C.S. through midgut

Figure A7 24 h chick embryo

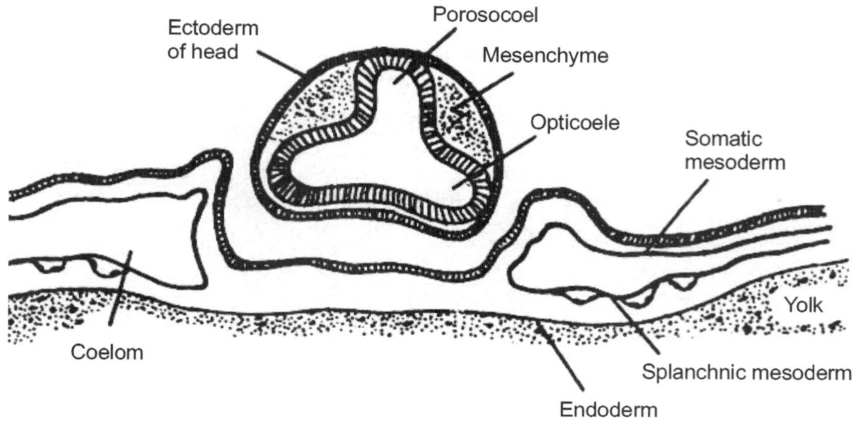

a) C.S. through brain (neural tube)

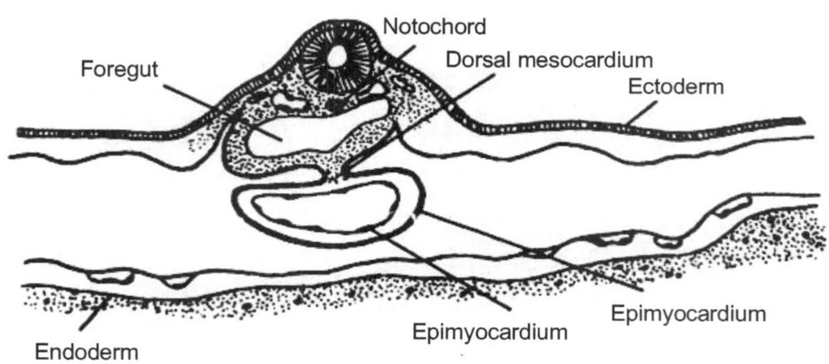

b) C.S. through heart

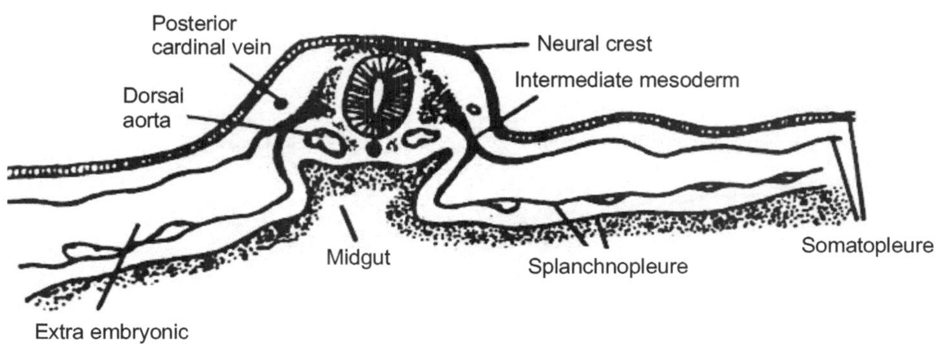

c) C.S. through somites

Figure A8 32 h chick embryo

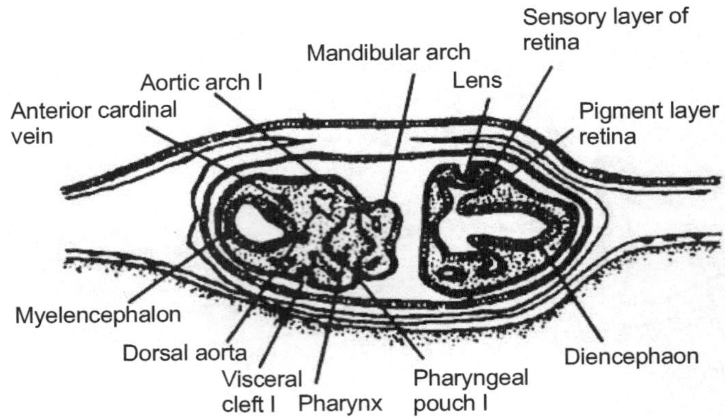

a) C.S. through the head

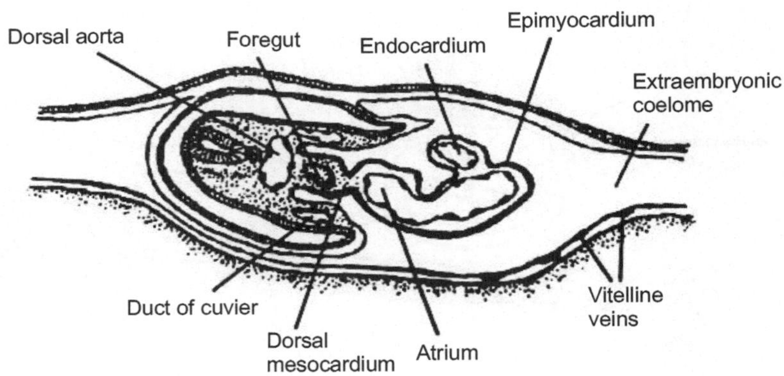

b) C.S. through heart

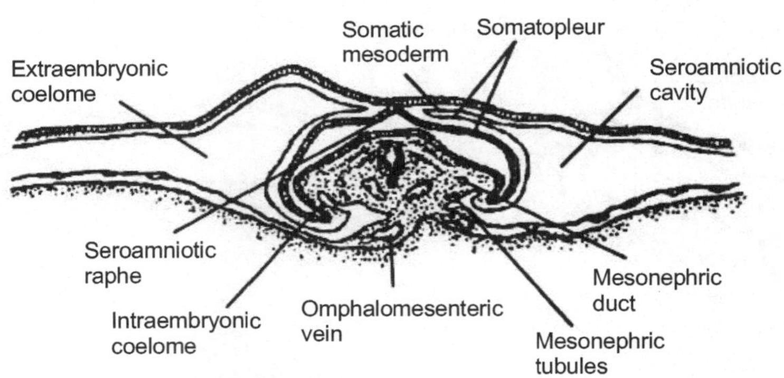

c) C.S. through gill arches

Figure A9 48 h chick embryo

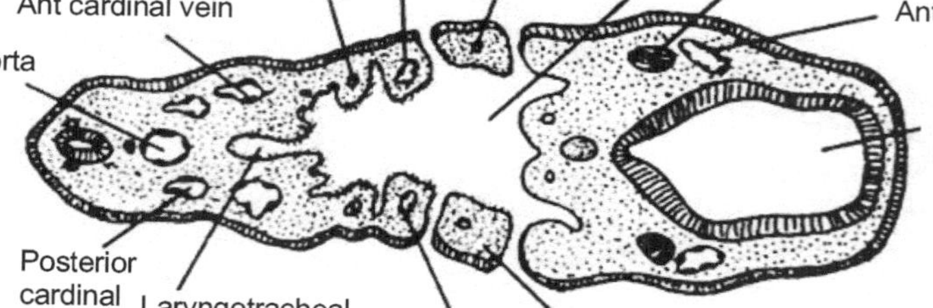

a) C.S. through gill arches

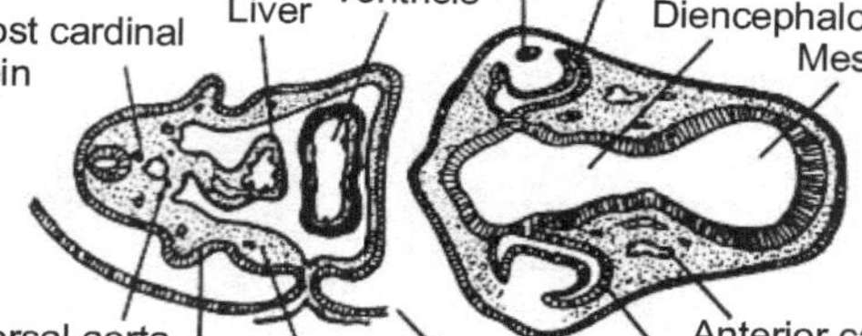

b) C.S. through trunk

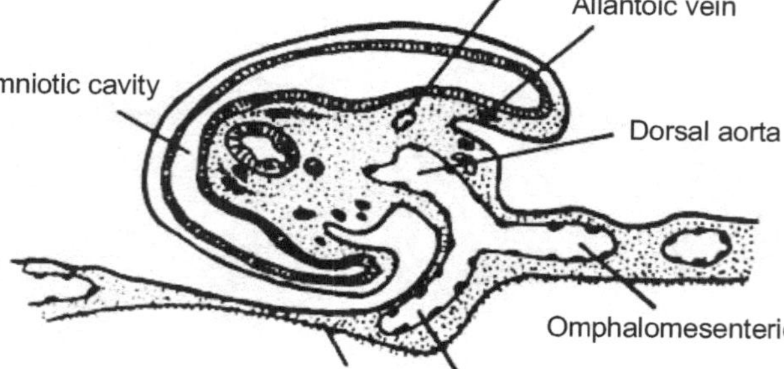

c) C.S. through tail

Figure A10 72 hrs chick embryo

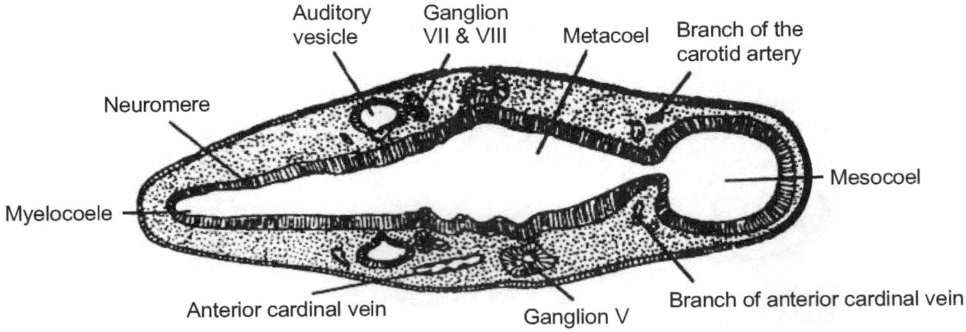

a) C.S. through head

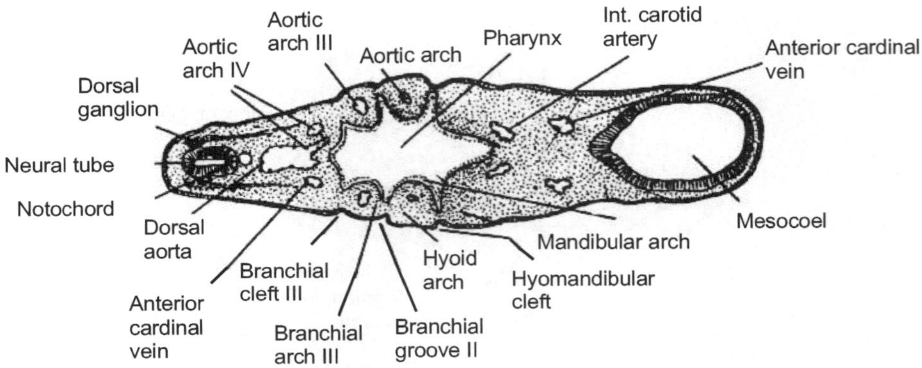

b) C.S. through aortic arches

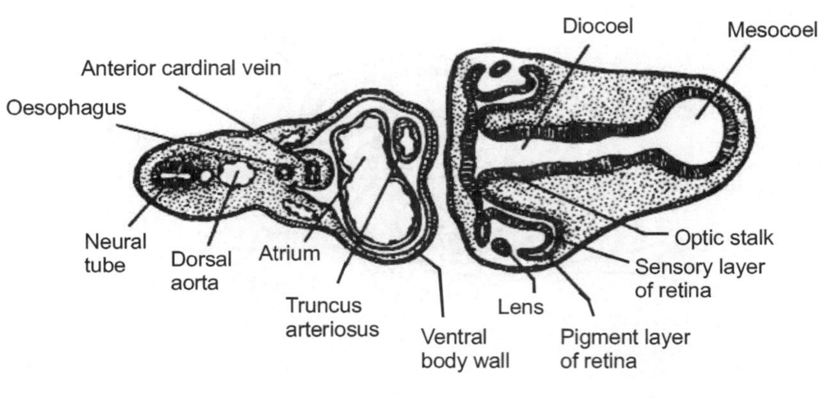

c) C.S. through heart and optic cup

Figure A11 96 h chick embryo

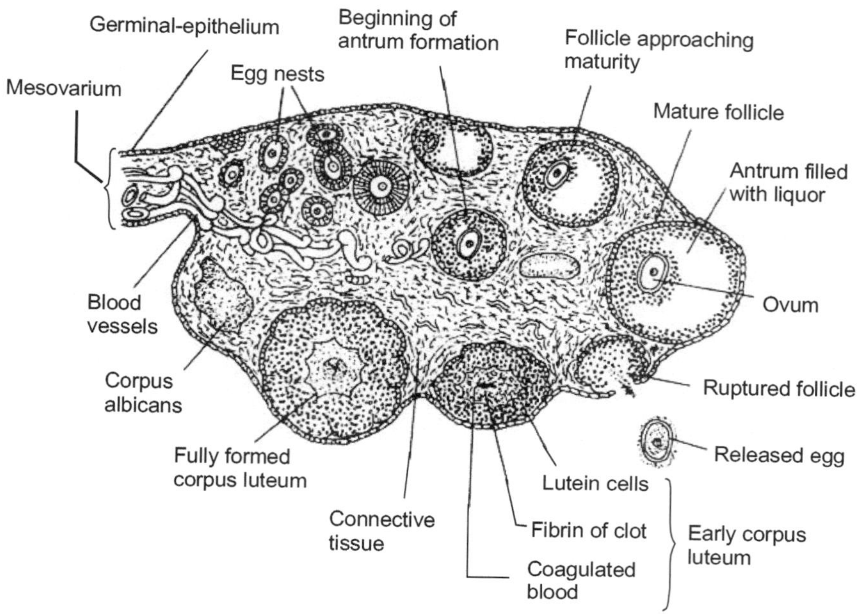

Figure A12 C.S. of ovary of mammal

1. Human sperm
2. Graafian follicle
3. C.S. of ovary of rat
4. Diffuse placenta (pig)
5. Cotyledonary placenta (sheep)
6. Zonary placenta (dog)
7. Discodial placenta (rat)

Glossary

Acrosome A compact mass found on the top of the nucleus of the sperm head and gives rise to a two-layered membrane covering the nucleus. It plays a prominent role in penetration of sperm into the ovum and in the activation of the egg for further development.

Allantoic circulation / Second extra-embryonic circulation The allantois after its development from the hindgut receives allantoic artery from the iliac branch of the dorsal aorta and returns the blood to the heart through the allantoic vein. This forms the allantoic circulation in the development of chick and also the second extra-embryonic circulation, the first being the vitelline circulation.

Allantois An extra-embryonic membrane developed from the splanchnopleure (endoderm and splachnic mesoderm) as an extension of hindgut and helps in respiration and in storing the excretory products in birds or participating in the formation of placenta in mammals.

Amniocentesis A specialized test during pregnancy by which a little quantity of amniotic fluid is removed from the amnion around the developing foetus for prenatal diagnosis of chromosomal abnormalities or foetal infections.

Amnion One of the foetal membranes in amniotes arising from somatopleure (ectoderm and endoderm) and encloses a cavity called amnion containing amniotic fluid which prevents desiccation of the embryo in chick or acts as a shock absorber preventing mechanical shocks in mammals.

Amphimixis The introduction of the male haploid chromosomes by the sperm into the egg, thus restoring the diploid number of chromosomes (maternal and paternal chromosomes) in the zygote.

Androgenesis The process in which the sperm activates the egg without the contribution of maternal genetic materials so that the offspring would have only paternal chromosomes.

Antifertilizin A chemical substance produced by the sperm and which counteracts with fertilizin from the unfertilized egg, thus forming a chemical lock which prevents the entry of more sperms (polyspermy) into the egg.

Antrum In mammals, the growing follicle develops a cavity called antrum which is filled with a fluid namely the follicular fluid in which the egg grows.

Arrhenotoky A type of parthenogenesis in which the eggs develop with only one reduction division (haploid egg) thus developing into haploid male individuals.

Axial filament The neck of the sperm contains the proximal and distal centrioles which lie at right angles to one another. Both the centrioles come out of the microcentrum in the cytoplasm of the spermatid and the distal centriole reaches the periphery and gives rise to the axial filament of the sperm tail.

Blastema or regeneration bud A large number of undifferentiated cells are formed under the epithelial covering from the adjoining tissues of the wound surface during regeneration and these cells with the epidermal layer constitute the blastema.

Brain Hormone (BH) The hormone secreted by the neurosecretory cells of the brain in insects and activates the thoracic glands to secrete moulting hormone.

Cell differentiation A process by which cells become specialized to perform specific functions, or it is the modification or the progressive specialization in structure and function of the cells. In other words, it is a sort of transformation of a more general homogeneous structure into a more specialized heterogeneous one during development.

Cell lineage or cytogeny The study of the developmental history of a cell in a cleaving egg or tracing the fate of particular blastomeres by artificial marking of blastomeres or by observation of cytoplasmic variations in different parts of the egg or naming of the blastomeres with the alphabet.

Chemodifferentiation/Morphogenetic substances The egg cytoplasm which is homogeneous in nature acquires complicated spatial structure due to accumulated substances of chemical reactions in definite parts of the egg and these substances are described as the morphogenetic substances as they exert a determining influence on future development of those parts and this phenomenon is called as chemodifferentiation.

Chorionic Villus Sampling (CVS) A kind of prenatal diagnosis by which a small amount of placental sample from the uterus is removed for the detection of genetic disorders in the foetus and can be carried out earlier than amniocentesis.

Cleavage The process of division of unicellular zygote by mitosis into a group of cells with decreased size namely blastomeres. It is otherwise called as segmentation which results in the formation of morula and blastula representing the final stage of cleavage.

Coeloblastula When the morula develops a cavity called blastocoel or segmentation cavity at the centre of cells forming the blasula, it is called coeloblastula in which the covering cells form the blastoderm as in the development of Amphioxus and frog.

Corpus luteum The mammalian follicle, after ovulation, is filled up with a solid body made up of connective tissue called corpus luteum which regresses and degenerates in the absence of fertilization. In the event of fertilization, it remains functional and acts as an endocrine gland concerned with implantation of ovum and early development.

Discoblastula In chick, the cleavage results in a disc-like blastoderm which becomes separated off from the underlying yolk thus enclosing a blastocoel that is restricted only to the disc-like region. Therefore the blastula is called as discoblastula.

Double monsters In rare occasions during the development of identical twins, the twins are joined or fused together at certain regions of the body. This condition is known as double monsters which includes two major types namely equal conjoined twins and unequal conjoined twins.

Ectoderm The outermost of the germ layers indicating the beginning of the tissue which covers the body surface and forms the central nervous system, the lens of the eye, cranial and sensory ganglia and nerves, pigment cells, epidermis, hair, mammary glands, etc.

Egg cortex The outer surface layer with the plasma membrane of the egg, which is more viscous, gelatinous and static with thickness varying from 2–3 μ containing characteristic cortical granules.

Emboly/Token invagination The process of inward movement of presumptive dermal, endodermal and chordamesodermal cells by the inherent property of cells or due to the movement of other cell groups.

Embryomata A kind of mixed tumour containing clearly differentiated organs or parts of organs representing all primary germ layers.

Embryonic induction The kind of stimulus received by the embryonic cells and tissues from the neighbouring tissues for the development into particular organs. Also called induction or induction interactions.

Embryonic knob/Cystoblastula In man, the cells of morula are arranged in such a way that they form a group called embryonic knob, the covering layer of which is called cyst. Therefore the blastula is called coeloblastula or blastocyst in which the blastocoel is in between the embryonic knob and the cyst.

Encephalon The anterior region of the neural tube that develops into brain and which differentiates into three primitive regions namely the forebrain or prosencephalon, the midbrain or mesencephalon and the hindbrain or rhombencephalon.

Endocardial tube The two delicate tubes between the endoderm and splanchnic mesoderm below the pharynx formed by the organization of the mesenchyme cells. These tubes unite to form a single heart tube, representing the beginning of the development of the chambered heart.

Endoderm The layer formed by the inward migration of cells along the archenteron and forming the digestive system, lining of digestive, respiratory and urinogenital systems and also glands like liver, pancreas, thyroid gland, parathyroid gland and so on.

Epiboly/Evagination The movement of presumptive neurectodermal cells which after multiplication and flattening become rearranged as the inner layer of the embryo.

Epimyocardium The covering mesodermal layer that surrounds the heart tube and which gives rise to the cardiac muscles.

Epimorphosis A type of reparative regeneration involving addition of parts to the remaining part of the organ as in the case of the regeneration of amphibian limb or of lost tail of the lizard or of wound healing.

Estrous/ Menstrual cycle The physiological cycle that begins with a period of sexual urge called estrous in all mammals except higher primates. Here, the uterine wall is prepared to receive the zygote. In the absence of fertilization, the uterine lining is shed within a short period known as metestrum which is followed by a period of rest and repair (diestrum). The wall of the uterus prepares once again for the estrous (proestrum). In humans, the estrous cycle occurs almost monthly and so it is known as menstrual cycle.

Evocators The chemical substances produced by the inductors as the products of cell metabolism especially as diffusible substances of protein nature that influence the differentiation of organs in the embryo.

Extra-embryonic coelom The extension of coelom between the serosa and amnion into which the allantois grows rapidly aiding in embryonic excretion.

Extra-embryonic membranes In vertebrates, only a portion of the fertilized egg develops into an embryo while the other parts around the area constitute the extra-embryonic regions which give rise to the various foetal membranes such as yolk sac, amnion, chorion or serosa and allantois which are collectively called as extra-embryonic membranes that play a major role in nutrition, respiration and excretion and in providing protection to the developing embryo.

Fate map A chart showing the fate of different parts of an early embryo or the position of presumptive germinal areas in the blastula. Its understanding is highly essential for the correct interpretation of gastrula in the developing eggs.

Fertilization cone At the time of sperm entry into the egg, the acrosomal substance dissolves the egg membrane and forms a conelike structure to which the sperm head comes in contact and is drawn into the egg. This is called fertilization cone.

Fertilization The coming together and union of two opposite sex cells namely male gamete (spermatozoa) and female gamete (ovum or egg) resulting in the formation of zygote or fertilized egg.

Fetoscopy A procedure to obtain blood and skin samples from the foetus for prenatal diagnosis of diseases like sickle cell anaemia, haemophilia, galactosaemia, chronic granulomatous disease and so on.

Follicle stimulating hormone (FSH A hormone secreted by the anterior pituitary and controls the sertoli cells of testis and the granulosa cells of ovary. It also stimulates the spermatogonial divisions and induces the growth of the follicle in the ovary.

Gametogenesis At sexual maturity, animals produce two specialized sex cells called gametes namely egg or ovum or female gamete and the sperm or spermatozoon respectively by females and males. This process is called gametogenesis.

Gastrulation An active process by which the single-layered blastula is transformed into a double-layered gastrula enclosing a cavity called blastocoel or archenteron opening to the outside by blastocoel.

Germ layers A group of cells that are arranged in layers, namely ectoderm, endoderm and mesoderm, and developed during animal embryogenesis, which through various cell lineages develop into all parts of adults via organogenesis.

Germplasm It produces germ cells in the gonads during embryonic development and it may be either gonadial or extragonadial in origin.

Gradient It is the spatial distribution and gradual changes of physical or chemical quantity in the vegetal and animal poles of eggs (animal gradient and vegetal gradient), the interaction of which determines the fate of each cell during cleavage.

Graafian follicle The developing egg which is covered by both follicular membranes (theca externa and theca interna) and egg membranes (basement membrane, membrane granulosa and zona pellucida) in mammals.

Gynogenesis The process in which a sperm activates an egg without contributing the genetic material and where the resulting embryo would possess only maternal chromosomes.

Head process The prospective notochordal cells during the gastrulation of chick embryo converge on the Hensen's node, sink through it and pass directly forward as a head process which consists of a thick central mass of cells destined to give rise to notochord and somatic mesoderm.

Implantation A process in which the blastocyst during the development of mammalian egg, moves to the uterus and gets attached to the uterine wall under the influence of ovarian hormones namely estrogen and progestrone.

Included fetuses A condition in which one member of a pair of conjoined twins lags behind the other during very early development and becomes encased in the body of the normal twin ('Foetus in Fetu').

Invagination The infolding or inpushing of blastodermal cells in which a region of blastoderm is pushed into the blastocoel as the inner layer and it may be either a process of active or passive infolding.

Involution 'Rolling in' or 'turning in' of cells which move and arrange along the inner margin of the blastopore. This rolling of the blastodermal cells into the blastocoel, forming the inner layer is called as involution.

Juvenile Hormone (JH) or Neotenin An insect hormone secreted from the corpora allata, which acts directly on the epidermal cells and retains the larval features, thus maintaining the larval characters.

Lateral mesoderm The ventral continuation of the mesoderm consisting of two sheets namely outer somatic mesoderm and inner visceral or splanchnic mesoderm and the cavity between these two sheets is the coelom or body cavity.

Luteinizing hormone (LH) The hormone secreted by the anterior pituitary, which stimulates synthesis and secretion of androgens, for the stimulation of spermatogenesis. It also induces ovulation and formation of corpus luteum inside the follicle in combination with follicle stimulating hormone.

Membranous labyrinths The structure which is formed by unequal expansions and constrictions of optic vesicle. Its lower part differentiates into the sacculus with cochlea or lagena and the upper part, into the utriculus with semicircular canals of the internal ear.

Mesoderm The layer of cells that develops from the inwardly migrating cells of gastrula as an additional layer between ectoderm and endoderm and forms coelom, skeletal muscles, skeleton, dermis of skin, connective tissue, uninogenital system, heart, blood, lymph cells, spleen, etc.

Metamorphosis A process by which the adult individual develops from a larva through a number of successive changes or alterations.

Metathetely A neotenous condition in which the individuals possess a number of infantile characters with capacity of reproduction.

Heteromorphosis The process in which the removal of one organ would result in the formation of another organ. Hetromorphosis is a rare phenomenon and is seen in some crustaceans.

Morphallaxis A reparative regeneration in which the adult is capable of producing new individuals from the body pieces involving reorganization of the remaining part of the body as in hydra, planaria and earthworm.

Morphogenesis The progressive formation of various tissues, organs and organ systems with changes in shape and organization in an orderly and sequential manner during the development of an organism.

Morphogenetic movements The movement of cells in embryos that result in many changes in the structure due to the rearrangement of blastomeres. These movements are due to the integrated migration of cells which are irreversible in embryos. As these cellular movements bring about new forms with new shapes in the embryo, they are known as morphogenetic movements.

Mosaic/Determinate development In some invertebrates, the eggs contain a mosaic of different cytoplasmic regions each of which has its own characteristic position and fate. Such eggs are called mosaic eggs and their development is known as mosaic or determinate development.

Moulting Hormone (MH) or Ecdysone The hormone produced by the prothoracic glands of insects and that initiates the changes in the epidermis leading to growth and deposition of new cuticle and casting of the old cuticle in combination with brain hormone.

Myotome The upper part of the mesoderm constitutes the myotome which gives rise to an outer sheath dorsally called dermatome and another plate at the lower end from the inner side called sclerotome, a supporting sheath around the notochord.

Neoteny/Paedogenesis The ability of an individual to reproduce before attaining adulthood leading to precocious reproduction in larval stages.

Nephrotome The cells that arise as a separate unit by rapid proliferation of the upper region of the somatic mesoderm and which gives rise to the kidney tubules.

Neural induction The influence of the differentiation and development of the nervous system by the roof of the archenteron of the embryo.

Neurocoel / Neutenteric canal In the elongated gastrula, the dorsal ectodermal surface at the centre becomes flattened and slightly depressed forming the medullary or neural plate which rolls upwards and fuses to form the neural tube enclosing the longitudinal canal called neural canal or neurocoel. The neurocoel is connected to the archenteron by a short canal namely neurenteric canal and opens to the outside by the neuropore.

Neurula The developmental stage in which the neural plate appears in the embryo as a centrally depressed and flat ectodermal surface on the dorsal region of the elongated gastrula.

Omphalomesenteric veins The developing simple heart tube divides posteriorly into two large vessels in front of the developing liver. These are omphalomesenteric veins that enter into the yolk, thus aiding the vitelline circulation.

Oogenesis The formation of eggs or ova from the primordial germ cells in the ovary of female animals.

Optic cup The optic vesicle which arises from the ventro-lateral region of the diencephalon differentiates into double walled optic cup, the outer thin layer of which forms the pigment layer of the eye and the inner thick layer becomes the neurosecretory layer or retina.

Ovulation The process of shedding of ovum during the breeding season. After maturation, the ovum is released periodically into the body cavity, transported into the oviduct and then to the outside as in non-mammals or to the uterus in mammals.

Parthenogenesis The development of an egg into an embryo without fertilization. The female gamete develops into an organism without genetic contribution from the male gamete (sperm).

Placenta A complex structure formed by the foetal membranes and uterine mucosa for physiological interchange between the mother and embryo in mammals.

Polarity The unequal distribution of the egg constituents like yolk, pigments, RNA and other cellular organelles in the fully developed advanced oocytes establishing two opposite poles namely animal and vegetal poles.

Poleplasm Immediately after fertilization, eggs of some worms get accumulations of special protoplasmic substances at vegetal and animal poles. These protoplasmic masses are called poleplasm, which slightly differ from the rest of the protoplasm in physicochemical composition and determines the normal development of the embryo.

Preblastema The accumulation of cells at the surface of a wound from the interior of the body and growing of the epithelial cells of the skin as a covering over the surface of the wound during regeneration.

Presumptive organ-forming areas During development, a particular area of the embryo would develop into a specific organ and so the cells in that area constitute the presumptive organ-forming areas or organ-specific areas.

Previtellogenesis The preparative stage of the oocyte prior to the deposition of yolk, in which the oocyte undergoes tremendous increase in volume of the nucleus and cytoplasm due to accumulation of nucleoprotenis and DNA.

Primary organizer The dorsal lip or the chordamesoderm of the gastrula, which influences the development of the forebrain and the optic region at the anterior end of the embryo.

Primitive streak An area of linear thickening formed on the surface of blastoderm of chick during gastrulation due to rapid growth of cells and cellular proliferation on the early blastodisc with a groove flanked on both sides by two primitive ridges with a primitive pit anterioly and primitive plate posterioly. It plays an important role in the formation of notochord and mesoderm.

Prothetely A type of neoteny in which the young ones become sexually active with incomplete adult characters.

Regeneration The ability of an organism to repair or renew or replace the damage in the body at varying degrees, and may include the replacement of the loss of an organ, a major part of the body or the whole organism, or simply wound healing.

Regulative/Indeterminate development In the egg of vertebrates, all the cytoplasmic parts of the blastomeres in early stages during cleavage are 'totipotent' or 'equipotential' and can regulate in order to replace the damaged parts. These eggs are called as regulative eggs and their development is known as regulative or indeterminate development.

Secondary organizer While the development of optic vesicle depends on the primary organizer (chordamesoderm), the optic vesicle induces the development of lens from the overlying ectoderm of the embryo, thus forming the secondary organizer.

Seroamniotic junction In amniotes the amnion arises as folds of somatopleure (ectoderm and somatic mesoderm) from all directions and all these folds meet at a point and form a structure called seroamniotic junction containing four membranes of which the outer two layers form the serosa and the inner two layers form the amnion.

Serosa/Chorion An embryonic membrane (serosa in birds and chorion in mammals) which develops from somatopleure (ectoderm and somatic mesoderm) and helps in respiration in chick embryo or takes part in the formation of placenta in mammalian embryo.

Sexual photoperiodicity The activity of gonads can be controlled and regulated by the ratio of light to dark period in each day. This periodicity in light controlling the sexual cycle via the nervous system is sexual photoperiodicity which is most prevalent in birds and few mammals.

Spermatogenesis The formation of sperms from the primordial germ cells found in the seminiferous tubules of testis of male animals.

Spermiogenesis The process of transformation of spermatids having haploid number of chromosomes into functional sperms through a number of changes.

Symmetry This is due to the regional cytoplasmic variations in the egg due to qualitative differences in the chemical composition of the part of the egg or the nature of the substances contained in parts of the egg namely morphogenetic substances.

Teratogenesis Refers to the interference with the normal development of either embryo or foetus resulting in abnormalities in newborns, more specifically morbidity and mortality among inborns.

Teratogens/Teratogenic agents The toxic substances which induce abnormal development in foetuses.

Teratology The study of any abnormality in internal organs or congenital defects or malformations that arise during the course of development.

Teratoma Any kind of mixed tumours in the tissues or fragmentary parts of organs derived from more than one germ layer but without normal architectural arrangement.

Thelytoky A kind of parthenogenesis in which the developing ovum retains the diploid number of chromosomes by the loss of reduction division or restoring the diploid number by fusing with one of the polar bodies. As a result, the developing individuals are all diploid in nature.

Vitelline circulation / Second extra-embryonic circulation A pair of vitelline arteries from the dorsal aorta enter the yolk sac from which the blood is collected by vitelline veins. The capillaries of veins and of the vitelline arteries become connected, thus forming the vitelline circulation. As the yolk lies outside the embryo, this is an extra-embryonic circulation.

Vitelline membrane A thin transparent membrane found closely applied to the underlying plasma membrane in the eggs of insects, molluscs, amphibians and birds and is formed by mucopolysaccharides and some fibrous proteins.

Yolk plug During the gastrulation of frog's egg, all the yolk cells are hidden by the pigmented cells after the formation of blastoporal lips except at the region of blastopore where they can be seen from the outside in the form of a mass called yolk plug.

Yolk sac A foetal membrane formed by the splanchnopleure (endoderm and splanchnic mesoderm) around the egg yolk in chick embryo in order to digest yolk and pass it on to the embryo through the vitelline circulation.

References

Adiyodi, Adiyodi, K.G., and Rita, G. Adiyodi. 2000. *Reproductive Biology of Invertebrates.* John Wiley and Sons Ltd.

Balinsky, B.I. 1970. *An introduction to Embryology,* 3rd Edn. W.B. Saunders Company, Philadelphia.

Berrill, N.J. 1971. *Developmental Biology.* McGraw-Hill Book Company, New York.

Donald, A.E. 1978. *An Introduction to Developmental Biology.* Blackie and Sons Ltd., Glasgow.

Gerald Schatten. 2005. *Current topics in Developmental Biology.* Academic Press, USA.

Jain, P.C. 2007. *Elements of Developmental Biology.* Vishal Publishing Co., Delhi.

Nelson, O.E. 1953. *Comparative Embryology of Vertebrates.* The Blackistan Company, Inc., New York.

Patten, B.M. 1964. *Foundation of Embryology*, McGraw-Hill Book Company, New York.

Saunders, J.W. 1970. *Pattern and Principles of Animal Development*, McMillon., London.

Scott F.Gilber. 2006. *Developmental Biology,* 8th Edn. Sinaur Associates, Inc., Suderland, MA.

Slack, J.M.W. 2005. *Essential Developmental Biology,* 2nd Edn. John Wiley and Sons, Inc.

Wolpert, L., Beddington, R., Jessel, T., Lawrence, P., Meyerowitg, E. and Smith, J. 2002. *Principles of Development,* 2nd Edn. Oxford University Press.

INDEX